Electronic Fetal Monitoring
Concepts and Applications

2nd Edition

Cydney Afriat Menihan, CNM, MSN, RDMS
Nurse Midwife and Perinatal Consultant
Wakefield, Rhode Island

Ellen Kopel, RNC, MS
Nurse Educator and Perinatal Consultant
Sarasota, Florida

D1341507

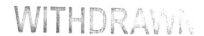
Wolters Kluwer | Lippincott Williams & Wilkins
Health
Philadelphia · Baltimore · New York · London
Buenos Aires · Hong Kong · Sydney · Tokyo

Senior Acquisitions Editor: Margaret Zuccarini
Editorial Assistant: Edward Slama
Production Project Manager: Cynthia Rudy
Director of Nursing Production: Helen Ewan
Senior Managing Editor / Production: Erika Kors
Art Director: Joan Wendt
Manufacturing Coordinator: Karin Duffield
Production Services / Compositor: Aptara, Inc.
Printer: R.R. Donnelley–Willard

2nd edition

9 8 7 6 5 4 3 2 1

Library of Congress Cataloging-in-Publication Data

Menihan, Cydney Afriat.
 Electronic fetal monitoring : concepts and applications / Cydney Afriat
Menihan, Ellen Kopel. — 2nd ed.
    p. ; cm.
 Includes bibliographical references and index.
   ISBN-13: 978-0-7817-7011-8
   ISBN-10: 0-7817-7011-4
 1. Fetal heart rate monitoring. I. Kopel, Ellen. II. Title.
 [DNLM: 1. Fetal Monitoring—methods. 2. Heart Rate, Fetal—physiology.
 WQ 209 M545e 2008]
 RG628.3.H42M44 2008
 618.3'2075—dc22
                                                          2007010581

LWW.com

DEDICATION

To Marilyn Lapidus, who laid the foundation and set the standard for fetal monitoring education and who provided us with extraordinary personal and professional opportunities—our heartfelt thanks.

Cydney and Ellen

To Jack, for sharing his strength and wisdom, para siempre y un día más.

Cydney

To Zachary, my reason for everything.

Ellen

CONTRIBUTORS

REBECCA F. CADY, RNC, BSN, JD
Partner
Grace, Hollis, Lowe, Hanson & Schaeffer, LLP
San Diego, California

PATRICIA ROBIN McCARTNEY, RNC, PhD, FAAN
Clinical Professor
School of Nursing
University at Buffalo
The State University of New York
Buffalo, New York

KATHLEEN RICE SIMPSON, RNC, PhD, FAAN
Perinatal Clinical Nurse Specialist
St. John's Mercy Medical Center
St. Louis, Missouri
Clinical Professor
Saint Louis University School of Nursing
St. Louis, Missouri

REVIEWERS/CONSULTANTS
To The First Edition

LINDA GOODWIN, RNC, MEd
Manager, Family Birthplace & Family
  Beginnings
Group Health Hospitals
Seattle and Redmond, Washington

JOHN F. HUDDLESTON, MD
Professor and Director
Division of Maternal–Fetal Medicine
Department of Obstetrics and Gynecology
University of Florida
Health Sciences Center/Jacksonville
Jacksonville, Florida

MARILYN R. LAPIDUS, RNC, BSN, JD
GE Medical Systems Information
  Technologies
Milwaukee, Wisconsin

JAMI STAR, MD
Associate Professor
Obstetrics and Gynecology
Brown University School of Medicine
Staff Maternal–Fetal Medicine Specialist
Department of Obstetrics and Gynecology
Women and Infants Hospital of Rhode
  Island
Providence, Rhode Island

CHRIS WOOD
Software Engineer
GE Medical Systems Information
  Technologies
Annapolis, Maryland

REVIEWERS/CONSULTANTS
To The Second Edition

CYNTHIA BELEW, CNN, MS
Assistant Clinical Professor
University of California, San Francisco/
    San Francisco General Hospital
Nurse–Midwifery Education Program
San Francisco, California

BONNIE FLOOD CHEZ, MSN, RNC
Perinatal Clinic Nurse Specialist/Consultant
Tampa, Florida

WENDY E. COLGAN, RNC, BSN
Staff Nurse III
Sutter Medical Center of Santa Rosa
Santa Rosa, California

WENDY HEIBEL, RN, BSN
Clinical Nurse Specialist
Malcolm Grow Medical Center
Andrews Air Force Base, Maryland

WASHINGTON C. HILL, MD, FACOG
Chairman, Department of Obstetrics and
    Gynecology
Director, Maternal–Fetal Medicine
Sarasota Memorial Hospital
Sarasota, Florida

CATHERINE H. IVORY, RNC, MSN
Women's Services Clinical Nurse Specialist
Mountain States Health Alliance
Johnson City Medical Center
Johnson City, Tennessee

BRIAN JACK, MD
Associate Professor and Vice Chair
Department of Family Medicine
Boston University School of Medicine
Boston, Massachusetts

MONA BROWN KETNER, RN, MSN
Perinatal Outreach Education Coordinator
Wake Forest University School of Medicine
Department of Obstetrics and Gynecology
Winston-Salem, North Carolina

SUSAN GRIFFITHS KNOWLES, RNC, BSN, CCAP
Clinical Manager/Clinical Educator
Overlake Hospital Medical Center
Bellevue, Washington

LISA A. MILLER, CNM, JD
President
Perinatal Risk Management and Education
    Services
Chicago, Illinois

LETTIE J. PRIMEAUX, RNC, BSN
Hill-Rom Company
Clinical Information Specialist–WatchChild
Marietta, Georgia

SUSAN K. WEIMER, RN
Clinical Nurse
Medical University of South Carolina
Charleston, South Carolina

LINDA GIVEN WELCH, CNM, MS
Certified Nurse–Midwife
Evanston Hospital
Instructor, Clinical Obstetrics and Gynecology
Feinberg School of Medicine, Northwestern
    University
Chicago, Illinois

FOREWORD

Electronic fetal heart rate monitoring has become the standard of care for assessing fetal well-being in both the antepartum and intrapartum settings, despite controversy about the efficacy and validity of this technique. The story is well known: A new technology that holds promise for identifying the fetus who is developing pathologic acidemia is introduced into clinical practice. Initial observational studies document a decrease in intrapartum stillbirth in settings that use electronic fetal heart rate monitoring for women in labor (Yeh, Diaz, & Paul, 1982). Then the technology is rapidly integrated into practice before clinical trials can assess how well it really works. The 1980s and 1990s saw a plethora of randomized controlled trials, and ultimately a meta-analysis (Alfirevic, Devane, & Gyte, 2006), all with consistent results: electronic fetal heart rate monitoring during labor is associated with a decrease in newborn seizures, no change in perinatal mortality or cerebral palsy, and an increase in cesarean and operative vaginal deliveries (Alfirevic et al., 2006). It was frustrating, and we entered the 21st century asking: Why doesn't electronic fetal heart rate monitoring improve the health of women and their newborns?

You have to ask the right question to get the right answer. In the six years since this book was first published, research in this field has narrowed the focus and chipped away at the problem. We have asked: What fetal heart rate characteristics are associated with fetal acidemia (Parer, King, Flanders, Fox, & Kilpatrick, 2006)? We have looked at second stage patterns (Sheiner et al., 2001); the length and depth of bradycardias (Williams & Galerneau, 2003); and the relationship between specific fetal heart rate patterns and umbilical artery pH and base excess values (Sheiner et al., 2001). Useful knowledge about the clinical significance of fetal heart rate patterns, how they evolve, and the strength of association between specific patterns and newborn acidemia is finally emerging.

However, the adoption of evidence-based clinical care practices is always a challenge with its own set of problems. Many of the questions being asked today focus on identifying a successful strategy for effecting change in practice patterns so that evidence-based care practices can be instituted (Fox, Kilpatrick, King, & Parer, 2000; Simpson, James, & Knox, 2006). We have some components of the solution for fetal heart rate monitoring interpretation. We have agreed on definitions for various fetal heart rate characteristics (NICHD, 1997; ACOG, 2005; AWHONN, 2006). We have consensus about those intrapartum events that can lead to cerebral palsy (ACOG, 2003). Now, with these clear definitions as "bookends," we can turn our attention to education and dissemination of this knowledge.

This second edition of *Electronic Fetal Monitoring: Concepts and Applications*, by Cydney Afriat Menihan and Ellen Kopel, is the comprehensive tool we need. It includes basic information about the physiology of the fetal heart rate and about electronic fetal monitors. The sections on fetal heart rate interpretation reflect all the current evidence for clinical management of specific fetal heart rate patterns. The chapter on competence validation summarizes the value of several teaching modalities—information important to nursing, midwifery, and medicine.

We know today that expert clinicians integrate information from a variety of sources (Benner, 1984). The exercises in electronic fetal monitoring that make up the bulk of this book are designed to foster excellence in clinical judgment. These exercises include clinical scenarios with fetal heart rate tracings. They are realistic in the presentation of several hours for each case. Perhaps as important, the cases involve nurses, midwives, and physicians, and thus are valuable teaching tools for every member of the obstetric health care team.

Ben Franklin said, "Nothing is more fatal to health than over care of it." Evidence-based interpretation of fetal heart rate patterns has been seriously hampered by significant variation in definition of terms and variation in care practices. We will not overcome these hurdles until we have interdisciplinary consistency and effective communication. This book is one of the best places to start.

Tekoa L. King, CNM, MPH
Associate Professor
Department of Obstetrics, Gynecology and Reproductive Sciences
University of California at San Francisco

REFERENCES

American College of Obstetricians and Gynecologists. (2005). Intrapartum fetal heart rate monitoring. *Practice Bulletin No. 62.*

American College of Obstetricians and Gynecologists & American Academy of Pediatrics. (2003). *Neonatal encephalopathy and cerebral palsy: Defining the pathogenesis and pathophysiology.* Washington, DC: American College of Obstetricians and Gynecologists.

Alfirevic, Z., Devane, D., & Gyte, G. M. L. (2006). Continuous cardiotocography (CTG) as a form of electronic fetal monitoring (EFM) for fetal assessment during labour. *Cochrane Database of Systematic Reviews,* Issue 3, Article No. CD006066. DOI: 10.1002/14651858.CD006066.

Association of Women's Health, Obstetric and Neonatal Nurses. (2006). *Fetal heart monitoring principles and practices.* (3rd ed.). Dubuque, IA: Kendall Hunt.

Benner, P. (1984). *From novice to expert: Excellence and power in clinical nursing practice* (pp. 13–34). Menlo Park, NJ: Addison-Wesley.

Fox, M., Kilpatrick, S., King, T., & Parer, J. T. (2000). Fetal heart rate monitoring: Interpretation and collaborative management. *Journal of Midwifery & Women's Health, 45,* 498–507.

National Institute of Child Health and Human Development Research Planning Workshop. (1997). Electronic fetal heart rate monitoring: Research guidelines for interpretation. *American Journal of Obstetrics and Gynecology, 17,* 1385–1390; *Journal of Obstetric, Gynecologic, and Neonatal Nursing, 26,* 635–640.

Parer, J. T., King, T. L., Flanders, S., Fox, M., & Kilpatrick, S. (2006). Fetal acidemia and electronic fetal heart rate patterns: Is there evidence of an association? *Journal of Maternal and Fetal Neonatal Medicine, 19,* 289–294.

Sheiner, E., Hadar, A., Hallak, M., Katz, M., Mazor, M., & Shoham-Vardi, I. (2001). Clinical significance of fetal heart rate tracings during the second stage of labor. *Obstetrics & Gynecology, 97,* 747–752.

Simpson, K. R., James, D. C., & Knox, G. E. (2006). Nurse–physician communication during labor and birth: Implications for patient safety. *Journal of Obstetric, Gynecologic, and Neonatal Nursing, 35,* 547–556.

Williams, K. P., & Galerneau, F. (2003). Intrapartum fetal heart rate patterns in the prediction of fetal acidemia. *American Journal of Obstetrics and Gynecology, 188,* 820–824.

Yeh, S. Y., Diaz, F., & Paul, R. H. (1982). Ten year experience of intrapartum fetal monitoring in Los Angeles County/University of Southern California Medical Center. *American Journal of Obstetrics and Gynecology, 143,* 496–500.

PREFACE

As of this writing, it remains unclear whether electronic fetal monitoring (EFM) is truly beneficial to perinatal outcome. The intent in developing an electronic means of evaluating fetal well-being was to prevent intrapartum asphyxia, thereby reducing neonatal morbidity and mortality. The incidence of intrapartum death and neurologic injury was specifically targeted. While evidence-based practice is fundamental in contemporary health care delivery, neither the public nor the clinical community in the 1960s and 1970s was as focused on prospective, randomized, controlled trials. EFM became available before sufficient testing defined its capabilities (as did other medical devices, pharmaceuticals, and practices).

Critics maintain that there has been no significant change in neonatal morbidity since the introduction of EFM. In regard to the rate of neurologic injury, however, we now understand that other causes of cerebral palsy (CP) exist and that less than 10% of cases are attributable to intrapartum events (Nelson & Ellenberg, 1986; Blair & Stanley, 1988; ACOG and AAP, 2003). It has been suggested that perhaps the wrong end point was chosen for determining the value of EFM (Paul, 1994; Parer & King, 2000). If the majority of CP is attributable to causes other than fetal hypoxia, how can EFM be measured for success against its incidence?

Factors that contributed to fetal and neonatal mortality and morbidity in the late 1960s and early 1970s were different than the challenges faced today. Neonatology was just emerging as a subspeciality and neonatal intensive care units were a rarity. In most cases, little or no attempt was made at saving the extremely premature fetus or neonate, as there was little means of support available postnatally. It wasn't until progress in mechanical ventilation of the neonate in the 1970s and the advent of surfactant in the 1980s that great advances in neonatal outcomes began to occur. Neonatal care has steadily improved and continues to do so, and premature infants who didn't survive 30 years ago now do. Unfortunately, a certain percent do sustain permanent damage. These factors set the scenario for the current manifestation of neonatal morbidity and mortality.

Cesarean birth rates are another source of issue when evaluating the impact of EFM. In 1988, 20 years after the introduction of EFM, cesarean birth rates reached an unprecedented 24.7% (United States Department of Health and Human Services, 2000). This increase in cesarean birth rate was attributed to EFM by many opponents of the technology and this opinion remains an issue of debate. It is necessary to understand that it wasn't until the late 1980s that a movement toward attempting vaginal birth after cesarean (VBAC) arose. Prior to that time, nearly all women who had cesarean births were relegated to repeat cesarean delivery. The trend toward VBAC was driven by multiple sources—many women wanted the opportunity to deliver vaginally, an alternative that was believed by many care providers to be safe and preferable to cesarean birth. Also, the reduced expenditure of a vaginal delivery versus a cesarean birth was appealing to insurance providers. The change in obstetric practice to promoting vaginal birth after cesarean led to a steady decline in repeat cesarean birth rates from 1989 to 1996. By 1996, cesarean rates had declined to 20.7%, as the VBAC rate increased by 50% (Menacker & Curtin, 2001). Concern over the rate of uterine rupture and corresponding rise in poor neonatal outcome (McMahon, Luther, Bowes, & Olsham 1996; Sachs, Kobelin, Castro, & Frigoletto, 1999), however, mandated greater attentiveness from providers (ACOG, 1999; ACOG, 2004) and led to a sharp decline in the rate of VBAC. According to the latest available data, in 2004 VBAC rates had fallen by 67% and the cesarean birth rate had increased 40% from the 1996 figures (Martin et al., 2006).

Other contemporary influences on cesarean birth rates include the popularity of labor induction (Simpson, 2002) and the growing demand for cesarean delivery on maternal request. A 45% decline in the use of forceps and vacuum extraction (Martin et al., 2006) and vaginal breech delivery (Hannah et al., 2000; Martin et al., 2006) from 1996 to 2004 and rising numbers of multiple and preterm births are other current contributing factors. Rather than focusing on EFM as the primary cause of increased cesarean birth rates, it is more reasonable to recognize the multifactorial composition of this problem.

While the rate of neurologic injury has not changed in 30 years, we must consider that the etiologies are different. If we correct for the number of children who have neurologic damage as the result of more contemporaneous concerns (such as prematurity and uterine rupture), we suspect the incidence of neurologic damage directly resulting from intrapartum asphyxia may have decreased significantly.

It is also important to consider that many more pregnancies that once would have been considered ill-advised due to their high-risk nature are now attempted. Advances in general medicine and the subspeciality of perinatology have furthered care of patients with diabetes, hypertension, cardiac defects and insufficiencies, HIV/AIDS, and autoimmune diseases. Societal changes have also impacted the patient population in obstetrics. More women of a later maternal age are having children. The ever-changing popularity of various recreational drugs affects fetuses in ways we recognize and in those we likely will not fully understand for years to come. Alcohol and tobacco also continue to challenge perinatal health. While progress has been made in providing access to perinatal care, there are still financial and cultural barriers to overcome.

Clearly, the most positive effect of EFM is that the fetus is now accepted as a patient "to whom the perinatal team has a definitive duty" (Paul, 1994). The most significant and direct contribution of EFM is the reduction in the rate of intrapartum stillbirth (Vintzileos et al., 1995). Rarely does a fetus die unexpectedly during the labor process, as occurred in decades past. Unfortunately, it is true that some practitioners rush to verdict at the first hint of fetal compromise, performing assisted or operative delivery before exhausting all means of assessing fetal well-being. However, adjunct methods of assessment are available to be utilized in the presence of a nonreassuring tracing, making diagnosis of fetal compromise more accurate and intervention more appropriate. Used appropriately, EFM is a very effective screening tool.

Most critics have expectations of EFM that are far from reasonable. The greatest misconception about EFM is the belief that it is a diagnostic tool. EFM is useful only as a screening tool, comparable in utility to a manometer. If a patient's blood pressure were to exceed normal limits, we would never presume to know, based solely upon that reading, whether she has hypertensive disease or is just having a stressful day. As with all good screening tests, the fetal monitor is highly predictive of negative results (~98%). What the fetal monitor does not do well is predict fetal distress. When the FHR pattern is suggestive of hypoxia, it is falsely positive nearly 90% of the time (Low, Victory, & Derrick, 1999).

Thacker and Stoup have supported that auscultation of the fetal heart rate is comparable to EFM in regard to outcomes (2000). Auscultation is also purported to have the benefit of allowing more personalized patient care, as the focus is toward the patient rather than a machine and is preferred by some patients and care providers. The financial benefit of each method is also fodder for argument. The equipment used for auscultation is much less expensive than an electronic fetal monitor. This technique does, however, require a 1:1 nurse to fetus ratio, a factor that may counterbalance the savings on capital equipment with increased labor expenditures. AWHONN (2000) and AAP ACOG and (2002) support the use of intermittent auscultation during labor.

The purpose of this book is not to promote one method of assessment over another. Certainly, each clinical situation must be approached on an individual basis. The fact remains that EFM is the most common obstetric procedure, utilized in more than 85% of all live births in the United States (Martin et al., 2003). Our aim is to educate clinicians who use EFM to any degree in their practice to employ this method of assessment appropriately and effectively.

Cydney Afriat Menihan
Ellen Kopel

REFERENCES

American Academy of Pediatrics & American College of Obstetricians and Gynecologists. (2002). *Guidelines for perinatal care* (5th ed.). Washington, DC: ACOG.

American College of Obstetricians and Gynecologists. (1999). Vaginal birth after previous cesarean delivery. *ACOG Practice Bulletin*, 54. Washington, DC: Author.

———. (2004). Vaginal birth after previous cesarean delivery. *ACOG Practice Bulletin*, 54. Washington, DC: Author.

American College of Obstetricians and Gynecologists & American Academy of Pediatrics. (2003). *Neonatal encephalopathy and cerebral palsy: Defining the pathogenesis and pathophysiology.* Washington, DC: ACOG.

Association of Women's Health, Obstetric and Neonatal Nurses. (2000). *Clinical position statement: Fetal assessment.* Washington, DC: Author.

Blair, E., & Stanley, F. J. (1988). Intrapartum asphyxia: A rare cause of cerebral palsy. *Journal of Pediatrics, 12*(4), 515–519.

Hannah, M. E., Hannah, W. J., Hewson, S. A., Hodnett, E. D., Saigal, S., & Willan, A. R. (2000). Planned caesarean section versus planned vaginal birth for breech presentation at term: A randomised multicentre trial. Term Breech Trial Collaborative Group. *Lancet, 356*(9239), 1375–1383.

Low, J. A., Victory, R., & Derrick, E. J. (1999). Predictive value of electronic fetal monitoring for intrapartum fetal asphyxia with metabolic acidosis. *Obstetrics and Gynecology, 93,* 285–291.

Martin, J. A., Hamilton, B. E., Sutton, P. D. (2003). Births: Final data for 2002. *National Vital Statistics Reports 52*(10). Hyattsville, MD: National Center for Health Statistics.

Martin, J. A., Hamilton, B. E., Sutton, P. D. (2006). Births: Final data for 2004. *National Vital Statistics Reports, 55*(1). Hyattsville, MD: National Center for Health Statistics.

McMahon, M. J., Luther, E. R., Bowes, W. A., & Olshan, A. F. (1996). Comparison of a trial of labor with an elective second cesarean section. *New England Journal of Medicine, 335,* 689–695.

Menacker, F., & Curtin, S. C. (2001). Trends in cesarean birth and vaginal birth after previous cesarean, 1991–99. *National Vital Statistics Reports, 49*(13). Hyattsville, MD: National Center for Health Statistics.

Nelson, K. B., & Ellenberg, J. H. (1986). Antecedents of cerebral palsy: Multivariate analysis of risk. *New England Journal of Medicine, 315,* 81–86.

Paul, R. (1994). Electronic fetal monitoring and later outcome: A thirty-year overview. *Journal of Perinatology, 14*(5), 393–395.

Parer, J., & King, T. (2000). Fetal heart rate monitoring: Is it salvageable? *American Journal of Obstetrics and Gynecology, 182,* 282–287.

Sachs, B. P., Kobelin, C., Castro, M. A., & Frigoletto, F. (1999). Risks of lowering cesarean-delivery rate. *New England Journal of Medicine, 340*(1), 54–57.

Simpson, K. R. (2002). Association of Women's Health, Obstetric and Neonatal Nurses Practice Monograph. *Cervical ripening and induction and augmentation of labor* (2nd ed.). Washington, DC: AWHONN.

Thacker, S. B., & Stoup, D. F. (2000). *Continuous electronic heart rate monitoring for fetal assessment during labor.* Cochrane Database System Rev 2000; 2:CD0000063.

United States Department of Health and Human Services. (2000). *Healthy People 2010.* Retrieved October 2006 from http://www.healthypeople.gov/Document/HTML/Volume2/16MICH.htm#_Toc494699664

Vintzileos, A. M., Nochimson, D. J., Guzman, E. R., Knuppel, R. A., Lake, M., & Shifrin, B. S. (1995). Intrapartum electronic fetal monitoring versus intermittent auscultation: A meta-analysis. *Obstetrics & Gynecology, 85*(1), 149–155.

CONTENTS

1 Maternal–Fetal Physiology of Fetal Heart Rate Patterns

The rationale for electronic fetal monitoring (EFM) is based on the knowledge that when normal metabolic processes are interrupted, either by a lack of oxygen (O_2) or an inability to expel end products, the subsequent accumulation of acids may damage all or part of the living system.

Fetal well-being depends on adequate functioning of sources and suppliers of oxygen and waste removal mechanisms. These include the maternal system, the placenta, the uterus, and the umbilical cord. At this time, the relationship between specific fetal heart rate (FHR) patterns and fetal acidemia is supported by observational studies only. However, the relationship appears to be strong (Parer, King, Flanders, Fox, & Kilpatrick, 2005, p. 292). This chapter explains the physiology of the maternal–fetal unit and relates its functioning to FHR patterns. The specific FHR patterns mentioned are detailed in Chapter 3.

Maternal Oxygenation

The maternal respiratory system is the primary source of oxygen for the fetus. If the maternal oxygen supply or oxygen-carrying capacity is diminished, fetal oxygenation is certain to be decreased. This can occur in conjunction with any maternal respiratory, circulatory, hemolytic, or cardiac condition that affects maternal oxygenation (Parer, 1997, 1998). Examples of these include, but are certainly not limited to, asthma, pulmonary embolus, pulmonary edema, pneu-

monia, hypertension, hypotension, anemia, sickle cell disease, and various forms of cardiac decompensation or insufficiency. To maintain optimal or even sufficient fetal oxygenation, maternal oxygenation must be adequately maintained and supported.

FHR patterns that result from a decrease in maternal oxygenation may include any or all of the following: late decelerations, fetal tachycardia, and/or decreased FHR baseline variability. Fetal bradycardia may also occur in response to a prolonged event. The physiologic basis of the late deceleration pattern is believed to originate with a decrease in oxygen available to the fetus, most commonly due to a decrease in the amount of oxygen perfused to the fetus through the placenta. The hypoxic fetus responds to the decrease in oxygen transfer across the placenta that normally occurs during uterine contractions by slowing its heart rate. The FHR then continues at a decreased pace until after the contraction has ended and uterine perfusion returns. It is only after blood flow to the fetus has fully resumed (when the uterus has relaxed) that the FHR returns to its baseline rate. The occurrence of this process is demonstrated by the presence of late decelerations in the FHR tracing.

As the fetus becomes hypoxic, rising levels of CO_2 stimulate the chemoreceptors and increase sympathetic activity, causing the FHR baseline to rise. Due to the effects of these same compensatory mechanisms, loss of variability in the FHR baseline usually accompanies fetal tachycardia.

Placental Circulation

The placenta is the organ that connects the maternal and fetal systems and performs many of the same functions for the fetus that its lungs will later assume in extrauterine life. The fetus relies on the placenta for transfer of oxygen and nutrients and removal of waste products. The placenta accomplishes this through the villi, fetal tissue that projects into maternal blood circulating in the intervillous space. It is through these projections that transfer of oxygen, carbon dioxide, and nutrients occurs. Oxygenated blood from the mother is carried to the placenta by the uterine arteries. Blood enters the intervillous space under positive arterial pressure, bathes the fetal villi, and then drains back to the maternal veins (Fig. 1–1).

A microscopic layer of fetal trophoblasts in the placenta serves as a filter, permitting the exchange of nutrients and waste products between the maternal and fetal systems without fetal and maternal blood cells coming into contact with one another. The passage of nutrients and waste products across this membrane occurs due to six mechanisms: facilitated diffusion, passive diffusion, active transport, bulk flow, pinocytosis, and breaks in the system (Table 1–1). Deoxygenated blood is carried from the fetus to the placenta through the two umbilical arteries. These umbilical arteries split off into smaller capillaries that traverse the fetal villi. The villi project into the intervillous space, where maternal and fetal blood supplies exchange necessary gases (ie, oxygen and carbon dioxide) and nutrients. After this transaction, oxygenated blood is carried back into fetal circulation by way of a single umbilical vein.

Due to vasoconstriction, blood flow across the intervillous space is diminished during uterine contractions. This temporary reduction in perfusion forces the fetus to rely on any oxygen that might be available in its system until the contraction ends and normal blood flow resumes. The vast majority of fetuses show no change in their heart rate or acid–base status during contractions. When placental vasculature and circulation are compromised, however, the fetus is likely to be affected by these episodes of diminished placental blood flow. Examples of maternal health factors that contribute to diminished placental function include, but are not limited to type 1 diabetes, hypertension, and smoking. Other conditions that may compromise the oxygen–carbon dioxide transfer through the placenta include placenta previa, abruptio placentae, chorioamnionitis, postterm gestation, and intrauterine growth restriction.

Transient events, such as uterine hyperstimulation (eg, six or more contractions in 10 minutes) or maternal hypotension, also diminish placental blood flow and lead to the occurrence of late decelerations (American College of Obstetricians and Gynecologists [ACOG], 2005). Alleviating transitory causes of uteroplacental insufficiency usually allows the fetus to recover and subsequently remediates the FHR pattern. If the events that are initiating the late deceleration pattern occur repetitively or over a prolonged period of time, oxygen is quickly depleted and the late decelerations become accompanied by other nonreassuring signs, such as tachycardia, decreased variability, bradycardia, and loss of accelerations.

Since maternal and fetal blood supplies are maintained independently, it may be consequential when fetal cells enter the maternal system. If blood incompatibilities such as Rh, ABO, or other antigen factors are present, isoimmunization can result.

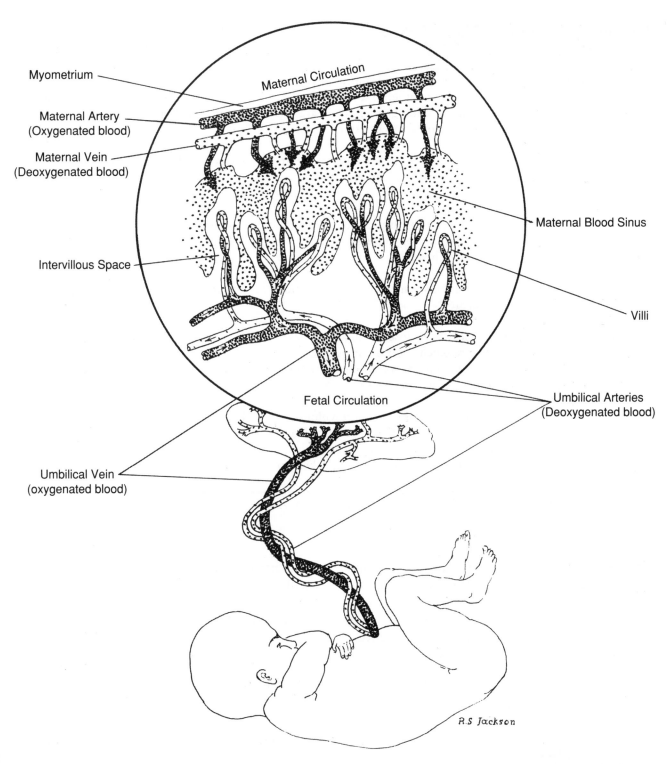

Figure 1–1. Maternal-placental-fetal exchange. (Adapted from: Afriat, C. I. (1989). *Electronic fetal monitoring.* Rockland, MD: Aspen.)

Table 1–1. MECHANISMS OF TRANSPORT

Mechanism	Description	Substances Exchanged
Passive diffusion	No energy required; substances pass from one area to another; transport based on concentration gradient from areas of high to low concentration	Oxygen, carbon dioxide, sodium, chloride, lipids, fat-soluble vitamins, some medications
Facilitated diffusion	Energy may be required; transport is faster than that based on concentration gradient; "pump"	Glucose, other carbohydrates
Active transport	Energy required; transport occurs against the concentration gradient; carrier molecules involved	Amino acids, water-soluble vitamins, large ions (calcium, iron)
Bulk flow	Transport based on hydrostatic or osmotic gradient	Water, dissolved electrolytes
Pinocytosis	Molecules are enclosed in small vesicles that are pinched off on one side of the placenta and traverse to the other side; contents are then released	Immunoglobulins, serum proteins
Breaks	Villi may break off within intervillous space, and contents may be extruded into maternal circulation; maternal intravascular contents may be taken up by fetal circulation	Fetal Rh-positive cells

Afriat, C. I. (1989). *Electronic fetal monitoring.* Rockland, MD: Aspen.

A break in the system, such as that which occurs during abruptio placentae, is a common means by which fetal and maternal blood mix. In addition to the potentially grave consequences such an insult may directly initiate, the resulting hemolytic effects on the fetus can be devastating. Sinusoidal FHR patterns (explained in Chapter 3) are most often attributable to Rh sensitization or other forms of fetal anemia (Rochard, Schifrin, Goupil, et al., 1976).

Uterine Blood Flow

The blood flow to and through the uterus is a key determinant in placental function. Approximately 10% to 15% of maternal cardiac output ($\sim$ 500 to 750 mL/min) flows through the uterus of the term gestation. Unlike the rest of the human vascular system, which can constrict and dilate under central nervous system (CNS) control, the uterine vascular bed is believed to constantly maintain maximum dilation. Only an increase in maternal cardiac output can improve uterine blood flow.

Because uterine blood flow is routinely decreased during contractions, a diminished amount of oxygen, carbon dioxide, and nutrients is exchanged between fetal and maternal blood during this time. This causes a loss of oxygen to the fetus and a buildup of carbon dioxide within the fetal circulation. Although a healthy, well-oxygenated fetus has a small reserve of oxygen from which to draw, this will be depleted quickly with repeated episodes of hypoxia. With each uterine contraction and subsequent decrease in perfusion, the fetus who is without reserve is placed in life-threatening circumstances.

Factors that contribute to decreased uterine blood flow are both iatrogenic and noniatrogenic

Table 1–2. CAUSES OF DECREASED UTERINE BLOOD FLOW

Etiology	Physiologic Effect
Iatrogenic	
Maternal supine position	Inferior vena cava compression, possible aortic compression, decreased venous return; decreased uteroplacental blood flow
Uterine hyperstimulation (induced)	Decreased uteroplacental blood flow
Regional anesthesia	Maternal hypotension and decreased uteroplacental blood flow
Valsalva maneuver (closed-glottis "pushing")	Decreased fetal oxygenation (Simpson & James, 2005)
Noniatrogenic	
Abruptio placentae	Alteration of placental vasculature, chronic placental change, decreased uteroplacental blood flow
Pregnancy-induced hypertension	
Chronic hypertension	
Uterine hyperstimulation (spontaneous)	
Smoking	
Substance abuse	
Malnutrition	
Pregnancy-induced hypertension	Maternal vasoconstriction, decreased uteroplacental blood flow
Chronic hypertension	
Smoking	
Substance abuse	
Collagen-vascular disease	
Abruptio placentae	Decreased functional placenta surface area due to calcifications, infarctions
Type 1 diabetes	
Postdate pregnancy	
Smoking	

(Table 1–2). The noniatrogenic causes include fetal hemorrhage secondary to abruptio placentae, placental deterioration, hypertension, hypotension, autoimmune disease, smoking, tachysystole, and tetanic contractions. Those that are of iatrogenic etiology commonly occur even though they are often within control of the perinatal team. For example, administration of oxytocin and other uterotonic agents can lead to tetanic contractions and/or uterine hyperstimulation. Uterine hyperstimulation may cause late or prolonged decelerations even in the well-oxygenated fetus, as a result of the extended period during which uteroplacental blood flow is diminished. In most of these situations, the fetus will have enough oxygen in reserve to recover from the loss of blood flow. A fetus who is experiencing chronic placental deterioration, however, may not have the ability to recover from an iatrogenic insult such as hyperstimulation. Tocolytic agents, such as terbutaline, may be used to treat FHR decelerations in the presence of uterine hypertonus or hyperstimulation. They may also be used in the absence of uterine hyperstimulation when an abnormal FHR pattern occurs in response to uterine activity. The neonate's condition may benefit from the improvement in uterine blood flow (ACOG, 2005).

The administration and management of regional anesthesia can contribute to diminished uteroplacental blood flow. It is of fundamental importance to support maternal circulation and prevent hypotension before, during, and after the administration of medications. Maternal hypotension can cause late decelerations due to the resulting decrease in blood flow to the uterus. The reduction in uterine blood flow potentiates a decrease in blood flow through the uterine arteries, subsequently decreasing blood flow across the placenta. Positioning the patient in the maternal supine position is a common, but avoidable, cause of hypotension. The Valsalva maneuver (ie, maternal breath holding with expulsive efforts during second-stage labor) is another practice to be considered. Various studies have indicated that the resulting maternal hemodynamic effects may decrease fetal oxygenation (AWHONN, 2000).

The Umbilical Cord

Oxygen-rich blood is carried to the fetus from the placenta through the umbilical vein. Deoxygenated blood is carried away from the fetus by two umbilical arteries. Changes in the blood flow through the umbilical cord can impact FHR. Pressure exerted on the umbilical cord can compress the umbilical vein and the umbilical arteries (Ikeda, Murata, Quilligan, et al., 2000).

If the umbilical cord is only partially compressed, as occasionally happens during uterine contractions, it is possible for the umbilical vein to be occluded while the arteries remain patent because the walls of the umbilical vein are thinner and more easily compressed than the walls of the arteries. When the umbilical vein is occluded, the flow of oxygen-rich blood to the fetus is diminished. This results in a sympathetic response in the fetus because the change in oxygenation stimulates the chemoreceptors to effect a transient increase in the FHR. It also causes the fetus to become hypotensive secondary to hypovolemia, which stimulates the fetal baroreceptors to trigger an increase in the FHR.

If the umbilical cord becomes further compressed, the umbilical arteries become occluded and the fetal baroreceptors are stimulated by the resulting increase in fetal blood pressure. This causes a parasympathetic response and the FHR drops abruptly, resulting in a variable deceleration of the FHR (explained further in Chapter 3).

As the contraction wanes, cord compression may be progressively alleviated, leaving only the umbilical vein occluded. The fetal chemoreceptors and baroreceptors again produce a sympathetic response and transiently accelerate heart rate. These brief accelerations, which can precede, follow, or occur on both sides of a variable deceleration, are part of the variable deceleration pattern and are referred to as *shoulders*. This is a benign finding usually associated with moderate FHR baseline variability.

If the fetus is already experiencing compromise, the response to cord compression may be quite different. There may be no acceleration present as the cord is compressed, only the occurrence of a variable deceleration. The variable deceleration is likely to fall far below the FHR baseline in this instance. Additionally, the FHR baseline will likely be tachycardic and have little variability. In an attempt to recover from the variable deceleration to its baseline rate, the compromised fetus first raises its heart rate above the baseline and then effects a very gradual return to baseline rate. These accelerations that occur as part of the variable deceleration pattern are referred to as *overshoots*. When overshoots are present, there is usually minimal or absent FHR baseline variability. Overshoots are considered to be a nonreassuring sign in the term fetus because this pattern is associated with autonomic nervous system (ANS) impairment (Schifrin, Hamilton-Rubenstein, & Shields, 1994). This is explained further in Chapter 3.

Chemoreceptors and Baroreceptors

Chemoreceptors and baroreceptors factor significantly in CNS control over the autonomic activities of heart rate and respiratory effort (Chaffee & Greisheimer, 1969). Stimulation of either type of receptor can effect a change in the FHR in response to gas or pressure changes in the fetal circulation.

Chemoreceptors

Chemoreceptors are nerve receptors in blood vessels that sense the chemical makeup of the surrounding environment. A change in the pH of the blood causes the chemoreceptors to initiate afferent nerve impulses to either speed up or slow down respiratory activity or heart rate. Acid–base balance is further explained later in this chapter.

S T O R K   B Y T E :

My heart is beating faster—either something really excited me or my chemoreceptors just kicked in!

Baroreceptors

Baroreceptors are sensors that are highly sensitive to changes in the pressure of the blood against vessel walls. Arterial baroreceptors are located in the walls of the aortic arch and the carotid bodies. If the arterial pressure rises above normal levels, the baroreceptors signal the cardiac system to slow the FHR. Stimulation of the baroreceptors causes vasodilation and a lowering of the arterial blood pressure. If the arterial pressure begins to fall below normal levels, the baroreceptors receive less stimulation and a reflex increase in the FHR results. At the same time, a vasoconstriction in the peripheral blood vessels occurs, causing arterial blood pressure to rise.

The venous system also has baroreceptors. These are located in the walls of the terminal portions of the venae cavae and the right atrium, with afferent fibers traveling to the vagus nerve. When baroreceptors in the veins are activated by high venous blood pressure, an increase in the FHR results.

S T O R K   B Y T E :

I can't take all this pressure!
  When arterial pressure increases, the baroreceptors slow my heart rate and cause vasodilation in order to decrease arterial pressure.

Central Nervous System

The anatomic portion of the CNS includes the brain and the spinal cord. The physiologic part includes the somatic (voluntary) nervous system and the autonomic (involuntary) nervous system. The somatic nervous system consists of nerve fibers that connect the CNS with structures of the body wall, such as the skin and skeletal muscles. The ANS consists of fibers that connect the CNS with smooth muscle, cardiac muscle, and the glands. It is the ANS that is directly responsible for changes in the FHR (Figure 1–2; Chaffee & Greisheimer, 1969).

The Autonomic Nervous System

Both structurally and functionally, the ANS may be divided into two parts: the sympathetic and parasympathetic nervous systems. The word *sympathetic* indicates a relationship between two parts whereby a change in one part affects the other. The parasympathetic nervous system functions to inhibit or oppose the effects of the sympathetic nervous system on specific organs (Table 1–3).

Parasympathetic Nervous System

The primary function of the parasympathetic nervous system is to coordinate activities related to the restoration and conservation of body energy and the elimination of bodily waste. Its major component, the vagus nerve, networks the brain and the heart (see Fig. 1–2). When the parasympathetic nervous system is activated, the vagus nerve carries the message from the cardoinhibitory center of the brain to the sinoatrial and atrioventricular nodes of the heart, telling them to decrease the rate of firing and transmission, thereby slowing the FHR. This communication commonly occurs when the fetal head is compressed—the resulting increase in intracranial pressure causes a decrease in cerebral blood flow, stimulating the parasympathetic nervous system to activate the vagus nerve and subsequently decrease the FHR. Potential initiators of this chain of events include cephalopelvic disproportion, fetal descent, cervical examination, forceps application, and/or the fetal head being pressed into the pelvis during contractions.

When the parasympathetic nervous system is stimulated in the adult, several responses occur. Motor responses include stimulation of the sphincter muscle of the iris, causing the pupils to contract; constriction of the bronchioles, causing difficulty with breathing; and stimulation of the intestines, stomach, and urinary bladder. Inhibitory responses also occur due to smooth muscle relaxation. This results in the dilation of the blood vessels of the salivary glands and external genitalia. The parasympathetic nervous system also controls secretory function by causing the stomach and pancreas to increase secretory activity and generate thin, watery saliva.

In short, stimulation of the parasympathetic nervous system in the adult causes the pupils to constrict (protecting the eyes from excessive light), gastrointestinal function to be promoted (so food energy can be taken into the body and stored for future use), heart rate to be slowed (so cardiac

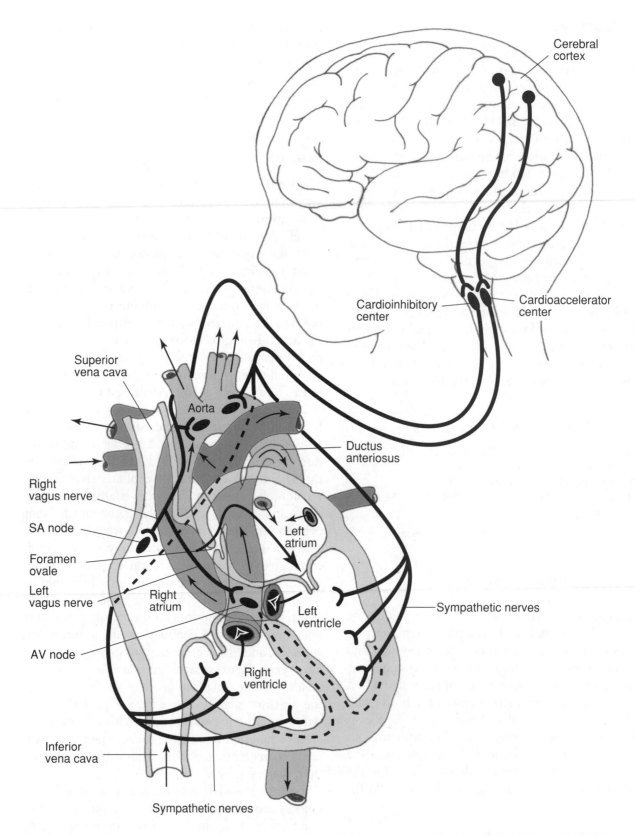

Figure 1–2. Central nervous system's control over heart rate. Note the baroreceptors, chemoreceptors, and pacemaker sites of the heart. Abbreviations: AV, atrioventricular; SA, sinoatrial.

Table 1–3. THE AUTONOMIC NERVOUS SYSTEM

Parasympathetic	Sympathetic
Pupillary constriction	Pupillary dilation
Production of watery saliva	Dry mouth
Bronchiole constriction	Increased lung capacity
Increased gastrointestinal activity	Decreased gastrointestinal activity
Increased bladder activity	Retention of bladder contents
Dry skin	Increased sweating, pilomotor muscle contraction (goosebumps)
Slowed heart rate	Increased heart rate
	Increased adrenal gland secretions
	Increased glycogenolytic function

muscle has the opportunity to rest), and bladder and bowel function to be regulated (so waste products are properly removed from the body). Similarly in the fetus, stimulation of the parasympathetic nervous system will cause a decrease in the FHR and may trigger release of meconium. Release of meconium can be a normal physiologic response and does not necessarily indicate fetal compromise.

S T O R K   B Y T E :

Easy on my cranium, please!
   Pressure on my head makes the parasympathetic nervous system lower my heart rate.

Sympathetic Nervous System

Changes in the external environment are responsible for stimulation of the sympathetic nervous system. The most commonly known effect that external factors have on the body is the sympathetic nervous system's "fight or flight" response to any situation perceived as an emergency. The sympathetic nervous system prepares the body for the intense muscular activity that may be involved in meeting the challenges of a stressful situation. When such motor functions in the adult are stimulated, the radial muscle of the iris contracts (dilating the pupils), the pilomotor muscles contract (causing goosebumps), and the smooth muscle in the sphincters of the gastrointestinal tract and the urinary bladder contract to retain their contents. The heart beats faster and more forcibly, and vasoconstriction of blood vessels occurs in the viscera and skin.

Relaxation of smooth skeletal and cardiac muscles causes blood vessels to dilate. In addition, the muscle in the walls of the gastrointestinal tract and urinary bladder relax, and the bronchioles dilate, making breathing easier. Stimulation of secretory functions increases the activity of the sweat glands and the secretion of epinephrine by the adrenal glands. Viscid saliva is produced, causing a feeling of dryness in the mouth. Stimulation of glycogenolysis facilitates the breakdown of glycogen to glucose, which is then released into the bloodstream to augment the available fuel source.

When the sympathetic nervous system is stimulated in the adult, the pupils dilate, saliva production decreases, adrenaline and glucose are produced, the gastrointestinal tract slows down, and cardiac and respiratory rates increase. Visceral and skin blood vessels constrict, whereas those in skeletal muscle, heart muscle, lungs, and brain dilate. These actions shunt blood to the vital organs. The fetus responds similarly when stimulated by loud noise, vibration, maternal abdominal palpation, scalp stimulation, or application of the spiral electrode.

S T O R K   B Y T E :

Hey, that tickles!
   Stimulating my sympathetic nervous system through sound or sensation causes my heart rate to increase.

Maintaining Balance

The actions and effects of the sympathetic nervous system counterbalance those of the parasympathetic nervous system. They function collaboratively to maintain a balance, unless one is sufficiently stimulated to override the other. This interaction is visually apparent in the maintenance of and changes in FHR baseline rate and variability, which is explained further in Chapters 2 and 3.

Development and Functioning of the Autonomic Nervous System

By approximately 32 weeks' gestation, the fetus' ANS is expected to be fully developed and capable of effecting predictable responses to various stimuli as demonstrated by changes in its heart rate. Many fetuses accomplish such development at an even earlier gestational age. The mature ANS is demonstrated by the presence of variations in the duration between each cardiac cycle. This normal occurrence of sinus arrhythmia is recognized as FHR baseline variability. The presence of variability in the FHR tracing is a visual display of the synergistic workings of the sympathetic and parasympathetic nervous systems. The fetal CNS is sensitive to changes in oxygen exchange with the maternal system and to its own carbon dioxide production and uses the ANS to effect actions intended to maintain a normal environment. The presence or absence of variability in the FHR, therefore, is the primary indicator of fetal oxygenation.

STORK BYTE:

An expression of gratitude. . .
   The presence of variability in my baseline heart rate indicates that I am well oxygenated, thank you very much!

Acid–Base Balance

The maintenance of proper acid–base balance within the human body is essential to well-being. When the maternal–uterine–placental exchange system is interrupted, the potential exists for fetal acidosis, which can lead to permanent damage or death. When fetal blood is analyzed, it is the blood from the fetal umbilical vein that reflects uteroplacental status. This is largely dependent on maternal condition. The composition of the blood from the umbilical arteries reflects uteroplacental status as well as fetal oxygenation (Pomerance, 2004).

The purpose of EFM is to screen for the development of hypoxia. The ability to distinguish reassuring FHR patterns from those that are not is essential to patient care. Direct and indirect measures of hypoxia (including fetal scalp blood sampling, fetal scalp stimulation, and vibra-acoustic stimulation) are valuable adjuncts to EFM in determining fetal status and are discussed in Chapter 5.

All chemical processes in the living cell involve the balance of hydrogen (H^+) and hydroxyl (OH^-) ions. The concentration of each of these elements in the body fluids determines the degree of acidity or alkalinity. If there are more hydrogen ions, the fluid is acidic; if there are more hydroxyl ions, the fluid is alkaline. The pH value is the means by which the measurement of hydrogen ion concentration is expressed. The amount of H^+ ions retained determines acid–base status: the greater the concentration of H^+ ions, the higher the acidity. The measurement of hydrogen ion concentration is inversely expressed as the pH (ie, the higher the hydrogen ion concentration, the lower the pH).

The body and all living cells are sensitive to changes in acidity and alkalinity. An alteration in the pH of blood affects the functioning of many cells. In the blood, there are buffer salts that keep the pH relatively constant. As a clinical example of alterations in pH status, consider the person who has experienced prolonged vomiting. Because there is significant loss of gastric fluid, which contains the acid *hydrogen chloride*, the blood becomes more alkaline and the person enters a state of alkalosis. Conversely, a person with lung disease who cannot exhale carbon dioxide as rapidly as it is produced accumulates this acid within the blood. As the pH value lowers, this person enters a state of acidosis. Alkalosis and acidosis can cause permanent damage to organs or progress to a fatal condition if the acid–base balance is not quickly restored.

Acids

The body produces two groups of acids: volatile acids (such as carbonic acid), and nonvolatile acids (such as lactic acid). Carbonic acid is formed by hydration of carbon dioxide. Alveolar ventilation regulates carbon dioxide levels in the adult and normally maintains a carbon dioxide partial pressure in the alveoli and arterial blood of 40 mm Hg. As a normal adaptive change, these pressures are altered during pregnancy. Because of her increased ventilation, a pregnant woman's carbon dioxide partial pressure is typically 30 to 32 mm Hg (Table 1–4). This allows the fetus to readily dispose of carbon dioxide by diffusion across the placenta, providing there is adequate intervillous and umbilical blood flow.

Nonvolatile acids are produced by anaerobic metabolism. Lactic acid is a major end product of anaerobic metabolism and is produced when the demand of muscles for oxygen during work exceeds the supply. When lactic acid accumulates, the need for oxygen is increased. This is usually experienced as feeling "out of breath," and the person in whom this is occurring responds by increasing her rate and depth of respiration. These increased respiratory efforts bring a greater amount of oxygen into the system, allowing for lactic acid to change into pyruvic acid and carbon dioxide through the process of aerobic metabolism. If the body is unable to accomplish this effectively and lactic acid continues to accumulate, muscle fatigue results. Excessive amounts of lactic acid depress the activity in muscle cells, leading to decreased muscle responsiveness.

In the adult, nonvolatile acids are excreted through the renal system. This process is slower than the rate of excretion of carbon dioxide, requiring hours rather than seconds to accomplish. The fetus disposes of nonvolatile acids by diffusion across the placenta. As in the adult, the process is slower than the diffusion of carbon dioxide.

Fetal Metabolism

Knowledge of acid–base balance should be applied to care of the fetus (Table 1–5). The normal fetal metabolic process begins as glucose is broken down into lactic acid. Oxygen is required to facilitate the next step, which is to convert lactic acid into carbon dioxide (CO_2) and water (H_2O). Carbon dioxide is a waste product of this process and is disposed of by the fetus through diffusion across the placenta into the maternal system. This is how the fetus produces energy.

Fetal Metabolism

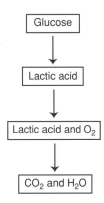

Buffers

If there is any interruption in blood flow to the uterus, across the placenta, or through the umbilical cord, fetal acid–base imbalance may result. Oxygen is necessary to complete the metabolic process by changing lactic acid into excretable end products. If fetal hypoxemia (decreased oxygen content in the blood) develops and is allowed to continue, hypoxia (decreased oxygen in the tissues) will result. Without oxygen, lactic acid is not broken down and begins to accumulate in the blood and the tissues. This buildup of lactic acid causes retention of hydrogen ions, an increase in their presence in the blood (acidemia), and an increase in their concentration in the tissues (acidosis). The fetus responds by activating its buffer system. Buffers are chemical substances that resist changes in the pH of a solution when an acid or base is added to it. Most buffers are comprised of a substance that is

Table 1–4. ADULT ACID–BASE PARAMETERS

pH	pO$_2$	pCO$_2$	Base Deficit
Nonpregnant Woman			
7.40	90–100 mm Hg	40 mm Hg	0
Pregnant Woman			
7.40	90–100 mm Hg	30–32 mm Hg	0

Table 1–5. FETAL ACID–BASE PARAMETERS*

pH	pO₂	pCO₂	Base Excess
Fetal Blood Sample			
7.25–7.40	18–22 mm Hg	40–50 mm Hg	0–11 mEq/L
*Venous Cord Sample** *			
7.25–7.45	17.2–40.8 mm Hg	26.8–49.2 mm Hg	0–11 mEq/L
*Arterial Cord Sample** *			
7.18–7.38	5.6–30.8 mm Hg	32.2–65.8 mm Hg	0–11 mEq/L

*Clinically significant fetal acidemia is defined as pH <7.00 for umbilical artery pH and <7.20 for scalp blood (ACOG, 2006, Gilstrap, 1999; Winkler et al., 1991). Normal fetal base deficit is 0 to 11 mEq/L. A base deficit >11 is considered potential metabolic acidosis (Helwig et al., 1996; Reis, Gabbe, & Petrie, 1999, ACOG, 2006).
**The umbilical venous blood gas always has a higher pH, a lower pCO₂, and a higher pO₂ than the umbilical arterial blood gas (Pomerance, 2004).

both weakly acidic and the salt of that substance. These pairs can react with relatively strong acids or bases and replace them with less harmful substances. These less volatile substances can then be eliminated from the body. Buffers are of primary importance in maintaining the proper ratio of hydrogen and hydroxyl ions in the body. Bicarbonate (HCO_3) is the most important buffer used by the fetus to normalize its environment.

When a scalp or cord pH sample is analyzed, information about how much HCO_3 was used by the fetus is expressed directly as a numeric value and also indirectly by the base deficit. Base deficit (referred to as base excess when reported as a positive integer) indicates the degree of metabolic acidosis. The higher the base deficit (or the lower the base excess), the greater the amount of buffer used. Because

bicarbonate is a buffer used to control metabolically produced acids, a high base deficit points to significant acidosis. Calculation of base deficit or base excess is based on pH and pCO_2; if pH and pCO_2 are within normal limits, the base deficit or base excess must also be (Pomerance, 2004).

In metabolic acidosis, the oxygen supply to the fetus is diminished over a period of time, causing an increase in the concentration of lactic acid. Bicarbonate is consumed in an effort to neutralize the buildup of acid. As this buffer base becomes depleted, the pH value continues to fall as the fetus becomes hypoxic. This can lead to permanent damage to tissue and organs. When the fetus is unable to excrete nonvolatile acids, its behavior is affected. This is demonstrated by a decrease in or lack of fetal movement, an absence of fetal tone, and a loss

Metabolic Acidosis

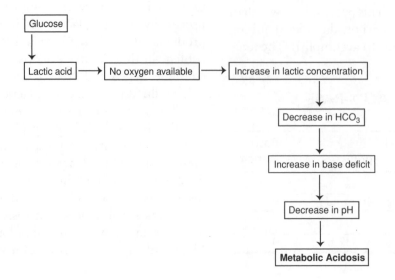

Table 1–6. METABOLIC ACIDOSIS

Parameter	Value	Reason
pH	Low; <7.20	Acidosis is present.
pCO_2	Normal; <60	No oxygen is present to allow conversion of lactic acid to CO_2.
pO_2	Low; <20	Lack of O_2 is the problem instigating the metabolic acidosis.
HCO_3	Low; <22	This buffer is used to neutralize metabolically produced acids.
Base excess	High; >8–11	Reflects amount of buffer used to neutralize acids.

of fetal breathing movements. A reduction in the amount of amniotic fluid may also occur if there is a prolonged period of lactic acid accumulation. Changes in the FHR tracing that may be observed include minimal or absent FHR baseline variability, tachycardia, a loss of accelerations, and, ultimately, terminal bradycardia (Table 1–6).

With respiratory acidosis, there is no production or accumulation of lactic acid. Respiratory acidosis occurs quickly and has the potential for rapid recovery. An example of this is the swimmer who holds his or her breath for a prolonged underwater swim. With breath holding, CO_2 accumulates and pH subsequently decreases. After resurfacing, the swimmer takes a big gasp of air. This causes heart rate and respirations to increase, promoting oxygen supply and consumption, and stabilizing the pH. In the fetus, respiratory acidosis may be reflected in the FHR pattern as a rise in the baseline FHR, a decrease in or loss of baseline variability, and a loss or diminution of accelerations. Usually, when the cause of the respiratory acidosis is corrected, the FHR experiences a relatively quick recovery. At delivery, a fetus with respiratory acidosis may have a low 1-minute Apgar score, but will usually respond to stimulation and oxygen administration and have a normal 5-minute Apgar score (Table 1–7).

It is possible for the fetus to experience respiratory and metabolic acidosis simultaneously. This condition is referred to as *mixed acidosis* and combines the worst values of each (Table 1–8).

Respiratory Acidosis

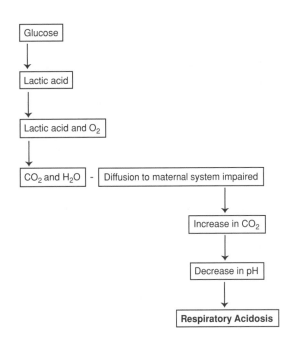

A variety of events can cause decreased perfusion to and through the uterus and placenta, negatively affecting fetal acid–base status. If the fetus is already compromised, even marginally, the risk of metabolic acidosis is even greater. It is of fundamental importance to continuously assess and support the maternal system's maintenance of optimal uteroplacental perfusion.

Assessment of Fetal Acid–Base Balance

EFM is used in both antepartum and intrapartum settings to assist the provider in determining whether the uterus is the optimal environment for

S T O R K   B Y T E :

Whom are you calling cute?
   Oh yes, respiratory acidosis is acute! But metabolic acidosis isn't so cute!

Table 1–7. RESPIRATORY ACIDOSIS

Parameter	Value	Reason
pH	Low; <7.20	Acidosis is present.
pCO_2	High; >60	Process continued through to production of this end product, which can't be excreted and is accumulating in the fetus.
pO_2	Normal; >20	Supply of O_2 is not the problem.
HCO_3	Normal; >22	Works against metabolically produced acids—not needed in this instance.
Base excess	Normal; <8–11	Measures buffers that work against metabolically produced acids—value is normal because buffers are not being used.

the fetus. EFM may be the sole means of assessing fetal status, or it may be used in conjunction with other techniques. Regardless of the reason for its initiation or the setting in which it is used, EFM's most beneficial feature is its capacity to display early signs of fetal compromise to the alert and discerning clinician.

Fetal Scalp Blood Sampling (Scalp pH)

In 90% of fetuses that demonstrate nonreassuring FHR patterns, no actual hypoxia/acidosis exists. Therefore, alternate methods of assessing acid–base status are needed to prevent unnecessary intervention (Low, Victory, & Derrick, 1999). Utilization of fetal scalp blood sampling in combination with EFM has been shown to decrease the number of cesarean births for fetal distress (Macones & Depp, 1996). Sampling of the fetal blood during labor is a technique that can provide a snapshot analysis of the acid–base status of the fetus who has a nonreassuring FHR pattern. This procedure is invasive to both the mother and the fetus; it involves puncturing the fetal scalp to obtain a small sampling of blood that is collected in a capillary tube and then analyzed for pH value. There are a number of limitations to this method of fetal assessment. Technical difficulties to be negotiated include mastery of the procedure, completion of the procedure on the laboring patient (who may not wish to remain still or who may experience discomfort), and positioning of the patient (what is optimal for the practitioner is often not the same in regard to promotion of maternal–fetal perfusion).

Table 1–8. MIXED ACIDOSIS

Parameter	Value	Reason
pH	Low; <7.20	Acidosis is present.
pCO_2	High; >60	What is converted to CO_2 can't be excreted and is accumulating in the fetus (respiratory acidosis).
pO_2	Low; <20	Lack of O_2 is instigating the metabolic part of the acidosis.
HCO_3	Low; <22	This buffer is being used to neutralize metabolically produced acids.
Base excess	High; >8–11	Reflects amount of buffer used to neutralize acids.

Other limitations exist in regard to processing of the fetal scalp blood sample. This includes lack of ability to distinguish between respiratory and metabolic acidosis. The laboratory result that is usually provided from the sample is the pH value, without benefit of the measurement of base deficit/base excess. Additionally, the timing of sampling affects the pH value. For example, a sample obtained during a deceleration or bradycardia will produce a lower value that is not accurately reflective of fetal status. Contamination of the sample with blood, meconium, or amniotic fluid may also alter results. Finally, blood obtained from caput may yield falsely low results.

Although fetal scalp blood sampling is performed much less frequently than in years past, it did leave a lasting contribution to EFM. Correlations made between particular FHR patterns and pH values led to improved understanding and interpretation of fetal status (Clark, Gimovsky, & Miller, 1984; 1982).

Scalp Stimulation

Based mainly on the work of Clark, Gimovsky, and Miller, manual stimulation of the fetal scalp has reduced the rate of fetal scalp blood sampling (1982, 1984). Initially, these researchers performed a retrospective study (N = 200) that revealed that no fetus who responded to a scalp pH sampling procedure with an acceleration (≥15 bpm × ≥15 seconds) had a scalp pH <7.21. In their 1984 prospective study (N = 100), they sampled fetuses with FHR patterns suggestive of acidosis by applying 15 seconds of gentle digital pressure to the fetal scalp followed by 15 seconds of pressure applied with an Allis clamp. Their results are summarized:

36/100 Acceleration with digital pressure	pH 7.19–7.40
15/100 No response to digital pressure, acceleration with Allis clamp	pH 7.23–7.33
49/100 No response to either stimulus	pH <7.20 (19) pH <7.23 (30)

The researchers reported the following impressions as conclusions of their study:

- Induced accelerations reflect a fetus with an intact autonomic nervous system.

- A fetus with the ability to demonstrate spontaneous or induced accelerations is not acidotic.

Based on these findings, the necessity for performing the fetal scalp blood sampling procedure has sharply decreased.

Fetal scalp blood sampling and scalp stimulation are procedures to be performed only when the FHR has recovered to baseline. The incidence of misleading results is greater if these procedures are done during a deceleration or bradycardia.

Umbilical Cord Blood Gas

New guidelines published by ACOG recommend umbilical cord arterial blood gases as the most objective method of assessing fetal metabolic condition at birth (2006). The recommendation is to obtain cord samples in certain circumstances (eg, newborns with low 5-minute Apgar scores or with abnormal FHR tracings). Umbilical cord gases with a pH <7.0 and a base deficit >12 mmol/L indicate a fetal metabolic acidosis possibly due to an intrapartum event and has an increased association with poor outcome (ACOG, 2006).

In conclusion, the entire clinical picture needs to be taken into account to accurately interpret the meaning of the FHR tracing. If the FHR tracing is reassuring, it is unlikely that metabolic acidosis is an issue. If the FHR tracing is nonreassuring, then steps must be taken to further evaluate fetal acid–base status.

REFERENCES

Afriat, C. I. (1989). *Electronic fetal monitoring.* Rockland, MD: Aspen.

American College of Obstetricians and Gynecologists. (2006). *Umbilical artery blood acid–base analysis.* ACOG Committee option 348. Washington, DC: Author.

American College of Obstetricians and Gynecologists (2005). *Intrapartum Fetal Heart Rate Monitoring.* ACOG Technical Bulletin 70. Washington, DC: Author.

Association of Women's Health, Obstetric, and Neonatal Nurses. (2000). *Second stage labor management: Promotion of evidence-based practice and a collaborative approach to patient care* [symposium]. Washington, DC: Author.

Chaffee, E., & Greisheimer, E. (1969). *Basic physiology and anatomy.* Philadelphia, PA: Lippincott.

———. (1982). Fetal heart rate response to scalp blood sampling. *American Journal of Obstetrics & Gynecology, 144,* 706.

Clark, S. L., Gimovsky, M. L., & Miller, F. C. (1984). The scalp stimulation test: A clinical alternative to fetal scalp blood sampling. *American Journal of Obstetrics & Gynecology, 148*(3), 274–277.

Gilstrap, L. (1999). Fetal acid–base balance. In Creasy, R. K., & Resnik, R. (Eds.), *Maternal–fetal medicine* (4th ed., pp. 331–340). Philadelphia, PA: W. B. Saunders.

Helwig, J., Parer, J., Kilpatrick, S., & Laros, R. (1996). Umbilical cord blood acid–base state: What is normal? *American Journal of Obstetrics and Gynecology, 174*(6), 1807–1812.

Ikeda, T., Murata, Y., Quilligan, E., Parer, J., Murayama, T., & Koono, M. (2000). Histologic and biochemical study of the brain, heart, kidney and liver in asphyxia caused by occlusion of the umbilical cord in near-term fetal lambs. *American Journal of Obstetrics and Gynecology, 182*(2), 449–457.

Low, J. A., Victory, R., & Derrick, E. J. (1999). Predictive value of electronic fetal monitoring for intrapartum fetal asphyxia with metabolic acidosis. *Obstetrics and Gynecology, 93*, 285–291.

Macones, G., & Depp, R. (1996). Fetal monitoring. In Wildschut, H., Weiner, C., & Peters, T. (Eds.), *When to screen in obstetrics and gynecology* (pp. 202–218). Philadelphia: W. B. Saunders.

Parer, J. T. (1997). *Handbook of fetal heart rate monitoring* (2nd ed.). Philadelphia: W. B. Saunders.

———. (1998). Effects of fetal asphyxia on brain cell structure and function: Limits of tolerance. *Comparative Bio-chemistry and Physiology, Part A. Molecular and Integrative Physiology, 119*(3), 711–716.

Parer, J. T., King, T., Flanders, S., Fox, M., & Kilpatrick, S. J. (2006). Fetal acidemia and electronic fetal heart rate patterns: Is there evidence of an association? *Journal of Maternal-Fetal and Neonatal Medicine, 19*(5), 289–294.

Pomerance, J. (2004). *Interpreting umbilical cord blood gases.* Pasadena, CA: BNMG.

Reis, E., Gabbe, S., & Petrie, R. (1999). Intrapartum evaluation. In Gabbe, S., Niebyl, J., & Simpson, J. L. (Eds.), *Obstetrics: Normal & Problem Pregnancies* (pp. 397–421). New York, NY: Churchill Livingston.

Rochard, F., Schifrin, B., Goupil, F., Legrand, H., Blottiere, J., & Sureau, C. (1976). Nonstress fetal heart monitoring in the antepartum period. *American Journal of Obstetrics and Gynecology, 126*(6), 699–706.

Schifrin, B., Hamilton-Rubenstein, T., & Shields, J. R. (1994). Fetal heart rate patterns and the timing of fetal injury. *Journal of Perinatology, 14*, 174–181.

Simpson, K. R., & James, D. C. (2005). Effects of immediate versus delayed pushing during second-stage labor on fetal well-being: A randomized clinical trial. *Nursing Research, 54*(3), 149–157.

2 Electronic Fetal Heart Rate Monitoring Equipment and Technology

To accurately interpret the data presented by the electronic fetal monitor, it is necessary to have a basic understanding of both the workings and the limitations of the equipment. The greatest effect on the data is produced by the mode of monitoring used. Information about both the fetal heart rate (FHR) and uterine activity may be gathered using sensors that are placed either internally or externally.

Acquisition of Fetal Heart Rate Data

Fetal Electrocardiogram (FECG)

Signal Processing

The most accurate means for assessing the FHR is through internal monitoring, currently accomplished by using the spiral electrode. The lead wires of the spiral electrode conduct the electrical signal of the fetal QRS waveform complex (FECG) to the electronic fetal monitor. From the FECG data, the electronic fetal monitor determines the FHR. The cardiotachometer is a component within the electronic fetal monitor that converts the FECG signal into the FHR. This processing is accomplished through the application of a mathematical equation:

$$FHR = \frac{60}{t}$$

Representing 60 seconds occurring per 1 minute

Representing the interval between successive QRS complexes

To determine the unknown factor of t to enter into this equation, the cardiotachometer measures the time elapsed between the R peaks of successive QRS complexes (Fig. 2–1).

Trending of Data

Once the factor of t is determined, it is then entered into the equation, $FHR = 60/t$. The product of this equation is the FHR, expressed in beats per minute (bpm). The FHR is then plotted on the FHR channel of the strip chart in bpm. Sinus arrhythmias are normal in the fetus and present as varying R–R intervals (t). Longer R–R intervals are represented by a slower FHR, whereas shorter R–R intervals are exhibited as a faster FHR. These fluctuations of the FHR from one beat to the next are recognized in the FHR tracing as *baseline variability*. (*Note:* Prior to the adoption of National Institute of Child Health and Human Development [NICHD] terminology [NICHD, 1997; American College of Obstetricians and Gynecologists (ACOG), 2005; Association of Women's Health, Obstetric and Neonatal Nurses (AWHONN), 2006] into clinical practice, this data [obtained only via internal monitoring] was further distinguished by use of the term *short-term variability*. Observation of the continuous recording of this data over a period of time allowed for even further determination of variations in the FHR baseline, previously known as *long-term variability*.)

Ultrasound

The FHR may also be determined from the signal acquired through use of external sensors. When properly placed on the maternal abdomen, the ultrasound transducer detects the movements of the

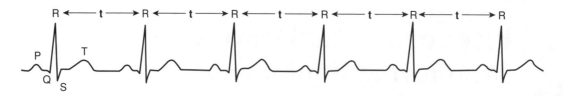

Figure 2–1. Fetal electrocardiogram.

fetal heart that occur with each beat. The ultrasound transducer contains crystals that transmit and receive high-frequency sound waves using the piezoelectric effect. The piezoelectric effect is the conversion of electrical energy into mechanical sound wave energy and vice versa. This is accomplished in the ultrasound transducer by the application of voltage to the crystals, which causes them to vibrate at a predetermined frequency. When this sound wave meets the fetal heart, its frequency becomes either compressed or stretched by the beating motion of the fetal heart and is reflected back to the crystals. The reflected sound wave is converted back into electrical energy at a frequency altered from the original transmitted frequency. The difference between the frequency of the sound wave that is transmitted and that which is reflected back is referred to as the Doppler shift. The Doppler shift frequency can be used to produce the audible sound that is recognized as the fetal heart beat and also provides the raw data from which the FHR can be determined by using the equation, FHR = 60/t.

Continual transmission and reception of sound waves to and from the ultrasound transducer is known as "continuous wave" ultrasound. This is accomplished by having certain crystals dedicated to emitting sound waves, whereas others only receive the reflected signal. Continuous wave ultrasound was used in early versions of the ultrasound transducer until it was replaced by pulse Doppler technology. Pulse Doppler ultrasound allows all of the crystals in the transducer to both send and receive sound waves. Each of the crystals inside the transducer is timed to transmit sound waves and then "standby" for a predetermined period (the amount of time it takes for the signal to be transmitted and reverberated). The crystals are then reactivated as receivers for the ultrasound signal as it is returned for processing. Pulse Doppler ultrasound makes it possible to monitor more than one fetus simultaneously. Because of the timing built into each crystal, the signal emitted by the ultrasound transducer for the purpose of evaluating one fetus will not be received by the ultrasound transducer that is tracking the second fetus.

Signal Processing

The external mode of monitoring requires different processes for identifying the factor of t for use in the equation, FHR = 60/t, than that which is used with internal monitoring. Determining the factor of t is very straightforward with internal monitoring—it is the time elapsed between the clearly identifiable, successive R peaks of the QRS complex. The raw data gathered by the ultrasound transducer do not contain such distinct reference points from which the factor of t may be figured. These data are created by electronically comparing the reflected ultrasound signal to the transmitted signal. The original signal is "subtracted" from the reflected signal, and the resulting waveform is representative of the motion of the fetal heart (Fig. 2–2). To facilitate determina-

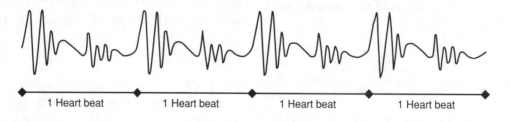

| 1 Heart beat | 1 Heart beat | 1 Heart beat | 1 Heart beat |

Figure 2–2. Raw waveform.

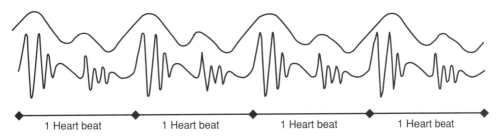

Figure 2–3. Waveform with filter applied.

tion of the factor *t,* the waveform is filtered to reduce the amount of high-frequency component. These filtered waveforms are irregularly shaped and lack an obvious common distinguishing element from which the timing of the occurrence of one waveform could be compared to that of the next (Fig. 2–3). To assist in converting these raw data into useful information, the monitor employs a method referred to as *autocorrelation.* Autocorrelation is a process of successively comparing waveforms to identify their similarities. Once such features are recognized, a template of the waveforms is created and is used as a comparison to incoming waveform data (Fig. 2–4). As correlations in the data are determined, the factor of *t* can be calculated from the peaks of the correlation function.

Trending of Data

Another difference of external versus internal monitoring is that information concerning the individual intervals between each successive fetal heart beat is not represented in the FHR tracing. Instead, once the factor of *t* is determined, it is applied in the equation FHR = 60/*t* and then averaged over several successive beats. It is only after this multiple beat average has been calculated that the FHR is determined and plotted on the strip chart. This averaging process is repeated continuously as data become available. Fluctuations in the FHR will be represented by varia-

tions in these averaged figures as the trend of the FHR is traced over a period of time. These variations are recognized by the clinician as *baseline variability.* (*Note:* Prior to the adoption of NICHD terminology [NICHD, 1997; ACOG, 2005; AWHONN, 2006] into clinical practice, fluctuations in the FHR obtained via external monitoring were further distinguished by use of the term *long-term variability.* Today, in accordance with current recommendations, the distinction between long- and short-term variability is no longer made. The visibly apparent fluctuations in the recorded trend of the FHR baseline [whether obtained internally or externally] are now simply referred to collectively as *baseline variability.*)

Limitations of Technology

Half-Counting and Double-Counting. The ultrasound transducer is able to recognize the FHR that is occurring within the range of approximately 50 to 180 bpm. As the FHR nears the outer limits of this range, it may be difficult to obtain a clear signal by external means. Occasionally, when the FHR nears the lower limits of the capacities of the ultrasound transducer, the electronic fetal monitor may begin to erroneously consider the motion data resulting from one heart beat to instead be that of two separate beats. This is exhibited by the intermittent trending of the FHR on the strip chart at twice the actual rate. Such an event is referred to as *double-counting*

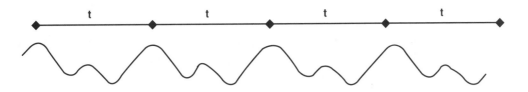

Figure 2–4. Resulting waveform.

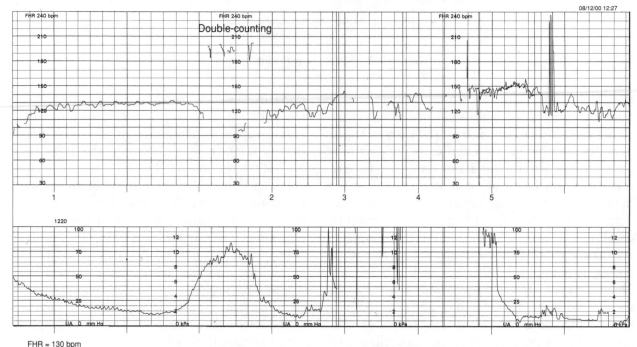

1) 08/12/00 12:20
   COMMENTS: DIFFICULT TO MONITOR FH DURING UCS. MD
   CONSULTED.
2) 08/12/00 12:23
   12:38 BP 131/71 M 94 P 70
   COMMENTS: FH AUDIBLE 90'S/100'S DURING UC.

3) 08/12/00 12:24
   116/118 EXTERNAL INOP
   COMMENTS: MD PRESENT TO PLACE INTERNAL MONITORS.
4) 08/12/00 12:25
   116/118 FECG EXTERNAL IUP
5) 08/12/00 12:26
   COMMENTS: SPIRAL ELECTRODE PLACED. 6 CMS NOW.

Figure 2–5. Double-counting.

(Fig. 2–5). If the FHR nears the upper limits of the capability of external monitoring, *half-counting* may occur. The monitor may only recognize every other section of motion data as a heart beat, thereby intermittently presenting the FHR at half the actual rate on the strip chart (Fig. 2–6). During the occurrence of both double-counting and half-counting, the audible signal will remain accurate and can be used as an indicator of the actual FHR. Internal monitoring may be selected as a remedy to either event because neither double-counting nor half-counting occurs during the use of this mode of monitoring.

Maternal Signal. The maternal pulse should be assessed and compared against the electronic fetal monitor's audible signal each time electronic fetal monitoring (EFM) is initiated or the mode of monitoring is changed (Murray, 2004; Doyle & Angelotti, 2004). The maternal heart rate may be transmitted by either mode of monitoring. The spiral electrode conducts electrocardiography (ECG) information to the electronic fetal monitor. In most cases, there are two sets of ECG data

> **S T O R K   B Y T E :**
> Pump up the volume! If there is a discrepancy between what you see on the strip chart and what you are hearing from the electronic fetal monitor, listen up! The sound of my heart beat is the definitive indicator of my actual heart rate.

available—fetal and maternal. The electronic fetal monitor recognizes the stronger of these two signals. As the spiral electrode is applied directly to the fetus, the FECG is expected to provide the stronger signal. If the spiral electrode is inadvertently applied to maternal tissue or to a fetus who is not alive, the maternal signal will appear stronger and, therefore, be the one that is transmitted (Fig. 2–7). The maternal signal may also be erroneously obtained when using the ultrasound transducer. When the transducer is placed over the maternal vessels, it will sense and record the movement data caused by pulsation (Fig. 2–8). The tracing of maternal heart rate is easily recog-

1) 05/23/99 11:25
   COMMENTS: PT REMAINS L SIDE WITH O2 ON.

2) 05/23/99 11:25
   BP 130/80 M 96 P118
   COMMENTS: T 101² ORAL.

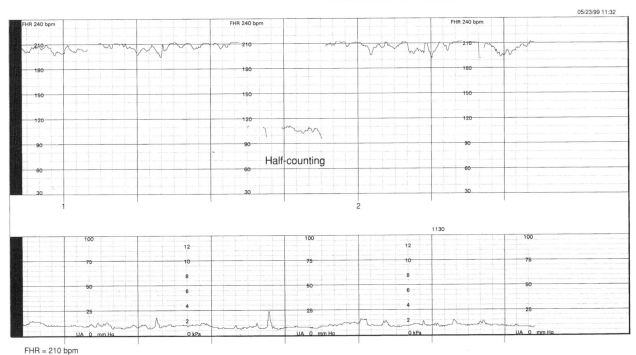

FHR = 210 bpm

Figure 2–6. Half-counting.

1) 03/24/01 15:20
   FM POWER ON 116 EXTERNAL INOP TOCO

2) 03/24/01 15:22
   COMMENTS: PT TRANSFERRED FROM TRIAGE TO LDR
   WITH DR PRESENT, SPIRAL ELECTRODE ON. U/S IN
   PROGRESS. P88. NO FHR, PT INFORMED. PT DISTRAUGHT,
   SOCIAL SVC. CONSULT ORDERED.

3) 03/24/01 15:25
   PT STATES HAVING FELT NO MOVEMENT SINCE LAST PM.

4) 03/24/01 15:27
   EFM DC'D NOW. OPTIONS FOR CARE EXPLAINED.

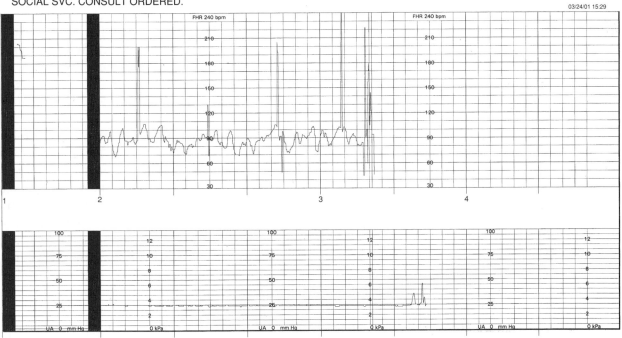

MHR = 90 bpm

Figure 2–7. Maternal heart rate acquired with spiral electrode.

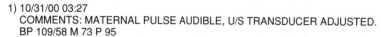

1) 10/31/00 03:27
    COMMENTS: MATERNAL PULSE AUDIBLE, U/S TRANSDUCER ADJUSTED.
    BP 109/58 M 73 P 95

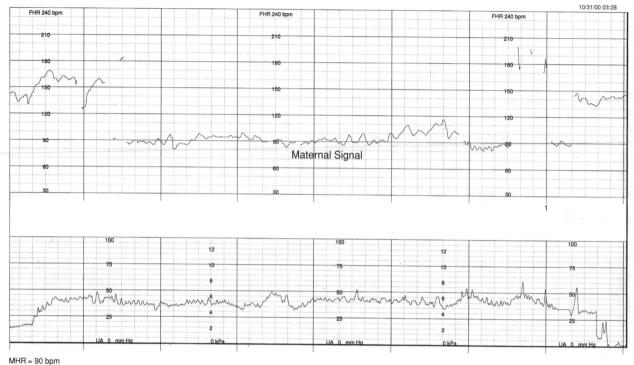

MHR = 90 bpm

Figure 2–8. Maternal heart rate obtained with ultrasound transducer.

nized by comparison of the maternal pulse to the monitor's audible signal. For documentation purposes, it is useful if the maternal heart rate can also be automatically obtained and printed or trended directly on the fetal strip chart.

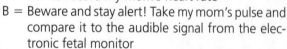

STORK BYTE:

The ABC's of EFM
A = Absence of my heart rate allows the electronic fetal monitor to record my mom's heart rate
B = Beware and stay alert! Take my mom's pulse and compare it to the audible signal from the electronic fetal monitor
C = Confirm the presence of my FHR by looking for cardiac activity with an ultrasound machine if you are in doubt

Dysrhythmia. The presence of a fetal dysrhythmia also poses a challenge to EFM. The rapid fluctuations in the FHR during a dysrhythmia make it extremely difficult to capture the FHR sig-

nal using an ultrasound transducer. A fetoscope, stethoscope, or M (motion)-mode sonography would provide better data. Internal monitoring may also be an option, although, with some types of dysrhythmias, it may be difficult to continuously observe the FHR baseline. If internal monitoring is being used, the electronic fetal monitor may be connected to a standard ECG recorder to observe the FECG and assist in diagnosis of the type of dysrhythmia.

It is important to recognize the difference between the presence of a dysrhythmia and the occurrence of artifact. Artifact occurs when there is interference in the FECG signal being transmitted by the spiral electrode. This can occur at the application site in instances of incomplete application or when there is a large amount of hair on the fetal head. Such interference of signal transmission commonly occurs when the spiral electrode is applied without first rupturing membranes. Artifact can also occur when the connection of the spiral electrode to the transducer, or the transducer to the electronic fetal monitor, is interrupted. This can occur in relation to maternal activity. For instance, artifact may be noted to occur simultaneously with events such as contractions, as the patient seeks comfort and moves her body in ways that interrupt the signal. Unlike dysrhythmias, artifact appears in the FHR tracing as disorganized deflections of varying lengths above or below the FHR signal. Although dysrhythmias may appear either continuously or intermittently on the strip chart, depending on their etiology, they maintain uniformity in their appearance. Dysrhythmias present as organized deflections of equal or similar lengths that occur at regular intervals to form a pattern. Also, the conspicuously irregular sounding beat of a dysrhythmia usually serves as an audible indicator to the clinician that this condition is present. More than one type of dysrhythmia may be present. Dysrhythmias are explored in further detail in Chapter 3.

Common Challenges to Signal Acquisition

Although frequent assessment and adjustment of the ultrasound transducer should be considered standard practice, there are some additional variables to consider that may necessitate an increase in the frequency of these activities. These include maternal size, shape, positioning, and activity level as well as fetal position, fetal activity, gestational age, and multiple gestation. It may prove difficult, for instance, in some cases of increased maternal body habitus to obtain the FHR externally and may, therefore, be necessary for the nurse to be available at the bedside to manually direct the positioning of the ultrasound transducer. This type of attention may also be required with variations in maternal and fetal activity and positioning to obtain an adequate signal.

S T O R K   B Y T E :
Tag, you're "it"! I like to move around a lot and so does my mom. That means you have to come and find me by adjusting the transducers!

Gestational age must also be considered when performing EFM (AWHONN, 2006). Not only does the preterm fetus pose a challenge to moni-

toring, but the clinician must also evaluate the type, value, and utility of the information being obtained. In cases of extreme prematurity, when the objective is simply to affirm presence of a FHR and the rate itself, it may be more prudent to assess the fetus with a fetoscope, hand-held Doppler, or by sonographic examination. An awareness and understanding of fetal physiology and growth are necessary to assist the clinician to evaluate the FHR using methods and parameters that are appropriate to gestational age.

Monitoring of the multiple gestation incorporates many of the considerations discussed previously. Unique to this situation, however, is the necessity to ensure that each of the fetuses is actually being monitored. Most electronic fetal monitors that are capable of monitoring multiple fetuses simultaneously are also equipped with the technology to allow the clinician to visually distinguish between two or more fetal heart rates or to alert the clinician to investigate when the FHR tracings have marked similarities.

S T O R K   B Y T E :
Who's who? With multiples, we all need to be heard!
   Do you know how to work your equipment to distinguish between each of our FHR tracings?

Acquisition of Uterine Activity Data

The significance of the FHR data as presented on the strip chart is interpreted with respect to concurrent uterine activity. Uterine activity data also carry import as a parameter in various clinical situations. Uterine activity may be determined with either internal or external sensors.

Intrauterine Pressure Catheter (IUPC)

The most accurate measure of uterine activity is accomplished internally, through the use of an intrauterine pressure catheter (IUPC). The IUPC provides information regarding the strength, frequency, and duration of contractions. It also measures the uterine resting tone, the tension of the uterine muscle between contractions. The IUPC may be of either the fluid-filled or sensor-tipped varieties. Both types of catheters measure hydrostatic pressure within the uterus and display the reading on the strip chart on a scale of 0 to 100 mm Hg (United States) and 0 to 13 kPa (used in some international settings). Since the IUPC is referenced to atmospheric pressure ("zeroed"), it provides an absolute measurement of intra-amniotic pressure. The techniques by which this zeroing is accomplished can vary significantly among types and brands of catheters. As with any technical equipment, information provided by the IUPC must be analyzed for accuracy and the catheter adjusted accordingly. Palpation of contractions and uterine resting tone is a simple technique that can be helpful in affirming that the data provided by the IUPC are consistent with actual uterine activity.

Tocotransducer

Uterine activity may also be measured externally, with the use of a tocotransducer. The tocotransducer houses a sensor that detects changes in myometrial tone, such as that which occurs during a contraction. Although the tocotransducer is referenced and a baseline is established when this device is applied to the maternal abdomen, these are arbitrary settings because the tocotransducer is not equilibrated to atmospheric pressure. The tocotransducer, therefore, provides a relative rather than an absolute measurement of pressure. The clinical significance of this is that the height of the contractions as presented on the strip chart is not indicative of the strength of contractions, nor is uterine resting tone accurately represented. Although the tocotransducer is a useful tool for determining the approximate frequency and duration of contractions, it is necessary to palpate the maternal abdomen and query the patient to determine the strength of contractions and the uterine resting tone.

During the active phase of labor, adequate uterine activity is considered to be contractions that occur approximately every 2 to 4.5 minutes and measure 25 to 75 mm Hg in intensity (ACOG, 2003). Proper spacing of contractions allows the uterus to achieve a state of relaxation, thus ensuring optimal uteroplacental perfusion between contractions. Resting tone of the uterus between contractions should be 15 to 20 mm Hg and the uterus should palpate as

soft. The duration of contractions should be approximately 60 to 90 seconds.

It is important to take steps to avoid and/or remedy the occurrence of uterine hyperstimulation (six or more contractions in a 10-minute time frame [ACOG, 2005]) and hypertonus (single contraction lasting more than 2 minutes [ACOG, 2005]), regardless of whether the FHR is adversely affected. If hyperstimulation and/or hypertonus are allowed to persist, complications may occur that affect the mother and/or the fetus. Hyperstimulation and hypertonus may occur in response to induction/augmentation agents or may happen spontaneously. It may be necessary to discontinue or decrease induction/augmentation medications and/or administer tocolytics to decrease uterine activity.

S T O R K   B Y T E :

Don't forget about my main squeeze! If you don't know what Mom's uterus is doing, then you can't really tell what's happening with me.

Challenges to Signal Acquisition

Challenges to monitoring uterine activity externally include placement technique and maternal activity, positioning, and body mass. The performance and subsequent utility of the tocotransducer are highly dependent upon placement technique. The tocotransducer should be applied to the maternal abdomen in the area of the uterine fundus and where the contractions are most strongly palpated. It is important to ensure that the tocotransducer is secured tightly enough to acquire a signal, but not so much as to interfere with it or cause discomfort to the patient. Placement of the sensor portion of the tocotransducer over the umbilicus may also interfere with the signal. Frequent re-referencing and reapplication of the tocotransducer will likely be necessary if the patient is physically active during the monitoring session. The thickness of the patient's subcutaneous layer will also affect the uterine activity reading. Less maternal tissue between the uterus and the tocotransducer allows uterine activity to register more prominently on the strip chart. A greater amount of maternal tissue buffers the myometrial contraction from the tocotransducer and may blunt the appearance of uterine activity on the strip chart. Depending on the amount of tissue that is present, the effect may range from producing a less impressive looking trend of uterine activity on the strip chart to completely preventing the information from being presented. Information about uterine activity is integral in the interpretation of FHR patterns and assessment of maternal and fetal well-being. The acquisition and maintenance of these data are responsibilities inherent to the performance of EFM.

Presentation of Data

Chart Paper Speed

Once the FHR and uterine activity data have been acquired, a trend of the information is then presented on the strip chart. Factors that affect the appearance of these data include the paper speed and paper scaling. The paper speed affects the rate at which the paper moves through the recorder of the electronic fetal monitor, but does not alter the rate at which FHR and uterine activity information is

acquired and presented. Throughout the United States, the majority of institutions run their electronic fetal monitors at a paper speed of 3 cm/min. In other countries, however, the practice is to have the paper speed set at 1 or sometimes 2 cm/min. At this slower rate, the information presented on the strip chart takes on a compressed appearance. It is important to realize that, although the data look different at varying speeds, the significance of the information remains the same.

> **STORK BYTE:**
> Don't judge simply by appearance! If you don't like the look of my heart rate, do something to help me. Changing the way my heart rate appears does not change what I am trying to tell you about my condition.

Chart Paper Scaling

In the United States, most institutions use chart paper that trends the FHR on a 30- to 240-bpm scale, partitioned into 10-bpm vertical increments. Some countries use chart paper that trends

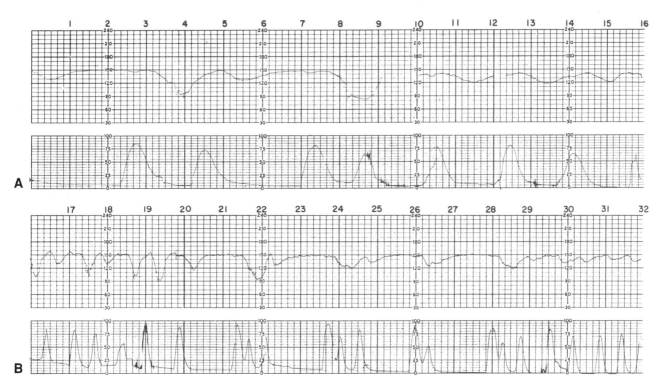

Figure 2–9. FHR tracings at different paper speeds. (**A**) Paper speed, 3 cm/min; spiral electrode. Late decelerations with no baseline variability are seen. (**B**) Paper speed, 1 cm/min; same tracing as in **A**. Note the differences in the shape of the decelerations and in the appearance of the variability. At this paper speed the FHR pattern would appear to be "better" than it actually is to a clinician accustomed to 3 cm/min paper speed.

the FHR on a 50- to 210-bpm scale. This type of chart paper apportions the vertical scaling into 20-bpm blocks. As with the selection of paper speed, these differences in paper scaling are a matter of preference. It is important, however, that an institution remain standardized once particular practices are established. When a clinician is familiar with interpreting data at a certain paper speed or scaling, education and a period of adjustment are required to perform analysis on a strip chart that is presented differently (Fig. 2–9). There is room for error in interpretation when one is not aware of or accustomed to different paper speed or scaling parameters. Part of the application technique for the electronic fetal monitor should, therefore, include ensuring that both the paper speed and paper scaling meet institutional standards.

Central Monitor Display

Another issue pertaining to visual interpretation is the discrepancy that may exist between the appearance of the strip chart at the bedside and its presentation on a central monitor system display. The dimensions of the strip chart may vary from the original when displayed on a computer screen, presenting a challenge to clinical interpretation. Additionally, the FHR tracing only has meaning when evaluated within the context of the entire clinical scenario. For this (and other patient care) reasons, it is necessary to perform regular assessments of the strip chart at the bedside. More information on electronic record keeping can be found in Chapter 8.

Summary

A complexity of issues surrounds the use of EFM equipment. As with any technology, the accuracy and utility of the information obtained through EFM rely on the skill and competency of the clinicians who operate the equipment and interpret the data. Means for evaluating such competency are addressed in Chapter 7.

SUGGESTED READINGS

American College of Obstetricians and Gynecologists. (2003). *Dystocia and the augmentation of labor.* ACOG Practice Bulletin 49. Washington, DC: Author.

——— (2005). *Intrapartum fetal heart rate monitoring.* ACOG Practice Bulletin 70. Washington, DC: Author.

Association of Women's Health, Obstetric and Neonatal Nurses. (2006). *Antepartum and intrapartum fetal heart rate monitoring: Clinical competencies and education guide.* Washington, DC: Author.

Boehm, F. H., Fields, L. M., Hutchison, J. M., Bowen, A. W., & Vaughn, W. K. (1986). The indirectly obtained fetal heart rate: Comparison of first and second generation electronic fetal monitors. *American Journal of Obstetrics & Gynecology, 155*(1), 10–14.

Carter, M. C. (1993). Signal processing and display—cardiotocographs. *British Journal of Obstetrics and Gynaecology, 100*(Suppl. 9), 21–23.

Divon, M. Y., Torres, F. P., Paul, R. H., & Yeh, S. (1985). Autocorrelation techniques in fetal monitoring. *American Journal of Obstetrics and Gynecology, 151*(1), 2–6.

Doyle, C., & Angelotti, T. (2004). Diagnosis of an unsuspected maternal hemorrhage via fetal heart rate tracing. *Journal of Clinical Anesthesiology 16*(6), 456–458.

Fukushima, T., Flores, C. A., Hon, E. H., & Davidson, E. C., Jr. (1985). Limitations of autocorrelation in fetal heart rate monitoring. *American Journal of Obstetrics and Gynecology, 153*(6), 685–692.

Herbert, W., Stuart, N. N., & Butler, L. S. (1987, July/August). Electronic fetal heart rate monitoring with intrauterine fetal demise. *Journal of Obstetric, Gynecologic, and Neonatal Nursing, 16,* 249–252.

Murray, M. (2004). Maternal or fetal heart rate: Avoiding intrapartum misidentification. *Journal of Obstetric, Gynecologic, and Neonatal Nursing, 33*(1), 93–104.

National Institute of Child Health and Human Development Research Planning Workshop. (1997). Electronic fetal heart monitoring: Research guidelines for interpretation. *Journal of Obstetric, Gynecologic, and Neonatal Nursing, 26*(6), 635–640.

Rabello, Y. A., Lapidus, M. R., & Paul, R. H. (1988). *Fundamentals of electronic fetal monitoring.* Wallingford, CT: Corometrics Medical Systems.

Overview: Modes of Monitoring FHR

	Internal (FECG) Signal source—Electrical	**External (Ultrasound)** Signal source—Motion
Indications	• Unsatisfactory external tracing • Abnormal/suspicious external tracing • Patient/practitioner preference	• Screening/fetal assessment • Antepartum/early labor, can be placed regardless of status of: — Membranes — Dilation — Station/presentation • Patient/practitioner preference
Advantages	• Accurate • Continuous • Variability • Patient comfort • No halving/doubling • Dysrhythmias	• Noninvasive • Easy to apply • Antepartum/early in labor
Limitations	• Requires: — Ruptured membranes — Adequate dilatation — Favorable station/presentation • Invasive to both patient and fetus	• Variability • Halving • Doubling • Maternal signal • Arrhythmias • Readjustment — Maternal/fetal activity — Maternal size/shape
Contraindications (relative)	• Presentation—Face, fontanelles, genitalia • Placenta previa; undiagnosed bleeding • Transmittable maternal infection • Need for maintenance of intact membranes • Patient refusal	• Patient refusal

Overview: Modes of Monitoring Uterine Activity

	Internal Intrauterine Pressure Catheter	**External** Tocotransducer

Indications	• Unsatisfactory external tracing
	 • Dysfunctional labor
	 • VBAC
	 • Patient/practitioner preference
		• Screening/fetal assessment
		 • Antepartum/early labor, can be applied regardless of status of:
		   — Membranes
		   — Dilation
		   — Station/presentation
		 • Patient/practitioner preference

Advantages	• Provides absolute measurement in mm Hg
	 • Provides information about:
	   — Strength, duration, and length of contraction
	   — Uterine resting tone
	 • Amnioinfusion
		• Noninvasive
		 • Easy to place
		 • Antepartum/early in labor
		 • Indicates frequency and length of contractions

Limitations	• Requires:
	   —Ruptured membranes
	   —Adequate dilation
	   —Favorable station/presentation
	 • Invasive to patient
		• Readjustment:
		   — Maternal/fetal activity
		   — Maternal size/shape
		 • Does not provide information about:
		   — Strength or exact duration of contractions
		   — Uterine resting tone

Contraindications	• Placenta previa, undiagnosed bleeding, suspected abruption	• Patient refusal

3 | Fetal Heart Rate Pattern Interpretation

Most screening techniques used within the field of medicine produce results to which a numeric value or descriptive name can be definitively assigned in an objective manner. The interpretation of fetal heart rate (FHR) patterns, however, bears the unusual distinction of being subjective and contextual in nature. This is due, in part, to the fact that interpretation of the FHR is based on visual assessment performed by individuals who possess varying degrees of experience and education. Interpretation has been further clouded by differing and, at times, conflicting opinion among experts in the practice of electronic fetal monitoring (EFM). Conflict of opinion exists over nomenclature, classification, and significance of EFM patterns. Such dissent exists both on the most insular level, as is frequently demonstrated between practitioners at the bedside, and also on a global level, as is evident by discrepancies in research and reports. For the purpose of clarity, the authors have chosen to utilize the terminology and classification system suggested by The National Institute of Child Health and Human Development (NICHD) Research Planning Workshop in 1997 (NICHD, 1997), and later adopted by the American College of Obstetricians and Gynecologists (ACOG, 2005) and the Association of Women's Health, Obstetric and Neonatal Nurses (AWHONN, 2006). Additional FHR patterns not addressed by the NICHD Workshop are otherwise referenced. The purpose of this chapter is to improve the reader's recognition of various FHR patterns.

Baseline Fetal Heart Rate

Baseline Rate

The normal fetus exhibits an overall constancy in its heart rate that can be considered comparable in nature to the resting heart rate of an adult. Most people maintain a certain average heart rate at rest. Although that rate changes with activity or excitement, it is expected to return to its usual rate when such stimuli are not present. This is also true of the fetus.

As explained in more detail in Chapter 1, the FHR is controlled by a number of mechanisms. These include the central nervous system (CNS), the autonomic nervous system (ANS), baroreceptors, chemoreceptors, and the endocrine system. As was also explained (see Chapter 2), the recorded trend of the FHR on the strip chart is calculated from the time intervals that elapse between successive beats of the fetal heart. Normally, this interval varies slightly from one beat to the next, causing a certain degree of fluctuation to appear in the trend of the baseline FHR. The bulk of these fluctuations, however, are contained within a constant range that is recognized as the FHR *baseline*. According to the NICHD (1997), "Baseline FHR is the approximate mean FHR rounded to increments of 5 bpm during a 10-minute segment, excluding periodic or episodic changes; periods of marked FHR variability; and segments of the baseline that differ by more than 25 bpm." For example, if the range of the baseline FHR is visualized to be 132 to 140 bpm, the mean FHR would be arrived at by adding these two integers (132 + 140)

29

and dividing the result by 2 (272 ÷ 2). The mean (in this case, 136) would then be rounded to the nearest increment of 5 (in this case, 135), if necessary. This is not intended to entail an intricate mathematical calculation, but rather a simple visual assessment and interpretation. It is also important to know that there are periods during which the FHR baseline cannot be assessed and/or interpreted. "In any 10-minute window, the minimum baseline duration must be at least 2 minutes or the baseline for that period would be indeterminate" (1997). In this case, one may need to refer to the previous 10-minute segment(s) to determine the baseline (NICHD, 1997).

The baseline is the first characteristic of the FHR to be evaluated, because it is the parameter against which all other facets of the interpretation process are based. The baseline is assessed only when the patient is not experiencing contractions and when the FHR is not exhibiting signs of periodic/episodic changes (ie, accelerations or decelerations, which will be detailed later in this chapter). It is necessary to have a minimum of 10 minutes of FHR recorded to determine the baseline. The FHR baseline is expected to be maintained between a range of numbers that are within the limits of 110 to 160 bpm (NICHD, 1997; ACOG, 2005) (Fig. 3–1).

Finding the FHR baseline is more than just looking at a segment of the strip chart and noting the lowest and highest points where the FHR was recorded. It requires critically evaluating the trend of the FHR at the appropriate times (between contractions and between periodic/episodic changes) to determine the integers between which the bulk of the relevant data are contained. Once the baseline FHR is initially identified for the particular portion of the tracing that is being evaluated, it is useful to reconfirm that finding at other points within the relevant segment of the tracing to ensure accuracy.

S T O R K   B Y T E :

Worth more than a passing glance. . . Correctly interpreting my baseline heart rate keeps you from missing other important characteristics of my heart rate pattern.

Variability

As has been mentioned in Chapters 1 and 2, there are normal physiologic variations in the time intervals that elapse between each fetal heart beat. When the FHR is displayed on the strip chart,

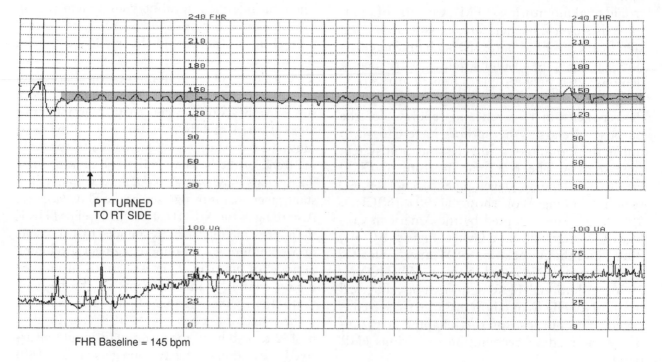

FHR Baseline = 145 bpm

Figure 3–1. FHR baseline.

these variations are visually apparent in the recorded trend of the FHR (see Appendix F). Fluctuation of the FHR baseline is referred to as *variability*. Variability is a component of baseline FHR data and, therefore, can only be assessed during the same time periods that it is appropriate to assess the baseline FHR (ie, between contractions and between periodic/episodic changes).

> ### STORK BYTE:
>
> Know me for who I am. . . FHR variability is a characteristic of my baseline heart rate. You can only assess it at times when my baseline can be assessed—and that's not during accelerations, decelerations, or contractions!

Moderate Variability

The presence of a moderate amount of variability indicates that the autonomic and central nervous systems of the fetus are well developed and well oxygenated. Its presence is also a reassuring indication that the fetus is maintaining a measure of tolerance to the changes in blood flow that occur during labor. A moderate amount of variability is considered to be fluctuation in the FHR baseline of as little as 6 bpm to as much as 25 bpm (Fig. 3–2).

Moderate variability is one of the most important and predictive aspects of the FHR recording. Even if decelerations are occurring, the presence of moderate variability is highly correlated with the *absence* of significant metabolic acidosis (Parer, King, Flanders, Fox, & Kilpatrick, 2006). Therefore, attention to and accurate assessment of variability are essential components in the practice of EFM.

Minimal Variability

It may be cause for concern if the FHR baseline appears to have a minimal ($\leq$5 bpm) or absent (no visible fluctuation) (NICHD, 1997) amount of variability, because this finding may signify the presence of fetal hypoxia/acidosis. It is important to put the finding of decreased variability within the context of the entire clinical picture, however, to accurately determine its meaning.

As discussed in Chapter 1, any condition or event that diminishes blood flow to the placenta deprives the fetus of adequate oxygenation and, if the resulting hypoxemia is sufficient to cause tissue hypoxia and metabolic acidosis, can create a loss of FHR baseline variability. Hypoxic causes of minimal or absent variability are related to diminished blood flow across the placenta or through the umbilical cord. Initially,

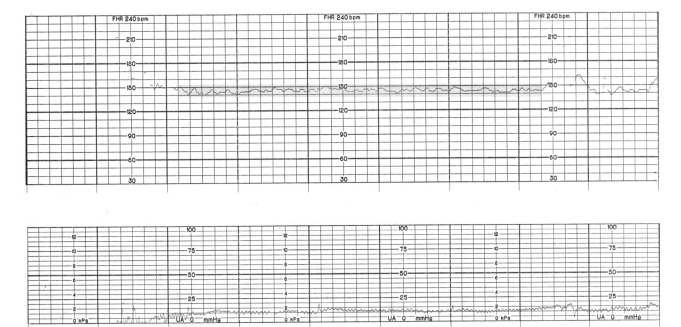

FHR Baseline = 145 bpm

Figure 3–2. FHR baseline with moderate variability.

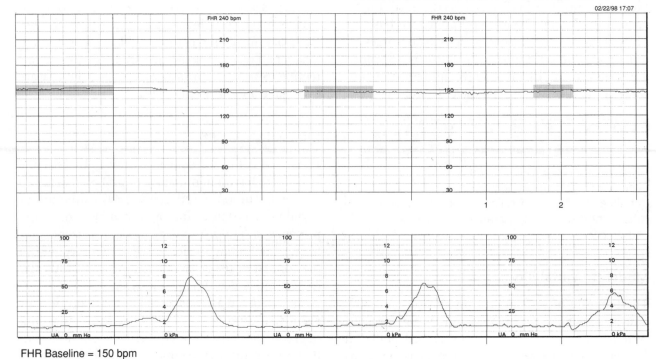

1) 02/22/98 17:05
    17:16 BP 133/58 M 85 P 84

2) 02/22/98 17:06
    COMMENTS: PT INDICATES UNDERSTANDING FOR NEED
    FOR P C/S, ANESTH IN FOR TOP OFF, PREP DONE
                                            02/22/98 17:07

FHR Baseline = 150 bpm

Figure 3–3. FHR baseline with minimal variability.

moderate variability may remain present, indicating that the fetus is effectively compensating for the diminished influx of oxygenated blood. If the cause of decreased perfusion is not corrected, however, variability eventually decreases. This is a warning sign, indicating that the fetus is losing its ability to tolerate or compensate for the stressors placed on it and is becoming hypoxic (Fig. 3–3).

The overall correlation between acidemia and minimal or undetectable FHR baseline variability in the presence of decelerations is only 23%. However, deepening of decelerations over time in association with minimal or undetectable FHR baseline variability may serve as an indicator for intervention (Parer et al., 2006).

Besides hypoxia/acidosis, there are other, more common reasons for the fetus to exhibit minimal baseline variability. These include fetal sleep, the effects of medications, an immature CNS, fetal dysrhythmias, and cardiac or CNS anomalies. Although fetal sleep is a common cause of minimal variability, it is necessary to remember that this is a transient state that should alternate with periods of moderate variability approximately every 20 to 40 minutes, and represents normal fetal physiologic function (Schifrin, 1990).

Medications that depress the maternal CNS are likely to produce similar effects on the fetal CNS. Although it is to be expected that variability will decrease after the administration of such medications, this effect on the fetus is temporary. Once the medication is metabolized and excreted, variability will return. It is, therefore, prudent to administer such medications only after fetal well-being has been established. Also, it is important to review the patient's medication history with her, because she may have knowingly or unknowingly exposed the fetus to a sedative or narcotic agent. Loss of variability secondary to medication effect does not require intervention.

The fetus who is less than 32 weeks' gestation may exhibit less variability, because the ANS may not yet be fully developed (see Chapter 1). It is important to note that, regardless of gestational age, once a fetus has exhibited a certain amount of variability, it has set a standard to which it should be held from that point forward.

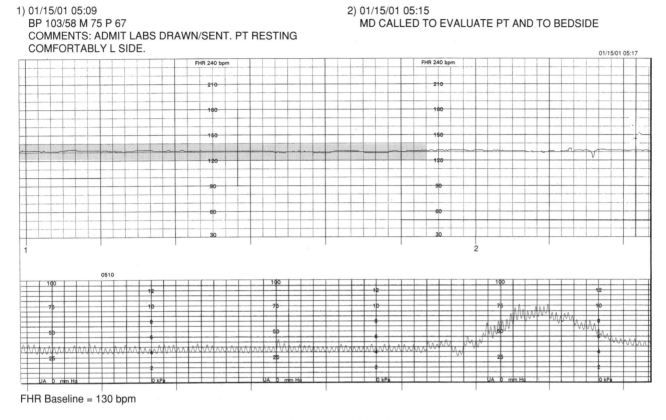

1) 01/15/01 05:09
BP 103/58 M 75 P 67
COMMENTS: ADMIT LABS DRAWN/SENT. PT RESTING
COMFORTABLY L SIDE.

2) 01/15/01 05:15
MD CALLED TO EVALUATE PT AND TO BEDSIDE

01/15/01 05:17

FHR Baseline = 130 bpm

Figure 3–4. FHR baseline with absent variability (secondary to fetal anomaly).

Minimal or absent variability is often noted in association with patterns of fetal dysrhythmia. It is also found in the FHR tracings of fetuses with anomalies that affect cardiac, CNS, or ANS functioning. If minimal or absent variability is persistent from the commencement of monitoring and its cause is not known, further investigation is needed (Fig. 3–4). If cardiac or CNS anomalies have not previously been ruled out by sonographic examination, it is advisable to have such testing performed.

Steps should be taken to remediate condition(s) suspected of causing minimal or absent variability. These include increasing fetal oxygenation by optimizing blood flow to and through the uterus, placenta, and umbilical cord. This is accomplished by promoting maternal cardiac and hemodynamic functioning (assess maternal vital signs and history; initiate therapies such as position changes and administration of medications, hydration, and oxygen as needed), uteroplacental perfusion (through maternal positioning and eliminating stress of uterine contractions), and blood flow through the umbilical cord (alleviate pressure through maternal positioning). Research utilizing fetal arterial oxygen saturation monitoring (a method of measuring fetal oxygenation directly) scientifically supported that an IV fluid bolus of 1,000 mL, the maternal lateral position, and oxygen administration of 10 L/min with a nonrebreather face mask for 15 minutes improves fetal oxygenation (Simpson & James, 2005). Not all instances of hypoxia can be alleviated with such interventions, but it is necessary to perform them in an attempt to oxygenate the fetus as much as possible. If minimal or absent variability is noted at the outset of the monitoring session and there are no other components of the FHR that can be considered reassuring (such as accelerations, which are discussed later in this chapter), then hypoxia should be ruled out. It is possible that a prior hypoxic insult has occurred (Phelan & Ahn, 1994; Schifrin, Hamilton-Rubinstein & Shields, 1994) (Table 3–1).

Marked Variability

The presence of more than 25 beats of fluctuation in the FHR baseline is known as *marked variability* (NICHD, 1997) (Fig. 3–5). This pattern is only usually seen intrapartum. Although marked

Table 3–1. MINIMAL OR ABSENT VARIABILITY

Possible Etiology: Uteroplacental insufficiency, cord compression

Hypoxic Causes (with metabolic acidosis)	Nonhypoxic Causes
• Cord prolapse/compression • Maternal hypotension • Uterine hyperstimulation • Abruptio placentae • Tachycardia • Dysrhythmia	• Prematurity • Fetal sleep • Medication effect • Fetal anomaly • Tachycardia • Dysrhythmia

Goal of Intervention	Rationale
Improve uteroplacental blood flow and perfusion through the umbilical cord	*Improving the amount and quality of blood flow to the fetus will assist with attempts at recovery*

Specific Interventions	Rationale
• Attempt to determine cause	Recognition of causative factors increases efficiency and validates necessity of response.
• If minimal or absent variability is associated with dysrhythmia, obtain sonographic evaluation	Structural examination of fetal heart, heart rate and rhythm, and observation for hydrops, ascites, and other abnormalities should be performed.
• Lateral positioning	Improve maternal circulation and perfusion to placenta; improve blood flow through the umbilical cord.
• Increase IV fluid rate unless otherwise contraindicated	Improve maternal circulation and perfusion to placenta; improve maternal hydration to potentiate greater amniotic fluid volume.
• Administer oxygen 8–10 L/min by mask	Hyperoxygenate maternal blood to increase fetal oxygenation.
• Discontinue oxytocin infusion; remove uterotonic agents; consider tocolytics	Eliminate additional stress of decreased blood flow during contractions until further assessment proves the fetus is not acidotic.
• Assess maternal vital signs	Maternal status directly influences FHR pattern.
• Palpate uterus	Palpation may be the most effective means of determining hyperstimulation.
• Observe tracing for previously reassuring signs such as accelerations and moderate variability	Accelerations and moderate variability suggest that the fetus was not sufficiently hypoxic to produce acidosis upon entering this episode.
• Initiate procedures to assist in determining fetal acid–base status, such as scalp stimulation and/or scalp blood sampling. Biophysical profile may also be indicated, depending upon the clinical situation	EFM is only a screening device. Adjunct means of assessment may be helpful in affirming suspicions and making a diagnosis.
• Consider internal monitoring	Internal monitoring with a spiral electrode may provide more accurate assessment.
• Observe for other nonreassuring signs such as rising baseline FHR; marked variability; presence of variable, late, or prolonged decelerations; or bradycardia	These are indicators that the fetal condition may be worsening; operative intervention may be necessary.

(continued)

Table 3–1. MINIMAL OR ABSENT VARIABILITY (*continued*)	
• Communicate FHR/UA pattern and interventions to care provider and personnel in charge, and document in medical record	Care provider should assess patient/fetal condition; charge personnel need to plan staffing accordingly and may provide expertise and assistance; medical record should reflect assessments and interventions.
• Prepare for delivery	If minimal or absent variability is found to be of hypoxic etiology and interventions are not effective, delivery of the fetus is indicated.

variability is sometimes caused by fetal activity or stimulation, it can also be a sign that the fetus is hemodynamically compromised or mildly hypoxemic (Parer, 1997). Once again, to put any finding in perspective, it is necessary to consider the entire clinical picture. Query the patient on her perception of fetal activity and attempt to objectively affirm and identify sources of the same. Ensure optimal blood flow to and through the uterus, placenta, and umbilical cord by promoting maternal cardiac and hemodynamic functioning (assess maternal vital signs and history; initiate therapies such as position changes and administration of medications, hydration, and oxygen, as needed). Promote uteroplacental perfusion through maternal positioning and eliminating stress of uterine contractions, and blood flow through the umbilical cord (alleviate pressure through maternal position changes) (Table 3–2).

1) 03/13/00 10:04
   COMMENTS: VE DONE AT THIS TIME BY DR. #1 WHO REMAINS IN RM AND IS VIEWING TRACING
   COMMENTS: PT REPOS FROM L TO R SIDE 03/13/00 10:04

2) 03/13/00 10:06
   COMMENTS: DR. #2 IN RM AT THIS TIME TRACING BEING VIEWED
   COMMENTS: TERB CALLED FOR IN RM 03/13/00 10:07

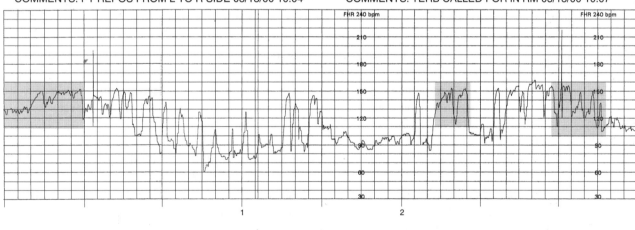

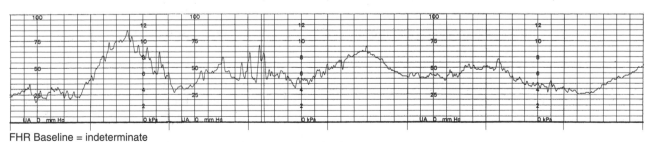

FHR Baseline = indeterminate

Figure 3–5. FHR baseline with marked variability.

Table 3-2. MARKED VARIABILITY

Possible Etiology: Uteroplacental insufficiency, cord compression

Hypoxic Causes	Nonhypoxic Causes
• Cord prolapse/compression • Maternal hypotension • Uterine hyperstimulation • Abruptio placentae	• Fetal activity • Fetal stimulation

Goal of Intervention	Rationale
Improve uteroplacental blood flow and perfusion through the umbilical cord	*Improving the amount and quality of blood flow to the fetus will assist with attempts at recovery*

Specific Interventions	Rationale
• Attempt to determine cause	Recognition of causative factors increases efficiency and validates necessity of response.
• Lateral positioning	Improve maternal circulation and perfusion to placenta; improve blood flow through the umbilical cord.
• Increase IV fluid rate unless otherwise contraindicated	Improve maternal circulation and perfusion to placenta; improve maternal hydration to potentiate greater amniotic fluid volume.
• Administer oxygen 8–10 L/min by mask	Hyperoxygenate maternal blood to increase fetal oxygenation.
• Discontinue oxytocin infusion; remove uterotonic agents; consider tocolytics	Eliminate additional stress of decreased blood flow during contractions until further assessment proves the fetus is not acidotic.
• Assess maternal vital signs	Maternal status directly influences FHR pattern.
• Palpate uterus	Palpation may be the most effective means of determining hyperstimulation.
• Observe tracing for previously reassuring signs such as accelerations and moderate variability	Accelerations and moderate variability suggest that the fetus was not sufficiently hypoxic to produce acidosis upon entering this episode.
• Initiate procedures to assist in determining fetal acid–base status, such as scalp stimulation and/or scalp blood sampling. Biophysical profile may also be indicated, depending upon the clinical situation	EFM is only a screening device. Adjunct means of assessment may be helpful in affirming suspicions and making a diagnosis.
• Consider internal monitoring	Internal monitoring with a spiral electrode may provide more accurate assessment.
• Observe for other nonreassuring signs, such as rising baseline FHR; minimal or absent variability; presence of variable, late, or prolonged decelerations; or bradycardia	These are indicators that the fetal condition may be worsening; operative intervention may be necessary.
• Communicate FHR/UA pattern and interventions to care provider and personnel in charge, and document in medical record	Care provider should assess patient/fetal condition; charge personnel need to plan staffing accordingly and may provide expertise and assistance; medical record should reflect assessments and interventions.
• Prepare for delivery	If marked variability is found to be of hypoxic etiology and interventions are not effective, delivery of the fetus is indicated.

Tachycardia

If the baseline FHR rises and is maintained above 160 bpm for 10 minutes or longer, this is considered to be a fetal tachycardia (NICHD, 1997). A fetal tachycardia may be maternal or fetal in origin. Common conditions that increase maternal heart rate (subsequently raising the FHR) include fever, dehydration, and medication effect. Remediation of the cause of the maternal tachycardia will usually assist the FHR in returning to normal range if the tachycardia is solely of maternal etiology.

S T O R K   B Y T E :

An ounce of prevention. . . Please pay attention to my baseline heart rate! If it is rising, do something to help me—even if my heart rate is still within normal limits!

Tachycardia may also result from hypoxia/acidosis, infection, and tachydysrhythmias. The onset of tachycardia or a rising baseline rate should be considered serious, because it is one of the first signs that the fetus is becoming hypoxic/acidotic. As described previously (see Chapter 1), when

there is decreased maternal–fetal perfusion, baroreceptors and chemoreceptors in the fetus trigger an increase in the FHR. In many instances, care providers do have influence over maternal–fetal exchange. This includes avoiding problems such as uterine hyperstimulation (Fig. 3–6) and maternal hypotension. In either of these cases, correcting the cause (eg, discontinuing oxytocin, removal/reversal of uterotonic agents, changing the maternal position) may improve fetal oxygenation and assist the FHR in recovery to normal range. In the event of infection or tachydysrhythmia, the usual means of intrauterine resuscitation should be employed (ie, position changes, increased maternal hydration and oxygenation, and decreasing stressors on the fetus such as contractions) in addition to any other medical or pharmaceutical remedies ordered (Table 3–3).

Bradycardia

A baseline FHR below 110 bpm for a period of 10 minutes or longer is termed a *bradycardia* (NICHD, 1997). This can occur in response to a variety of acute and chronic conditions that may be of hypoxic or nonhypoxic etiology. Also, just

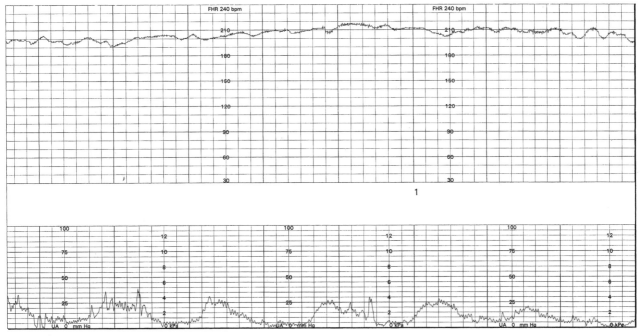

FHR Baseline = 205 bpm

Figure 3–6. FHR baseline tachycardia (with uterine hyperstimulation).

Table 3–3. TACHYCARDIA

Possible Etiology

Related to Maternal Conditions	Related to Fetal/Intrauterine Conditions
• Fever • Dehydration • Medication effect • Anxiety • Thyroid disease	• Chorioamnionitis • Hypoxia/acidosis • Dysrhythmia

Goal of Intervention	Rationale
Improve uteroplacental blood flow and perfusion through the umbilical cord	*Improving the amount and quality of blood flow to the fetus will assist with attempts at recovery*

Specific Interventions	Rationale
• Attempt to determine cause; assess patient history	Recognition of causative factors increases efficiency of response, allows prompt rule out and/or treatment of nonhypoxic causes (fever, dehydration, medication effects, anxiety).
• If tachycardia is associated with dysrhythmia, obtain sonographic evaluation	Structural examination of fetal heart, heart rate and rhythm, and observation for hydrops, ascites, and other abnormalities should be performed.
• Provide explanation, education, support, and comfort measures to patient and her support persons as needed	Maternal anxiety may cause catecholamine release, shunting blood away from the uterus.
• Ensure thyroid disease is under control	Thyroid-stimulating hormone can cross the placenta to the fetus and cause tachycardia.
• Lateral positioning	Improve maternal circulation and perfusion to placenta; improve blood flow through the umbilical cord.
• Assess maternal vital signs, especially temperature and pulse. Periodically reassess for maternal fever.	Maternal fever causes the fetus to become tachycardic. In cases of chorioamnionitis, the fetus often becomes tachycardic before maternal temperature rises. Maternal temperature should be reassessed frequently and treated.
• Increase IV fluid rate (bolus) unless otherwise contraindicated	Improve maternal circulation and perfusion to placenta; improve maternal hydration to potentiate greater amniotic fluid volume.
• Administer oxygen 8–10 L/min by mask	Hyperoxygenate maternal blood to increase fetal oxygenation.
• Discontinue oxytocin infusion, uterotonic agents; consider tocolytics	Eliminate additional stress of decreased blood flow during contractions until further assessment proves the fetus is not acidotic.
• Observe tracing for reassuring signs such as accelerations and moderate variability	Accelerations and moderate variability suggest that the fetus is not sufficiently hypoxic to produce acidosis.
• Initiate procedures to assist in determining fetal acid–base status, such as scalp stimulation and/or scalp blood sampling. Biophysical profile may also be indicated, depending upon the clinical situation	EFM is only a screening device. Adjunct means of assessment may be helpful in affirming suspicions and making a diagnosis.

(continued)

Table 3–3. TACHYCARDIA (*continued*)	
• Consider internal monitoring	Internal monitoring with a spiral electrode may provide more accurate assessment (rule out erroneous signals).
• Observe for other nonreassuring signs such as continuously rising baseline FHR; minimal, absent, or marked variability; presence of variable, late, or prolonged decelerations; bradycardia	These are indicators that the fetal condition may be worsening; operative intervention may be necessary.
• Communicate FHR/UA pattern and interventions to care provider and personnel in charge, and document in medical record	Care provider should assess patient/fetal condition; charge personnel need to plan staffing accordingly and may provide expertise and assistance; medical record should reflect assessments and interventions.
• Prepare for delivery	Emergent delivery is likely if FHR continues to rise or if other nonreassuring signs are present and interventions are not effective.

as it is understood that adults have varying degrees of normal, the same concept applies to the fetus. In some cases, FHR baseline less than 110 bpm that also has reassuring signs present (such as moderate variability and/or accelerations) may be accepted as normal for a particular fetus.

Hypoxic Etiology

The fetus suffering from untreated chronic deprivation of oxygen has a distinct, suspicious-looking tracing (Schifrin, 1990). Typically, either variable or late decelerations are present, denoting a decrease of blood flow through either the umbilical cord or the placenta. As the fetus becomes increasingly hypoxic, carbon dioxide accumulates in the fetal blood. This stimulates the chemoreceptors and causes a compensatory elevation in the FHR. As the increase in the FHR baseline continues, FHR baseline variability decreases and any periodic/episodic changes of the FHR that are present become less visually apparent. The final phase in this process is bradycardia, a terminal event in the case of prolonged fetal hypoxia or asphyxia.

This chain of events is rarely seen in its entirety, because surgical intervention usually preempts its completion. It is also possible for the early phases of progressive fetal compromise to be concealed from the clinician, because it may have occurred before admission. This clouds assessment of the FHR tracing, because there is no normal pattern to which comparison can be made and deviations identified. For instance, the patient may present for fetal monitoring with an FHR that is technically within normal limits and is without decelerations, but with a lack of both accelerations and variability also noted. Interpretation of such a tracing may be confounding and, therefore, it is imperative to determine promptly the status of fetal oxygenation. A biophysical profile may be useful for this purpose. Techniques such as scalp stimulation and/or fetal scalp blood sampling (discussed in Chapter 1) may be employed, as long as a deceleration or bradycardia is not in progress. These methods of evaluation may be helpful in determining whether the fetus is presenting having already sustained neurologic impairment.

Examples of hypoxic events related to bradycardia include cord prolapse/compression, maternal hypotension, uterine hyperstimulation, abruptio placentae, or uterine rupture. If the insult that initiated the bradycardia is acute and remediable in nature (such as cord compression, maternal hypotension, uterine hyperstimulation) and is identified and treated expeditiously, it is possible that the FHR will return to its normal range. If it does not, a promptly executed cesarean or assisted birth may be indicated.

Cord compression/occlusion can be precipitated by the actions or positioning of the fetus or by such conditions as nuchal cord, cord entanglement, short or knotted cord, occult or overt prolapse, oligohydramnios, or thick meconium. Transient compression of the cord due to fetal position or movement is usually corrected by altering maternal–fetal position. Cord entanglements are not as easily reversible, and hypoxia/acidosis can result. Although position changes may help in the instance of partial or occult prolapse, an overt prolapse requires emergent intervention. Prolonged or persistent cord compression can result in fetal bradycardia with minimal or absent variability. This type of FHR pattern may precede death in utero and is, therefore, extremely concerning (Fig. 3–7).

Although decreased oxygenation of the fetus is associated with acute episodes of bradycardia (resulting from events such as uterine hyperstimulation or maternal hypotension), variability will usually remain present, provided such occurrences are transient in nature. Once the insult is corrected and fetal oxygenation resumes, the FHR will usually recover to its prior baseline rate. Chronically decreased blood flow across the uteroplacental unit is also likely to result in FHR bradycardia. This ongoing instance of hypoxia is much more serious, however, as demonstrated by minimal or absent variability of the FHR baseline and the inability to recover with interventions (Fig. 3–8).

Bradycardia is the most common FHR change when uterine rupture occurs during a trial of labor after a previous cesarean birth. Before the onset of the bradycardia, FHR patterns have been reported to range from reassuring to those with variable or late decelerations and fetal tachycardia (Leung, Leung, & Paul, 1993; Menihan, 1998). This type of bradycardia is representative of fetal hypoxia and requires immediate intervention. In Leung's study, it was noted that fetal distress was the most common signal and that significant neonatal morbidity occurred if a fetal bradycardia lasted 18 minutes or longer before surgical intervention (1993). The rate of perinatal asphyxia after uterine rupture is reported to be 5.1% (Miller, Diaz, & Paul, 1994).

If a trial of labor is attempted after a previous cesarean birth, the onset of bradycardia should be seen as a red flag until proven otherwise. Although it is possible for bradycardia to result from other causes (such as those discussed previously in this chapter), the consequences of uterine rupture are severe enough to warrant preparation for operative

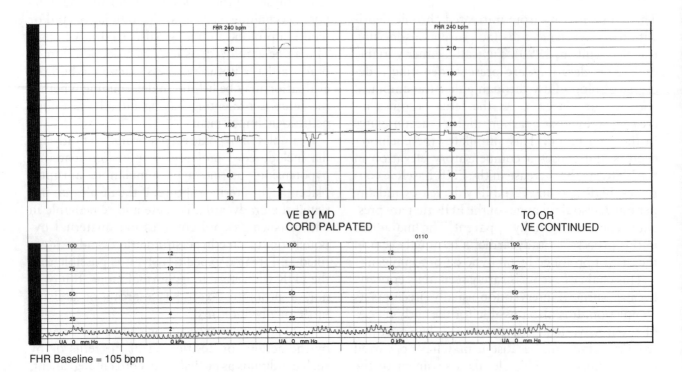

FHR Baseline = 105 bpm

Figure 3–7. FHR baseline bradycardia (with cord compression).

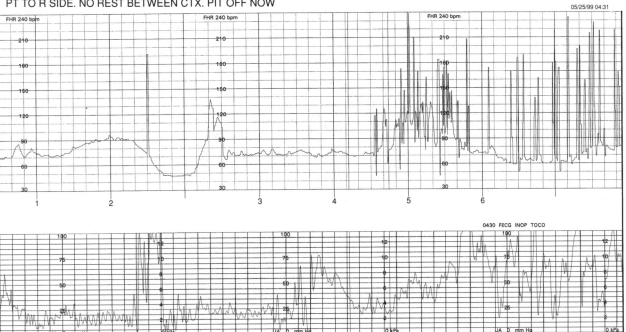

FHR Baseline = Indeterminate

Figure 3–8. FHR baseline bradycardia (with uterine hyperstimulation).

delivery if the bradycardia cannot be promptly reversed. In the event that the FHR does not recover with primary interventions (maternal position change, administration of intravenous fluids and oxygen, discontinuation of oxytocin, or removal of uterologic agents and/or the administration of tocolytics [Ingemarsson, Arulkumaran, & Ratnam, 1985]), expeditious cesarean delivery is indicated (Fig. 3–9).

Nonhypoxic Etiology

If the bradycardia is due to a nonhypoxic cause, such as vagal stimulation during the second stage of labor (Parer, 1997), the fetus can recover. In the second stage of labor, intense intracranial pressure occurs as the fetal head descends through the maternal pelvis and vagina. A second-stage bradycardia may be seen in the adequately oxygenated fetus as a normal response to stimulation of the vagus nerve. The key factor in recognizing the difference between hypoxic and nonhypoxic bradycardia is FHR baseline variability. In hypoxic cases of bradycardia, FHR baseline variability is minimal or absent, whereas, in nonhypoxic instances, it will usually remain moderate (Table 3–4).

Periodic/Episodic Changes of the Fetal Heart Rate

Various excursions of the FHR above or below the determined baseline become apparent during the analysis of FHR tracings. Although many of these changes occur directly in response to contractions, some may result from interventions performed by the care team, fetal movement, or maternal positioning, or they may arise spontaneously.

Accelerations

Spontaneous and Induced Accelerations

The term *acceleration* describes the occurrence of a transient increase in the FHR of an amplitude of

1) 02/06/01 03:30
   COMMENTS: VE BY MD, NO PROLAPSE, UNABLE TO
   ASSESS DILATION. PT C/O PAIN, ANESTHESIA CALLED
   FOR TOP UP.

2) 02/06/01 03:34
   STRIP REVIEWED BY RN; COMMENTS: MD ASSESSING
   TRACING. PT REPOSITIONED LEFT TO RT SIDE, O2
   REMAINS ON 8L VIA FACE MASK, IV FLUIDS REMAIN
   INFUSING, OR TEAM NOTIFIED

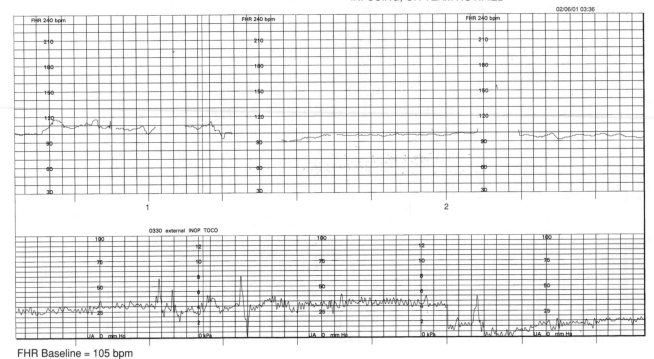

FHR Baseline = 105 bpm

Figure 3–9. FHR baseline bradycardia (with uterine rupture).

15 beats or greater above the FHR baseline, continuing for 15 seconds or longer (NICHD, 1997). If the baseline FHR is reported as a range of numbers, then the zenith of the acceleration should reach a point ≥15 beats greater than the upper limit of that range. The duration of the acceleration is assessed from the time the FHR departs from the baseline until its return. Most accelerations return to baseline within 2 minutes (Fig. 3–10).

Accelerations are an important finding because they indicate that the fetus has a functioning ANS and is not experiencing acidosis (Clark, Gimovsky, & Miller, 1984). Accelerations are an expected and reassuring event on the tracing of the fetus that is greater than 32 weeks' gestation. Accelerations often occur spontaneously, in relation to fetal movement or contractions (Figs. 3–11 and 3–12). They also may be induced by the application of a fetal acoustic stimulator to the maternal abdomen or by manual stimulation of the fetal head.

While the absence of accelerations can be a nonreassuring finding, this may also occur for rela-

> **STORK BYTE:**
>
> Functioning at full capacity. . . Accelerations of my heart rate tell you that I am getting enough oxygen and my neurologic system is healthy and mature.

tively brief periods of time due to fetal sleep (expected to last no longer than 40 minutes). Accelerations may be absent for longer periods due to the effects of medication, as can occur with narcotics, propanolol, and magnesium sulfate (Panayotopoulos et al., 1998; Sherer & Bentolila, 1998).

Uniform Accelerations

Some FHR accelerations maintain a very distinctive appearance and have a different etiology than spontaneous or induced accelerations. These are known as *uniform accelerations*. Uniform accelerations are a pattern of accelerations that present

Table 3–4. BRADYCARDIA

Possible Etiology: Uteroplacental insuffiency, cord compression

Hypoxic Causes	Nonhypoxic Causes
• Cord prolapse/compression • Maternal hypotension • Uterine hyperstimulation • Abruptio placentae • Uterine rupture	• Bradydysrhythmia • Vagal stimulation during the second stage of labor • Hypothermia (fetal dive reflex)

Goal of Intervention	Rationale
Improve uteroplacental blood flow and perfusion through the umbilical cord	*Improving the amount and quality of blood flow to the fetus will assist with attempts at recovery*

Specific Interventions	Rationale
• Attempt to determine cause	Recognition of causative factors increases efficiency of response.
• Be cognizant of patient history, particularly previous uterine surgery and/or cesarean birth	Patient with such history is at increased risk of uterine rupture.
• Maintain normal intrauterine temperature by assuring fluid used during amnioinfusion or for flushing fluid-filled intrauterine pressure catheter is at least room temperature. A blood warmer is an acceptable means of warming fluid to assure temperature	Infusion of cold fluid into the uterus may cause a parasympathetic response in the fetus (also known as a "dive reflex") that results in bradycardia.
• Vaginal examination	Check for cord prolapse. If prolapse is detected, lift presenting part off the umbilical cord and continue to do so until delivery of the fetus.
• Discontinue oxytocin infusion; remove uterotonic agents; consider tocolytics	Eliminate additional stress of decreased blood flow during contractions until further assessment proves the fetus is not acidotic.
• Positioning—left lateral, right lateral, knee–chest	Reposition until successful, giving each position a chance to take effect. Improve maternal circulation and perfusion to placenta; improve blood flow through the umbilical cord.
• Increase IV fluid rate (bolus) unless otherwise contraindicated	Improve maternal circulation and perfusion to placenta; improve maternal hydration to potentiate greater amniotic fluid volume.
• Administer oxygen 8–10 L/min by mask	Hyperoxygenate maternal blood to increase fetal oxygenation.
• Assess maternal vital signs	Maternal status directly influences FHR pattern.
• Palpate uterus	Palpation may be the most effective means of determining hyperstimulation.
• Observe tracing for previously reassuring signs such as accelerations, moderate variability	Accelerations and moderate variability suggest that the fetus was not sufficiently hypoxic to produce acidosis upon entering this episode.
• When FHR returns to baseline, initiate procedures to assist in determining fetal acid–base status, such as scalp stimulation and/or scalp blood sampling	EFM is only a screening device. Adjunct means of assessment may be helpful in affirming suspicions and making a diagnosis.

(continued)

Table 3–4. BRADYCARDIA (*continued*)

• Consider internal monitoring	Internal monitoring with a spiral electrode may provide more accurate assessment of the FHR (rule out erroneous signals).
• Consider sonographic evaluation	Direct visualization of the fetal heart may be helpful in ruling out artifactual signals (such as maternal heart rate, half- or double-counting) or fetal dysrhythmias. A biophysical examination may be done after the FHR has recovered to the baseline to assess fetal condition for signs of asphyxia/hypoxia.
• Observe for other previously nonreassuring signs such as rising baseline FHR; minimal, absent, or marked variability; presence of variable, late, or prolonged decelerations	These are indicators that the fetal condition had been progressively worsening before the bradycardia; operative intervention is likely.
• Communicate FHR/UA pattern and interventions to care provider and personnel in charge, and document in medical record	Care provider should assess patient/fetal condition immediately; charge personnel need to plan staffing accordingly and may provide expertise and assistance; medical record should reflect assessments and interventions.
• Prepare for delivery	If interventions are not effective and the bradycardia is of hypoxic etiology, emergent delivery is likely.

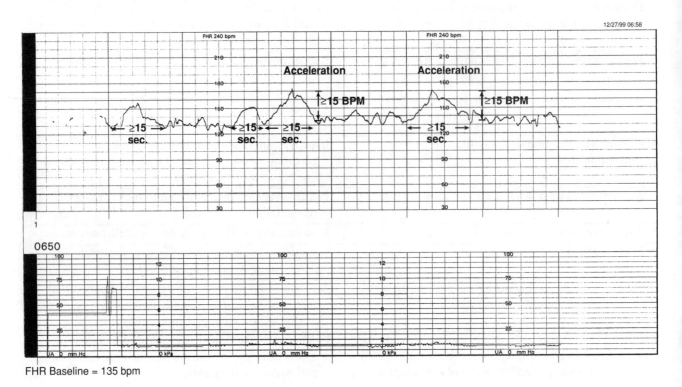

FHR Baseline = 135 bpm

Figure 3–10. Spontaneous accelerations (arrows denote 15 beats above, 15 seconds length).

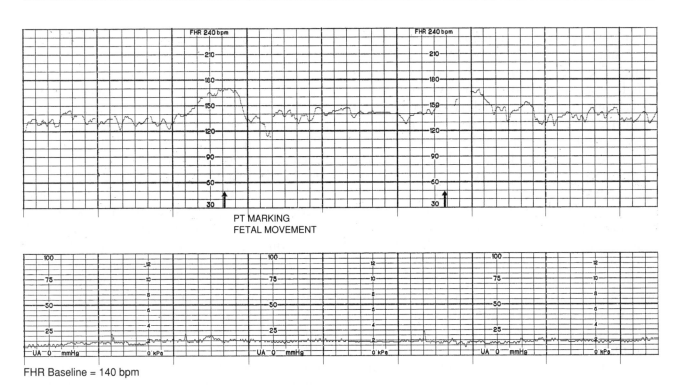

FHR Baseline = 140 bpm

Figure 3–11. Accelerations in response to fetal movement (↑).

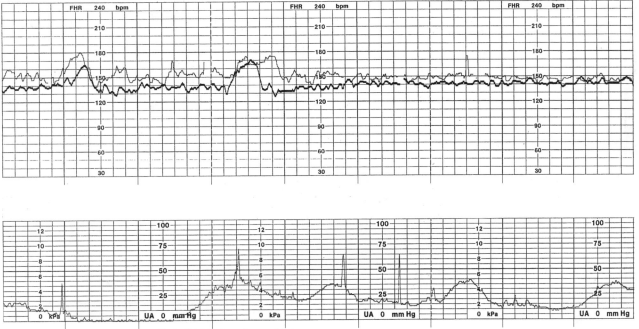

Twin A FHR Baseline = 130 bpm; Twin B FHR Baseline = 150 bpm

Figure 3–12. Accelerations of both fetal heart rates in a twin gestation.

simultaneously with contractions and maintain a very similar (uniform) shape with each occurrence. The presence of uniform accelerations is usually attributable to one of two conditions: breech presentation or mild cord compression (Schifrin, 1990). Although accelerations are considered a reassuring finding regardless of their etiology, for purposes of appropriate clinical management, it is necessary to understand what is precipitating their appearance.

When the fetus is in a breech position, contractions of the uterus may cause a sympathetic response as the fetal torso is stimulated. Concurrently, there is an absence of parasympathetic stimulation that would normally occur when the fetal head is pressed into the pelvis during contractions. These events result in a pattern of transient increases in the FHR during contractions known as uniform accelerations. If the position of the fetus has not been confirmed and a pattern of uniform accelerations is noted,

assessment for presentation is warranted (Schifrin, 1990).

Another reason for the appearance of uniform accelerations is that the umbilical cord may be in a position that makes it vulnerable to pressure during a contraction (Paul, Petrie, Rabello, & Mueller, 1979). The force exerted on the umbilical cord may be sufficient to inhibit flow through the umbilical vein, but not of a degree great enough to affect perfusion through the sturdier walls of the umbilical arteries. The subsequent decrease in blood flow to the fetus caused by compression of the umbilical vein during the contraction elicits a sympathetic response in the fetus. The resulting increases of the FHR noted to occur simultaneously with contractions are uniform accelerations (Fig. 3–13).

When uniform accelerations are present, it is important to also consider the possibility that maternal heart rate is being erroneously recorded (discussed in Chapter 2), especially if the baseline heart rate is in the lower ranges of normal or below

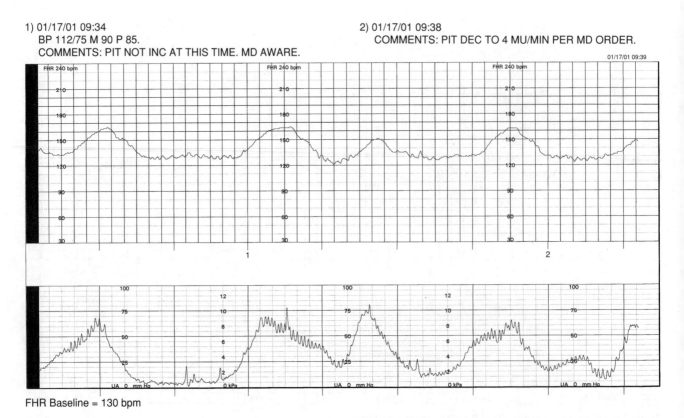

1) 01/17/01 09:34
   BP 112/75 M 90 P 85.
   COMMENTS: PIT NOT INC AT THIS TIME. MD AWARE.

2) 01/17/01 09:38
   COMMENTS: PIT DEC TO 4 MU/MIN PER MD ORDER.
   01/17/01 09:39

FHR Baseline = 130 bpm

Figure 3–13. Uniform accelerations of the FHR.

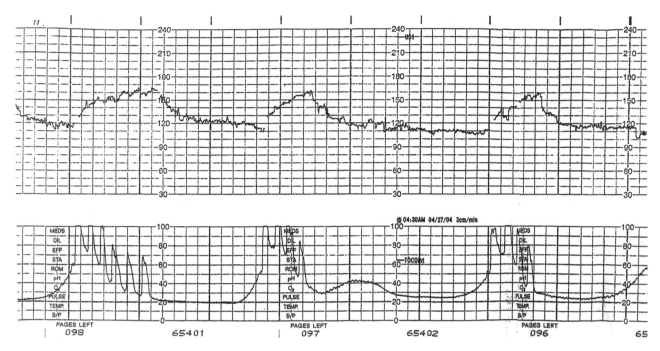

Figure 3–14. Maternal heart rate (MHR) showing increases during expulsive efforts.

what is expected for the FHR. If this is the case, the increase in a woman's heart rate that occurs as she experiences pain or exerts expulsive efforts during contractions could be mistaken for an acceleration of the FHR (Fig. 3–14). To eliminate confusion, palpate the maternal pulse and compare it to the monitor's audible signal. For documentation purposes, it is useful if the maternal heart rate can also be automatically obtained and printed or trended directly on the fetal strip chart. If there is any uncertainty, sonographic evaluation may be useful to visually confirm fetal cardiac activity.

Prolonged Accelerations

When accelerations of the FHR occur for a period greater than 2 minutes, but less than 10 minutes in duration, they are known as *prolonged accelerations* (NICHD, 1997). As with the accelerations discussed previously, prolonged accelerations peak at amplitude of at least 15 bpm above the FHR baseline. Their distinguishing characteristic, however, is their duration—an interval between 2 and 10 minutes. Prolonged accelerations

are a reassuring indication of fetal well-being (Fig. 3–15).

Accelerations and Fetal Maturity

As discussed previously, the premature fetus may not yet have developed full physiologic maturity, particularly in relation to ANS functioning. At less than 32 weeks' gestation, it cannot be assumed that the fetus has the capacity to produce accelerations of ≥15 bpm × ≥15 seconds. Therefore, in the fetus less than 32 weeks' gestation, accelerations may be satisfactory if there is a transient increase above the FHR baseline by ≥10 bpm that is sustained for ≥10 seconds duration (NICHD, 1997). This finding may be significant as an indicator of well-being in the preterm fetus that has not previously demonstrated the ability to accelerate its heart rate according to the 15 bpm × 15 seconds criterion.

Decelerations

Transient decreases in the FHR can occur in relation to the stress of contractions or can be triggered by other physiologic events. There are specific

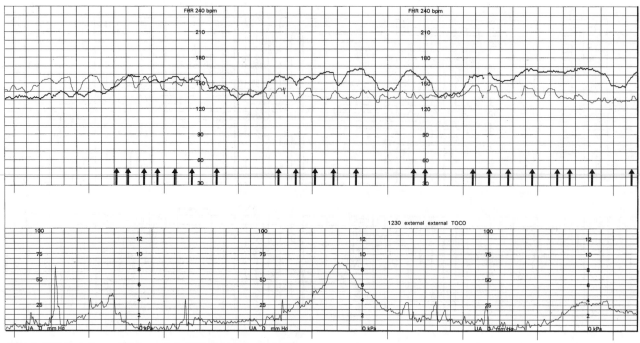

Twin A FHR Baseline = 135 bpm; Twin B FHR Baseline = 135 bpm

Figure 3–15. Prolonged accelerations. (Fetus "B," indicated by the heavier density tracing, responds to movement by accelerating its heart rate ≥2 minutes, but ≤10 minutes.)

criteria by which such changes of the FHR are evaluated for identification and clinical management purposes. These include:

Depth (measured in beats per minute)

Descent (time, in seconds, from the onset of the deceleration to its nadir)

Duration (length of the deceleration as measured from its onset to recovery)

Timing (in relation to/in the absence of contractions)

Other factors that are considered include shape, frequency of occurrence, and the amount of variability present in the FHR baseline.

Early Decelerations

Early decelerations are usually thought to result from compression of the fetal head (see Chapter 1). This pattern can occur with cephalopelvic disproportion, fetal descent, cervical examination, forceps application, or as a result of the fetal head being pressed into the pelvis during contractions. Early decelerations are often seen during the later phases of active labor. Pressure exerted on the fetal head during contractions stimulates the parasympathetic nervous system and subsequently slows the FHR. This is a normal physiologic event that does not require treatment (Fig. 3–16).

See Table 3–5 for the characteristics of early decelerations usually seen on visual assessment of the FHR tracing.

Late Decelerations

Late decelerations indicate basal fetal hypoxemia as a result of maternal, fetal, or placental conditions that impede the necessary provision of oxygen from the mother to the fetus. Late decelerations maintain many of the same visually apparent attributes as early decelerations; however, they are readily distinguishable by their timing in relation to contractions (Table 3–6) (Fig. 3–17).

As explained in Chapter 1, only a minimal to no amount of oxygen crosses the placenta during a contraction. The fetus who has experienced prolonged periods of hypoxia before the onset of contractions may already be compromised. Therefore,

Table 3–5. CHARACTERISTICS OF EARLY DECELERATIONS

Depth	Shallow; usually dropping no more than 15 beats below the FHR baseline
Descent	Gradual; onset to nadir ≥30 seconds (NICHD, 1997)
Duration	Usually about the same length as the contraction: greater than 15 seconds and less than 2 minutes
Timing	Simultaneous with contractions; early decelerations usually begin when the contraction starts, reach their nadir as the contraction reaches its peak, and are concluded by the time the contraction has ended (NICHD, 1997)
Shape	Uniform; most early decelerations appearing within proximity look similar to one another
Frequency of occurrence	Repetitive; appear with ≥50% of contractions
Variability in the FHR baseline	Usually moderate (6–25 beats of fluctuation)

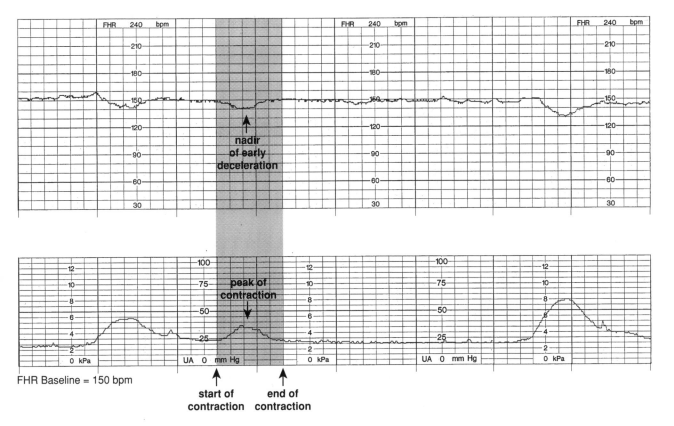

Figure 3–16. Early deceleration.

Table 3–6. CHARACTERISTICS OF LATE DECELERATIONS

Depth	Shallow; usually dropping no more than 15 beats below the FHR baseline
Descent	Gradual; onset to nadir ≥30 seconds (NICHD, 1997)
Duration	Usually about the same length as the contraction; greater than 15 seconds and less than 2 minutes
Timing	Offset from contractions; late decelerations usually begin after the contraction has started and reach their nadir after the contraction has reached its peak; the FHR does not return to baseline rate until after the contraction has ended (NICHD, 1997)
Shape	Uniform; most late decelerations appearing within proximity look similar to one another
Frequency of occurrence	Repetitive; appear with ≥50% of contractions
Variability in the FHR baseline	Moderate (6–25 beats of fluctuation), minimal (≤5 beats), or absent (no visible fluctuation)

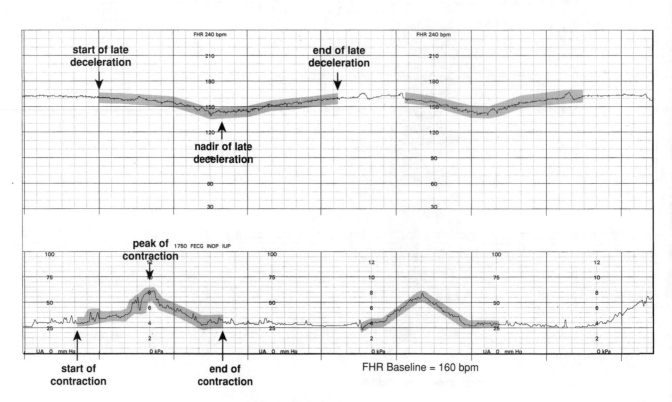

Figure 3–17. Late decelerations.

when contractions begin and blood flow diminishes, the FHR slows in response to the level of hypoxemia. The FHR remains lowered until the contraction ends and maternal–fetal exchange resumes. The FHR then slowly returns to the baseline rate.

S T O R K   B Y T E :

How much my heart rate slows down during late decelerations does not tell you how bad my problem is. Many times, I am in worse condition when my heart rate is falling below the baseline by only a few beats per minute.

Previously well-oxygenated fetuses also demonstrate late decelerations when faced with an acute decrease in oxygenation. This often occurs with uterine hyperstimulation due to oxytocin administration or maternal hypotension secondary to either supine positioning or administration of a regional anesthetic. In these instances, the response to contractions is similar to that of the chronically hypoxic fetus. If the contractions are occurring too close together, uteroplacental blood flow will remain diminished throughout the episode of hypertonus or hyperstimulation. If maternal blood pressure is low, there is decreased uteroplacental perfusion as blood is diverted to organs more critical to maternal survival (ie, maternal heart and brain) (Table 3–7).

Variable Decelerations

Variable decelerations are usually considered to occur in relation to compression of the umbilical cord. They have also been identified as resulting from head compression in the second stage of labor secondary to vagal stimulation (Ball, Parer, Caldwell, & Johnson, 1994). Any factor that inhibits the umbilical cord from floating freely (eg, actions or positioning of the fetus, monoamniotic multiple gestation, nuchal cord, cord entanglement, short or knotted cord, occult or overt prolapse, oligohydramnios, or thick meconium) may lead to the presence of variable decelerations. If the umbilical cord is compressed, blood flow into or out of the fetal circulation may be impeded. In response, the FHR drops abruptly. Once the cord compression/ occlusion is alleviated, the FHR usually returns to its normal baseline rate. If variable decelerations are repetitive, occur over a prolonged period of time, and do not respond to treatment, the fetus may become hypoxic.

Variable decelerations have a very different appearance from other types of decelerations. The abruptness of their onset and the sharp, deep decline of the FHR usually make them readily identifiable. The usual characteristics of variable decelerations are shown in Table 3–8 (Fig. 3–18).

S T O R K   B Y T E :

Hey, look at me! Sometimes I squeeze my umbilical cord just to get attention!

Variable decelerations can often be eliminated with position changes. Amnioinfusion is another effective means for remediating the variable deceleration pattern. Results are usually seen within half an hour of beginning this procedure. Amnioinfusion is often indicated in cases where cord compression due to decreased amniotic fluid or fluid thickened by meconium is an issue and expedient delivery is not indicated. Amnioinfusion is accomplished by the instillation of normal saline or lactated Ringer's solution into the uterine cavity through a device such as an intrauterine pressure catheter. This is accomplished by bolus dose or maintenance dose, with or without use of an infusion pump, and with or without use of a blood warmer, depending on hospital protocol. A number of variations of amnioinfusion technique exist and are effective. When properly performed, this intervention may be helpful in alleviating cord compression before the fetus experiences any further decline in status.

Shoulders

Variable decelerations possess another unique feature—they are the only type of deceleration pattern that, at times, includes an accelerative phase within the context of their occurrence. There are two specific acceleration patterns that can occur as part of the variable deceleration. These are known as *shoulders* and *overshoots*. Shoulders are brief accelerations of the FHR that may immediately precede or follow the

Table 3–7. LATE DECELERATIONS

Possible Etiology: Uteroplacental Insufficiency

Related to Maternal Conditions	Related to Fetal/Placental Conditions
• Hypertension/vascular disease • Cardiac status • Hypotension • Anemia • Diabetes • Smoking • Uterine hyperstimulation	• Postterm • Intrauterine growth restriction • Abruptio placentae • Chorioamnionitis • Placenta previa/hemorrhage

Goal of Intervention	Rationale
Improve uteroplacental perfusion	*Improving the amount and quality of blood flow to the fetus will assist with attempts at recovery*

Specific Interventions	Rationale
• Lateral positioning	Improve maternal circulation and perfusion to the placenta.
• Increase IV fluid rate (bolus) unless otherwise contraindicated	Improve maternal circulation and perfusion to placenta.
• Administer oxygen 8–10 L/min by mask	Hyperoxygenate maternal blood to increase fetal oxygenation.
• Discontinue oxytocin infusion; remove uterotonic agents; consider tocolytics	Eliminate additional stress of decreased blood flow during contractions until further assessment proves the fetus is not acidotic.
• Palpate uterus	Palpation may be the most effective means of determining hyperstimulation.
• Assess maternal vital signs	Maternal status directly influences FHR patterns.
• Observe for reassuring signs such as accelerations and moderate variability	Accelerations and moderate variability suggest that the fetus is not sufficiently hypoxic to produce acidosis.
• Initiate procedures to assist in determining fetal acid–base status, such as scalp stimulation and/or scalp blood sampling	EFM is only a screening device. Adjunct means of assessment may be helpful in affirming suspicions and making a diagnosis.
• Consider internal monitoring	Internal monitoring with a spiral electrode may provide more accurate assessment of the FHR.
• Consider BPP	BPP may be helpful in assessing for signs of hypoxia/asphyxia.
• Observe for other nonreassuring signs such as rising baseline FHR; minimal, absent, or marked variability; variable or prolonged decelerations; bradycardia	These are indicators that the fetal condition is worsening. If interventions are not improving fetal status, operative intervention may be necessary.
• Communicate FHR/UA pattern and interventions to care provider and personnel in charge, and document in medical record	Care provider should assess patient/fetal condition; charge personnel need to plan staffing accordingly and may provide expertise and assistance; medical record should reflect assessments and interventions.
• Prepare for delivery	If interventions are not effective and the late deceleration pattern continues, operative or assisted delivery may be performed.

Table 3–8. CHARACTERISTICS OF VARIABLE DECELERATIONS

Depth	Often deep; usually dropping at least 15 beats below the FHR baseline (NICHD, 1997)
Descent	Abrupt; onset to nadir <30 seconds (NICHD, 1997)
Duration	>15 seconds and <2 minutes (NICHD, 1997)
Timing	May occur in relation to stress placed on the umbilical cord during contractions and may also occur independently of contractions in response to other cord-related events
Shape	Irregular; variable decelerations appearing within proximity may appear similar to one another or they may take on different forms
Frequency of occurrence	Can appear singularly or in a repetitive fashion
Variability in the FHR baseline	Moderate (6–25 beats of fluctuation) to minimal (≤5 beats) or absent (no visible fluctuation)

decelerative phase of the variable deceleration and denote progressive amounts of pressure being placed on and removed from the umbilical cord, compressing the umbilical vein. When shoulders appear, there is usually a moderate amount of variability present in the FHR baseline as a reassuring sign of fetal status. If there is a shoulder on the concluding end of the variable deceleration, it returns rapidly to FHR baseline (Parer, 1997; Schifrin, 1990; Fig. 3–19).

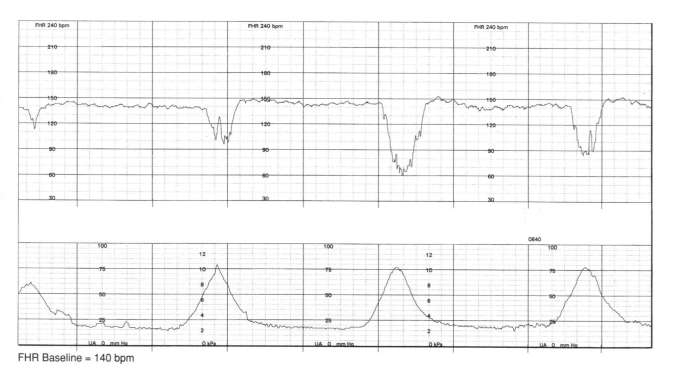

FHR Baseline = 140 bpm

Figure 3–18. Variable decelerations.

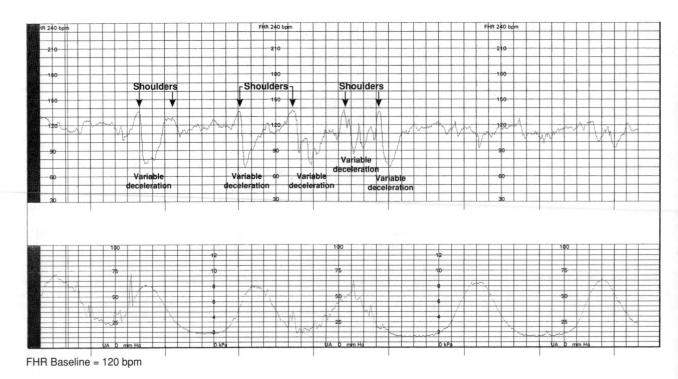

FHR Baseline = 120 bpm

Figure 3–19. Variable decelerations with shoulders.

Overshoots

Overshoots are another type of acceleration associated with variable decelerations. Overshoots appear as the FHR is attempting to resolve back to baseline from the variable deceleration. The compromised fetus, in an attempt to recover to baseline rate, raises its heart rate well above (overshoots) the baseline. When overshoots are present, variability in the FHR baseline is usually minimal to absent and there is no accelerative phase preceding the variable deceleration. The fetus usually maintains the overshoot for a fairly significant period of time before returning to baseline FHR (Fig. 3–20). Overshoots are considered to be a nonreassuring sign in the term or postterm fetus, because this pattern is associated with ANS impairment and significant hypoxia/acidosis (Schifrin & Clement, 1990). Overshoots are an anticipated response, however, when they present before maturity of the ANS has occurred or in the event that atropine has been administered to the mother (Schifrin, 1990; Schifrin, Hamilton-Rubinstein, & Shields, 1994) (Table 3–9).

Prolonged Deceleration

A prolonged deceleration is the most easily recognizable deceleration, characterized simply by its duration. Prolonged decelerations ($\geq$15 bpm below baseline) range in length from 2 to 10 minutes (NICHD, 1997) (Fig. 3–21). The span of the deceleration is measured from the point where the FHR falls from the baseline until its return to baseline FHR. The etiology of the prolonged deceleration is varied. It is related to any acute event that transiently interrupts maternal–fetal perfusion, such as cord compression, uterine hyperactivity, or maternal hypotension. Prolonged decelerations usually exhibit the characteristics shown in Table 3–10.

Because the insult initiating the prolonged deceleration is often unknown at the time of its occurrence, interventions are a compilation of those aimed at promoting intrauterine resuscitation with other nonreassuring FHR patterns and baseline changes. This strategy includes the following actions:

Decreasing stress on the fetus (eg, discontinuing oxytocin/removing uterotonic agents, administering tocolytics)

Promoting maternal oxygenation (eg, hyperoxygenation with O_2)

Promoting perfusion to and through the uterus, placenta, and umbilical cord (eg, maternal positioning, hydration, discontinuing oxytocin/

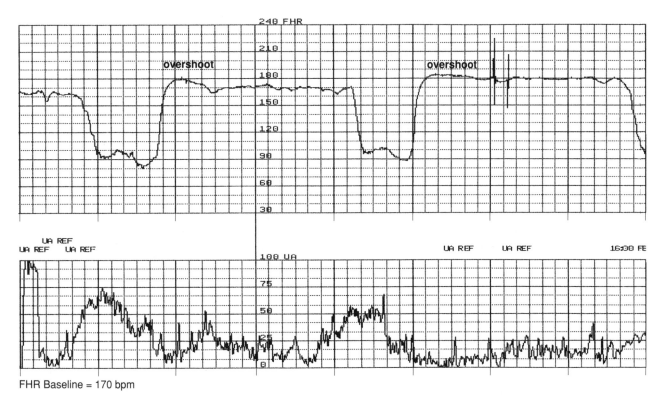

FHR Baseline = 170 bpm

Figure 3–20. Variable decelerations with overshoots.

removing uterotonic agents, administering to-colytics, vaginal assessment for cord prolapse and fetal descent (Table 3–11)

The following section focuses on less commonly occurring FHR patterns. Although they do not happen frequently, it is necessary to be familiar with such patterns to be able to react appropriately when one is encountered.

From Reassuring to Nonreassuring

The majority of women are admitted to labor and delivery with reassuring FHR patterns (ie, stable baseline rate that is within normal limits, moderate variability, accelerations present, and no decelerations). It is optimal to observe the FHR and take notice of any changes that begin to appear over time. If late and/or variable decelerations begin to develop, interventions (see Tables 3–7 and 3–9) to resolve these patterns should be employed. If the FHR continues to display these nonreassurring components despite intervention, the tracing should be closely monitored for other elements that may indicate the development or progression of fetal hypoxia. Such changes may include a slowly rising baseline, diminishment and/or the loss of variability, and worsening of deceleration patterns.

During the course of such progression, the FHR may temporarily settle into what can *appear* to be an improved pattern (stable rate that is still within "normal" limits, diminishment and/or disappearance of decelerations, but with variability minimal or absent) if considered only in the present context. When compared against an earlier recording of the FHR, however, it becomes evident that this is not a sign of recovery but rather of compromise. Fetal heart rate patterns indicative of fetal acidemia evolve over a reasonably long period of time. The literature supports approximately a 1-hour time frame for this progression to acidemia to occur, giving the providers ample time to make decisions and take action (Parer et al., 2006).

Preexisting Neurologic Injury

Two retrospective case studies have demonstrated that, when the FHR tracings of neurologically

Table 3–9. VARIABLE DECELERATIONS

Possible Etiology: Cord compression, vagal stimulation

Related to Maternal/Fetal Conditions	Related to Intrauterine Conditions
• Positioning • Second-stage labor • Copious fluid loss with rupture of membranes • Monoamniotic multiple gestation	• Oligohydramnios • Meconium • Cord entanglement • Nuchal cord • Short cord • Knotted cord • Prolapsed cord

Goal of Intervention	Rationale
Improve blood flow through the umbilical cord	*Alleviating stress on the umbilical cord will help it to float freely and not be compressed*

Specific Interventions	Rationale
• Vaginal examination	Check for cord prolapse. If prolapse is detected, lift presenting part off cord and continue to do so until delivery of fetus.
• Positioning—left lateral, right lateral, knee–chest	Improve maternal circulation and perfusion to placenta; improve blood flow through the umbilical cord.
• Increase IV fluid rate (bolus) unless otherwise contraindicated	Improve maternal circulation and perfusion to placenta; improve maternal hydration to potentiate greater amniotic fluid volume.
• Administer oxygen 8–10 L/min by mask	Hyperoxygenate maternal blood to increase fetal oxygenation.
• Amnioinfusion	Create cushioning for the cord and alleviate compression.
• Consider discontinuation of oxytocin infusion, uterotonic agents; consider tocolytics	Additional stress on the fetus of decreased blood flow during contractions may be too great when repetitive or severe variable decelerations are present. Decrease the stress of contractions on the fetus until further assessment proves the fetus is not acidotic.
• Do not ask patient to "push" with every contraction	Gives fetus a chance to recover/reoxygenate.
• Observe for reassuring signs such as accelerations and moderate variability	Accelerations and moderate variability suggest that the fetus is not sufficiently hypoxic to produce acidosis.
• Initiate procedures to assist in determining fetal acid–base status, such as scalp stimulation and/or scalp blood sampling	EFM is only a screening device. Adjunct means of assessment may be helpful in affirming suspicions and making a diagnosis.
• Consider internal monitoring	Internal monitoring with a spiral electrode may provide more accurate assessment of the FHR.
• Consider BPP	BPP may be helpful in assessing for signs of hypoxia/asphyxia.
• Observe for other nonreassuring signs such as rising baseline FHR; minimal, absent, or marked variability; overshoots; late or prolonged decelerations; or bradycardia	These are indicators that the fetal condition is worsening. If interventions are not improving fetal status, operative intervention may be necessary.

(continued)

Table 3–9. VARIABLE DECELERATIONS (continued)

• Communicate FHR/UA pattern and interventions to care provider and personnel in charge, and document in medical record	Care provider should assess patient/fetal condition if variable decelerations are repetitive or severe; charge personnel need to plan staffing accordingly and may provide expertise and assistance; medical record should reflect assessments and interventions.
• Prepare for delivery	If interventions are not successful and the variable deceleration pattern continues, operative or assisted delivery may be necessary.

damaged children were reviewed, several common features were present (Phelan & Ahn, 1994; Schifrin, Hamilton-Rubinstein, & Shields, 1994). Phelan noted that 69% of these children had nonreactive patterns from admission to delivery. Schifrin noted that all 44 children with cerebral palsy in his study showed persistently absent variability and small variable decelerations with overshoots from the onset of intrapartum monitoring.

Despite these findings, the care provider cannot rely solely on a nonreassuring or nonreactive FHR tracing as evidence that prior neurologic injury has occurred. Although the negative predictive value of EFM is quite high (~98%) when the FHR tracing is reassuring, it also has a high false-positive rate when the FHR tracing is suggestive of fetal compromise, thus prompting further investigation of fetal status (Fig. 3–22).

1) 02/13/01 13:30
   UTERUS BEGINNING TO RELAX PER PALPATION AND PT REPORT

2) 02/13/01 13:31
   UTERUS SOFT PER PALPATION

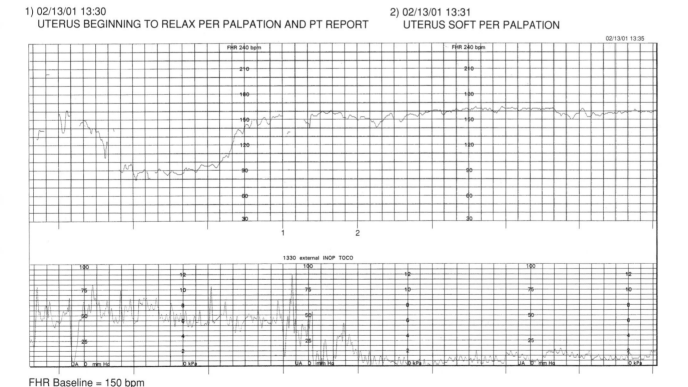

FHR Baseline = 150 bpm

Figure 3–21. Prolonged deceleration with hyperstimulation.

Table 3–10. CHARACTERISTICS OF PROLONGED DECELERATIONS

Depth	May be deep or shallow, depending on the etiology, but usually drop by ≥15 bpm below baseline (NICHD, 1997)
Descent	May be abrupt or gradual, depending on the etiology
Duration	Two minutes or longer but less than 10 minutes (NICHD, 1997)
Timing	May occur in relation to stress placed on the umbilical cord, uterine hyperactivity, maternal hypotension, changes in maternal hemodynamic/cardiac status
Frequency of occurrence	Can appear singularly or in a repetitive fashion
Variability in the FHR baseline	Moderate (6–25 beats of fluctuation), minimal (≤5 beats), or absent (no visible fluctuation)

Unusual FHR Patterns

Sinusoidal Pattern

When the rare sinusoidal pattern occurs, the FHR baseline rate remains stable and within normal range, but the tracing has an obviously unusual appearance. The predominant feature of the sinusoidal pattern is that the FHR baseline undulates across the strip chart, repetitively creating a constant, sine-wave-shaped form. These oscillations occur regularly, at a frequency of two to five times per minute with amplitude of 5 to 15 beats above and below the FHR baseline (Schifrin, 1990). The actual FHR baseline is indeterminate when a sinusoidal pattern is present. The FHR baseline variability is absent or minimal (Garite, 1988), giving the sinusoidal pattern its smooth shape. Usually, there are no periods during the FHR tracing with a sinusoidal pattern where the FHR appears normal (Figure 3–23). This pattern will not resolve spontaneously. The FHR tracing with a sinusoidal pattern may be complicated by additional nonreassuring elements, such as variable, late, or prolonged decelerations.

The possible etiologies of sinusoidal patterns include fetal anemia, fetal hypoxia, or maternal narcotic administration (see Chapter 1). Sinusoidal patterns are most commonly due to fetal anemia secondary to Rh isoimmunization. This was described as the causative factor in the original description of a sinusoidal pattern (Rochard et al., 1976). Fetal anemia can also result from other maternal–fetal blood incompatibilities, maternal trauma, abruptio placentae, placenta previa, or any fetal–maternal hemorrhage and can present as a sinusoidal pattern. In some cases (such as with blood–antigen incompatibilities), fetal transfusion by way of percutaneous umbilical blood sampling (PUBS) may temporarily resolve the anemia. Once the anemia is corrected, the FHR tracing will no longer appear sinusoidal. In these instances, it is often necessary to repeat this treatment numerous times during the antepartum. When a sinusoidal pattern is noted, a sonographic examination is performed to observe the fetus for ascites and/or hydrops. Other methods of fetal assessment are also employed to evaluate fetal oxygenation.

Sinusoidal patterns can result from severe fetal hypoxia. Lack of oxygen affects the fetal ANS, subsequently altering the fetal heart rhythm. In the majority of these cases, prompt delivery of the fetus is indicated, although it is recognized that some measure of neurologic damage to the fetus may have already occurred.

Most commonly observed is the sinusoidal tracing resulting from narcotic administration. When this occurs, the tracing is referred to as *pseudosinusoidal*, indicating that the causative nature of the sine-wave-shaped undulations is not pathologic. Pseudosinusoidal patterns were originally noted after the administration of alphaprodine

Table 3–11. PROLONGED DECELERATIONS

Possible Etiology: Uteroplacental insufficiency, cord compression

Goal of Intervention	Rationale
Improve uteroplacental blood flow and perfusion through the umbilical cord	Improving the amount and quality of blood flow to the fetus will assist with attempts at recovery

Specific Interventions	Rationale
• Attempt to determine cause	Recognition of causative factors increases efficiency of response.
• Vaginal examination	Check for cord prolapse. If prolapse is detected, lift presenting part off cord and continue to do so until delivery of the fetus.
• Positioning—left lateral, right lateral, knee–chest	Reposition until successful, giving each position a chance to take effect. Improve maternal circulation and perfusion to the placenta; improve blood flow through the umbilical cord.
• Increase IV fluid rate (bolus) unless otherwise contraindicated	Improve maternal circulation and perfusion to placenta; improve maternal hydration to potentiate greater amniotic fluid volume.
• Administer oxygen 8–10 L/min by mask	Hyperoxygenate maternal blood to increase fetal oxygenation.
• Discontinue oxytocin infusion; remove uterotonic agents; consider tocolytics	Eliminate additional stress of decreased blood flow during contractions by promoting uterine relaxation until further assessment proves the fetus is not acidotic.
• Palpate uterus	Palpation may be most effective means of determining hyperstimulation.
• Assess maternal vital signs, particularly BP for hypotension	Maternal status directly affects FHR pattern.
• Observe tracing for reassuring signs such as accelerations and moderate variability	Accelerations and moderate variability suggest that the fetus is not sufficiently hypoxic to produce acidosis.
• Initiate procedures to assist in determining fetal acid–base status, such as scalp stimulation and/or scalp blood sampling	EFM is only a screening device. Adjunct means of assessment may be helpful in affirming suspicions and making a diagnosis.
• Consider internal monitoring	Internal monitoring with a spiral electrode may provide more accurate assessment of the FHR.
• Consider BPP	BPP may be helpful in assessing for signs of hypoxia/asphyxia.
• Observe for other nonreassuring signs, such as rising baseline FHR; minimal, absent, or marked variability; presence of variable or late decelerations; progression to bradycardia	These are indicators that the fetal condition is worsening. If interventions are not improving fetal status, operative intervention may be necessary.
• Communicate FHR/UA pattern and interventions to care provider and personnel in charge, and document in medical record	Care provider should assess patient/fetal condition; charge personnel need to plan staffing accordingly and may provide expertise and assistance; medical record should reflect assessment and interventions.
• Prepare for delivery	If interventions are not successful and prolonged decelerations continue to occur, operative or assisted delivery may be performed.

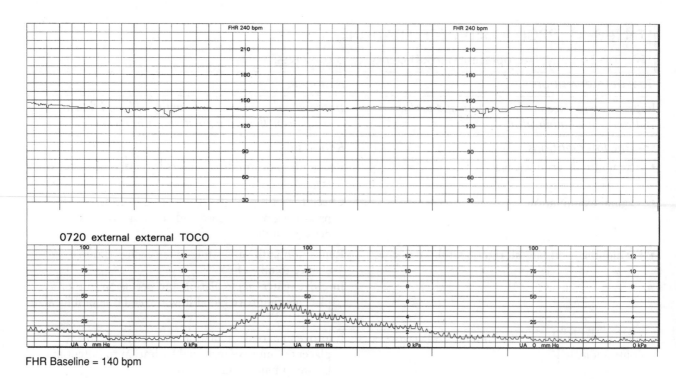

FHR Baseline = 140 bpm

Figure 3–22. Chronic hypoxemia.

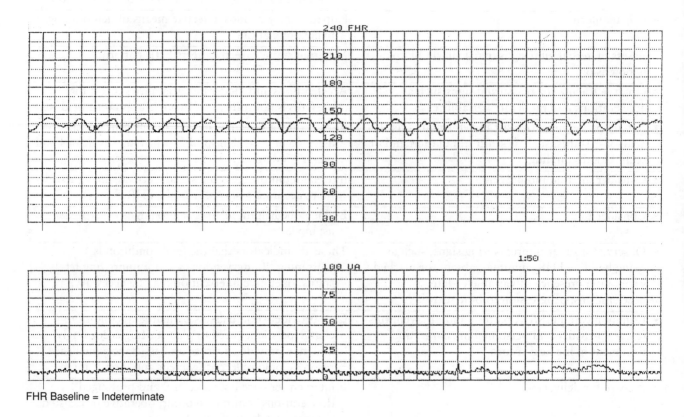

FHR Baseline = Indeterminate

Figure 3–23. Sinusoidal pattern.

and are commonly seen after the administration of butorphanol, morphine sulfate, and meperidine. Various illicit drugs also have this effect on the FHR. It is prudent to obtain a reassuring FHR tracing before dispensing pain medications so that, if a sinusoidal pattern ensues, it can be determined to have resulted from the narcotic rather than the onset of fetal hypoxia or anemia. The benign pseudosinusoidal pattern is usually distinguishable from the ominous sinusoidal pattern through careful history taking and assessment of the FHR tracing. Unlike the sinusoidal pattern, the pseudosinusoidal pattern usually has periods of normal FHR baseline, baseline variability, and other reassuring elements such as spontaneous or induced accelerations of the FHR (Fig. 3–24). The pseudosinusoidal pattern is corrected when the drug effects subside.

When a patient presents with a sinusoidal pattern, it is important to ascertain a complete maternal and prenatal history to rule out causes of fetal anemia or fetal hypoxia. Fetal scalp stimulation or vibra-acoustic stimulation can be done to elicit accelerations of the FHR (thus ruling out aci-

dosis). A fetal scalp blood sample for blood gas analysis may also be indicated. These techniques are discussed in greater detail in Chapter 1.

Fetal Dysrhythmias

Fetal dysrhythmias are a relatively rare occurrence, affecting about 1% of all pregnancies. Less than 20% pose a serious threat to fetal or neonatal well-being, and most (99%) disappear shortly (hours to weeks) after birth and are of no long-term consequence (Clement & Schifrin, 1987). Fetal dysrhythmias are recognizable on the strip chart as abrupt changes in rhythm or rate between beats (R–R interval) of the fetal heart. This is demonstrated in the recorded FHR as linear deflections above and/or below the FHR baseline, depending on the type of arrhythmia. These deflections appear in an organized fashion and may be present intermittently or continuously. Fetal dysrhythmias can only be recorded on the strip chart when the signal source is the FECG and the FHR is printed without the use of any type of artifact-elimination technology (Fig. 3–25). Diagnosis of the specific type of dysrhythmia cannot

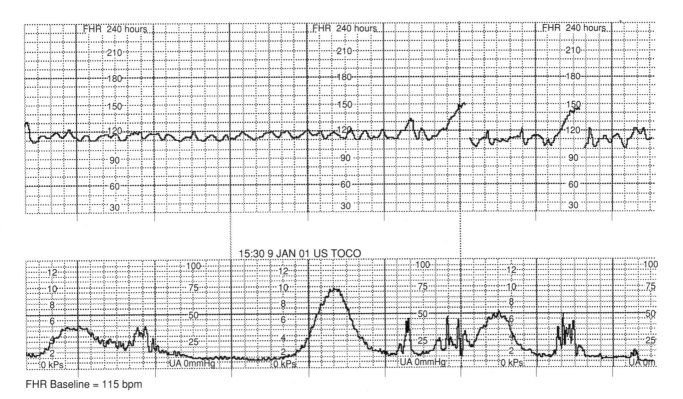

FHR Baseline = 115 bpm

Figure 3–24. Pseudosinusoidal pattern. The two accelerations occurring toward the end of this tracing negate the presence of a sinusoidal pattern.

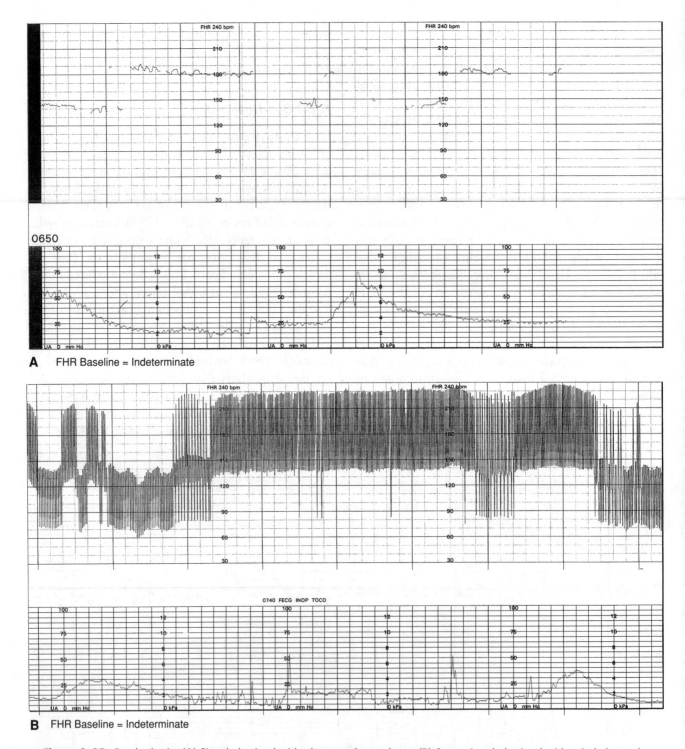

A   FHR Baseline = Indeterminate

B   FHR Baseline = Indeterminate

Figure 3–25. Dysrhythmia. (**A**) Signal obtained with ultrasound transducer. (**B**) Same signal obtained with spiral electrode.

be accomplished simply by looking at the FHR tracing (equipment issues are discussed in Chapter 2). This is most effectively accomplished either by FECG or M-mode ultrasound. A printout of the FECG waveform can usually be obtained by connecting the electronic fetal monitor to an adult ECG recorder. M-mode ultrasound can be used to visualize the fetal heart and record the rhythm. Usually, when an irregular FHR is noted, the patient is referred to a perinatologist for evaluation.

Once a diagnosis has been made, the risks and benefits of various treatment modalities are weighed. Depending on the type of dysrhythmia and its etiology, expectant management may be the chosen course of action. Other treatment modalities may include administration of antidysrhythmic drugs to the mother (usually orally) or to the fetus (through PUBS); use of steroids or other medications to decrease maternal antibodies; or delivery, with planned treatment of the neonate postnatally. During labor, scalp stimulation can be used to assess fetal oxygen status (Wax, Emmerich, & Eggleston, 1996).

Examples of Fetal Dysrhythmias

Premature Ventricular Contractions and Premature Atrial Contractions. Fetal dysrhythmias are most commonly associated with the following conditions: hydrops, hydramnios, intrauterine growth restriction, family history of congenital heart disease, maternal connective tissue disease, and maternal viral disease. Two of the most common types of fetal dysrhythmias are premature ventricular contractions (PVCs) and premature

atrial contractions (PACs). PVCs comprise more than half the cases of fetal dysrhythmia. These dysrhythmias are characterized by isolated extrasystoles and may be related to maternal usage of caffeine, tobacco, cocaine, alcohol, adrenergic drugs (pseudoephedrine), or beta-mimetic tocolytics. They are generally considered benign, but do warrant observation because up to 2% of fetuses with PVCs have structural anomalies and up to 1% may develop a sustained tachydysrhythmia causing risk for fetal hydrops (Simpson & Marx, 1994). PVCs may also lead to the dysrhythmic patterns of bigeminy (two PVCs occurring at a time) or trigeminy (three PVCs occurring at a time).

Fetuses with irregular FHRs seldom have significant structural heart defects. If congenital heart disease is diagnosed, however, it is important to rule out chromosomal abnormalities because there is a strong association between these two findings. Although atrial extrasystoles (PACs) (Fig. 3–26) appear to be benign, there is a chance they can precipitate supraventricular tachycardia (SVT), which is a more worrisome dysrhythmia (Copel, Liang, Demasio, Ozeren, & Kleinman, 2000).

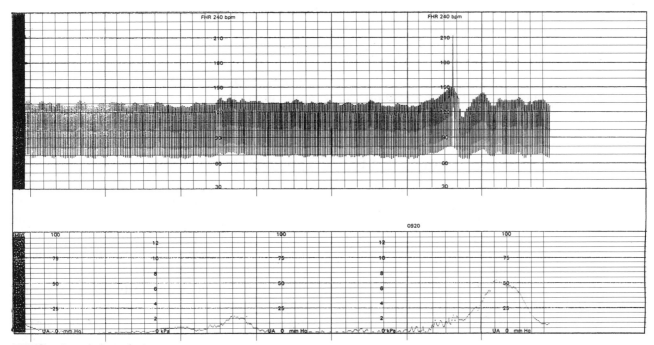

FHR Baseline = Indeterminate

Figure 3–26. Fetal extrasystoles.

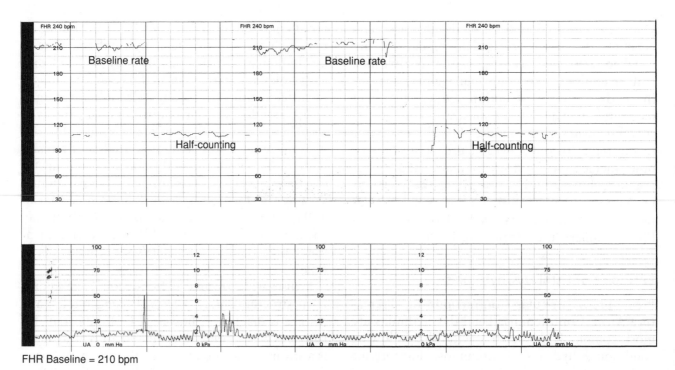

FHR Baseline = 210 bpm

Figure 3–27. Supraventricular tachycardia with half-counting. Signal obtained with ultrasound transducer, dysrhythmia later verified.

Supraventricular Tachycardia. Supraventricular tachycardia (SVT) is the most common serious fetal dysrhythmia. It is characterized by FHR baseline rate greater than 200 bpm, 1:1 atrial to ventricular activity, and a fixed R–R interval (little or no beat-to-beat variation) (Fig. 3–27). Most (~95%) of SVTs are caused by an electrical impulse that reenters the atrium from the ventricle, an etiology usually responsive to pharmacologic management (Kleinman & Copel, 1991). Only a small percentage (~5%) of SVTs have an atrial flutter/fibrillation or an ectopic atrial focus, which may require surgical intervention (Kleinman & Copel, 1991). Sustained SVT can lead to congestive heart failure or hydrops, and can put the fetus at risk for demise. Treatment modalities depend on etiology, gestational age, whether the condition is sustained or intermittent in nature, and whether hydrops has occurred. Fetuses with known SVTs or atrial flutter may be followed with antepartum testing as well as sonographic evaluation for signs of hydrops or ascites. Even in the presence of hydrops, chances of survival are 73% (Simpson & Sharland, 1998). Treatment usually includes administration of digoxin or other antiarrhythmic agents (such as procainamide) to the patient (to break the cycle of tachycardia) or delivery of fetus.

Bradydysrhythmia. As described earlier in this chapter, FHR baseline bradycardia is defined as FHR below 110 bpm for ≥10 minutes. The nonhypoxic types of fetal bradycardia that have been described in the literature include response to increased intracranial pressure (Parer, 1997) and fetal bradydysrhythmia (Copel, Friedman, & Kleinman, 1997).

A fetal bradydysrhythmia (Fig. 3–28) can result from cardiac anomalies, incomplete heart block associated with premature atrial contractions (PAC) or supraventricular tachycardia (SVT), or complete heart block. Diagnosis of the type of dysrhythmia is made by fetal echocardiography or M-mode ultrasound. In most situations, expectant management is recommended in consultation with a maternal–fetal medicine expert. In the presence of fetal hydrops or fetal heart failure, delivery may be indicated (Bayer-Zuoirello, Kanaan, Benner, Yu, & Gimovsky, 1995).

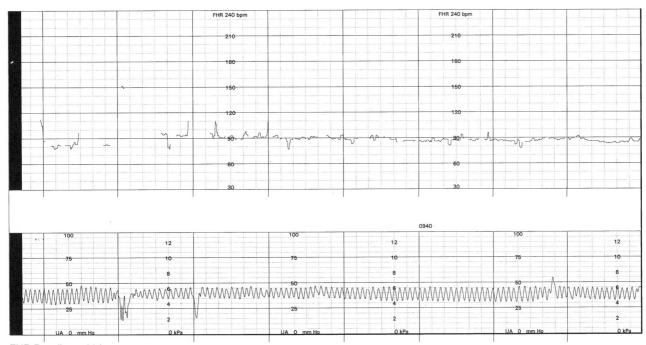

FHR Baseline = 90 bpm

Figure 3–28. Fetal bradydysrhythmia.

Atrioventricular block, also known as congenital heart block, is the most concerning bradydysrhythmia. It is characterized by a baseline FHR of 50 to 70 bpm. First-degree AV block is a rare occurrence, marked by a prolonged P–R interval and dropped beats. In second-degree AV block (Fig. 3–29), the rapid atrial beats are incompletely conducted to the ventricles, exhibiting as dropped beats. With third-degree AV block, there is complete atrioventricular dissociation, meaning that atrial beats are not conducted to ventricles. About half the fetuses with complete heart block have congenital heart disease, which is associated with poor outcome. If the heart is structurally normal, the outcome is more favorable. Maternal autoimmune disease (systemic lupus erythematosus, anti-SSA/Ro, anti-SSB/La) and viral disease (cytomegalovirus) are common causes of complete heart block when the fetal heart is structurally normal. Steroids or medications to decrease maternal antibodies may be used as treatment in these cases. The fetus must be observed for development of hydrops, an indicator of worsening prognosis.

The primary method of distinguishing between artifact and dysrhythmia is auscultation of the FHR and rhythm. As discussed in Chapter 2, when the spiral electrode is in use, interference with signal acquisition can occur. It is necessary to differentiate this event from the presence of a dysrhythmia. Auscultation of the FHR with a fetoscope or use of M-mode sonography can assist in this process by providing information about rate and rhythm. Artifact is usually visually discernible from dysrhythmia by its disorganized appearance and presence during events that disrupt the FECG signal, such as maternal movement or vaginal examinations (Fig. 3–30).

This chapter focused mainly on visual interpretation of the FHR tracing. To integrate this knowledge into practical clinical application, the practitioner must comprehend the underlying physiology of each FHR pattern and subsequently apply this knowledge in the form of appropriate interventions at the bedside. It is important to know that not every FHR pattern can be definitively categorized or described using existing nomenclature. Some patterns occur so infrequently that they are

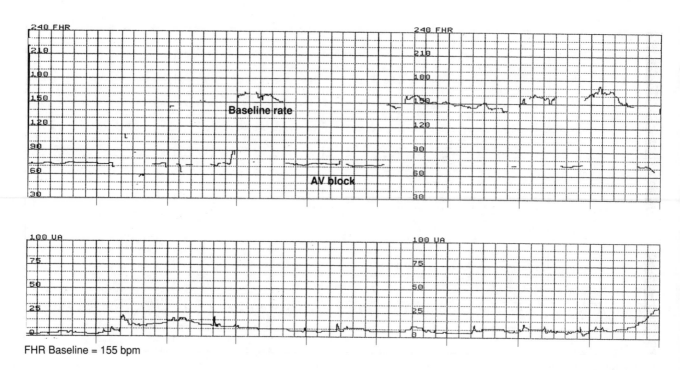

FHR Baseline = 155 bpm

Figure 3–29. Atrioventricular block.

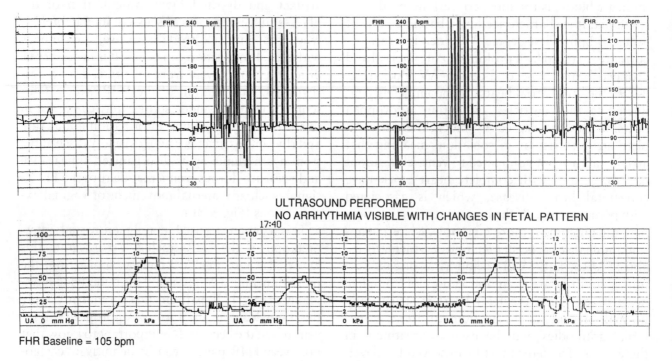

ULTRASOUND PERFORMED
NO ARRHYTHMIA VISIBLE WITH CHANGES IN FETAL PATTERN

FHR Baseline = 105 bpm

Figure 3–30. Artifact.

described in the literature as case reports. Most FHR tracings, however, can usually still be categorized as either reassuring or nonreassuring by examining individual recognizable components.

REFERENCES

American College of Obstetricians and Gynecologists. (2005). *Intrapartum fetal heart rate monitoring.* ACOG Practice Bulletin 70. Washington, DC: Author.

Association of Women's Health, Obstetric and Neonatal Nurses. (2006). *Antepartum and intrapartum fetal heart rate monitoring: Clinical competencies and education guide.* Washington, DC: Author.

Ball, R. H., Parer, J. T., Caldwell, L. E., & Johnson, J. (1994). Regional blood flow and metabolism in ovine fetuses during severe cord occlusion. *American Journal of Obstetrics and Gynecology, 117*(6), 1549–1555.

Bayer-Zuoirello, L. A., Kanaan, C. M., Benner, R., Yu, C., & Gimovsky, S.L. (1995). Fetal heart rate monitoring casebook: Persistent bradycardia. *Journal of Perinatology, 15*(6), 514–516.

Clark, S. L., Gimovsky, M. L., & Miller, F. C. (1984). The scalp stimulation test: A clinical alternative to fetal scalp blood sampling. *American Journal of Obstetrics and Gynecology, 14*(3), 274–277.

Clement, D., & Schifrin, B. (1987). Diagnosis and management of fetal arrhythmias. *Perinatal/Neonatal, 11,* 9–20.

Copel, J., Liang, R., Demasio, K., Ozeren, S., & Kleinman, C. (2000). The clinical significance of the irregular fetal heart rhythm. *American Journal of Obstetrics and Gynecology, 182,* 813–819.

Copel, J. A., Friedman, A. H., & Kleinman, C. S. (1997). Management of fetal cardiac arrhythmias. *Obstetrics & Gynecology Clinics of North America, 24*(1), 201–211.

Garite, T. (1988, May). Sinusoidal pattern from anemia. *Contemporary OB/GYN,* 42–46.

Ingemarsson, I., Arulkumaran, S., & Ratnam, S. S. (1985). Single injection of terbutaline in term labor. I. Effect on fetal pH in cases with prolonged bradycardia. *American Journal of Obstetrics and Gynecology, 153*(8), 859–865.

Kleinman, C. S., & Copel, J. A. (1991). Electrophysiological principles and fetal antiarrhythmic therapy. *Ultrasound Obstetrics and Gynecology, 1,* 286–297.

Leung, A., Leung, E., & Paul, R. (1993). Uterine rupture after previous cesarean delivery: Maternal and fetal consequences. *American Journal of Obstetrics and Gynecology, 169*(4), 945–949.

Menihan, C. (1998). Uterine rupture in women attempting vaginal birth following prior cesarean birth. *Journal of Perinatology, 18*(6), 440–443.

Miller, D., Diaz, F., & Paul, R. (1994). Vaginal birth after cesarean: A 10 year experience. *Obstetrics and Gynecology, 84*(2), 255–259.

National Institute of Child Health and Human Development Research Planning Workshop. (1997). Electronic fetal heart monitoring: Research guidelines for interpretation. *Journal of Obstetric, Gynecologic, and Neonatal Nursing, 26*(6), 635–640.

Panayotopoulos, N., Salamalekis, E., Kassanos, D., Vitoratos, N., Loghis, C., & Batalias, L. (1998). Intrapartum vibratory acoustic stimulation after maternal meperidine administration. *Clinical and Experimental Obstetrics and Gynecology, 25*(4), 139–140.

Parer, J. (1997). *Handbook of fetal heart rate monitoring* (2nd ed.). Philadelphia, PA: W. B. Saunders.

Parer, J. T., King, T., Flanders, S., Fox, M., & Kilpatrick, J. (2006). Fetal acidemia and electronic fetal heart rate patterns: Is there evidence of an association? *Journal of Maternal-Fetal and Neonatal Medicine, 19*(5), 289–294.

Paul, R. H., Petrie, R. H., Rabello, Y. A., & Mueller, E. A. (1979). *Fetal intensive care.* Wallingford, CT: Corometrics Medical Systems.

Phelan, J., & Ahn, M. O. (1994). Perinatal observations in forty-eight neurologically impaired term infants. *American Journal of Obstetrics and Gynecology, 171*(2), 424–431.

Rochard, F., Schifrin, B., Goupil, F., Legrand, H., Blottiere, J., & Sureau, C. (1976). Nonstressed fetal heart monitoring in the antepartum period. *American Journal of Obstetrics and Gynecology, 126*(6), 699–706.

Schifrin, B. (1990). *Exercises in fetal monitoring.* St. Louis MO: Mosby–Year Book.

Schifrin, B., Hamilton-Rubinstein, T., & Shields, J. (1994). Fetal heart rate patterns and the timing of fetal injury. *Journal of Perinatology, 14*(3), 174–181.

Sherer, D. M., & Bentolila, E. (1998). Blunted fetal response to vibroacoustic stimulation following chronic exposure to propanolol. *American Journal of Perinatology, 15*(8) 495–498.

Simpson, J., & Sharland, G. (1998). Fetal tachycardias: Management and outcome of 127 consecutive cases. *Heart, 79,* 576–581.

Simpson, K. R., & James, D. C. (2005). Efficacy of intrauterine resuscitation techniques in improving fetal oxygen status during labor. *Obstetrics and Gynecology, 105,* 1362–1368.

Simpson, L. L., & Marx, G. R. (1994). Diagnosis and treatment of structural fetal cardiac abnormality and dysrhythmia. *Seminars in Perinatology, 18*(3), 215–227.

Wax, J., Emmerich, M., & Eggleston, M. (1996). Intrapartum fetal atrial bigeminy—Diagnostic and therapeutic role of the fetal scalp stimulation test. *American Journal of Obstetrics and Gynecology, 174,* 1649–1650.

4 | Antepartum Fetal Assessment

The methods and means for assessing the fetus during the antepartum are selected based on gestational age, patient history and presentation, patient and practitioner preferences, and available technology. The purpose of antepartum testing is to screen for adequacy of uteroplacental function and to determine whether the fetus can safely remain in utero. It is important to consider that antepartum tests currently available are very effective for predicting fetal well-being but are not capable of making definitive diagnosis of fetal hypoxia/acidosis. See Table 4–1 for conditions indicating the need for antepartum surveillance. Antepartum surveillance is also indicated for other conditions affecting or suspected to affect the maternal–fetal unit. The American Academy of Pediatrics (AAP) and American College of Obstetricians and Gynecologists (ACOG) have issued research-based guidelines that delineate testing criteria and procedures (AAP & ACOG, 2002; ACOG, 1999).

Nonstress Test (NST)

The nonstress test (NST) involves the application of an electronic fetal monitor (EFM) to the maternal abdomen for the purpose of evaluating the fetus' ability to perform a specified number of accelerations within a specified period of time. If the fetus is able to accomplish this task, the test is deemed *reactive*. If the fetus is not able to produce the desired amount of fetal heart rate (FHR) accelerations within the allotted time frame, the test is considered to be *nonreactive*. The fetus is typically given up to 40 minutes to produce a reactive NST. This is to allow for the possibility that the time of testing might coincide with a period of fetal sleep. The NST is noninvasive and relatively easy to perform. Activities that affect fetal movement patterns and uteroplacental perfusion, (eg, maternal nutrition, hydration, smoking habits, medication effects, positioning, and time of day) should be considered when performing the NST.

The occurrence of two or more accelerations, each rising to ≥15 beats above the FHR baseline and lasting for a period of ≥15 seconds, accomplished within a 20-minute time frame constitutes a reactive NST (AAP & ACOG, 2002; ACOG, 1999; Bishop, 1981). A detailed explanation of accelerations is provided in Chapter 3. It is expected that the fetus should be able to meet these criteria by 32 weeks' gestation. Although some fetuses are able to produce a reactive NST as early as 24 to 28 weeks' gestation, there is a high false-positive rate (as much as 50%) in this population (Bishop, 1981). Between 28 and 32 weeks' gestation, there is a 15% chance that the NST will be nonreactive, because the fetal autonomic nervous system may not have reached the maturity necessary to accelerate the fetal heart per NST criteria (Druzin, Fox, Kogut, & Carlson, 1985; Lavin, Miodovnik, & Barden, 1984). When such development is exhibited at an early age, however, it is expected that the fetus will continue to achieve a reactive result during all subsequent monitoring sessions.

S T O R K   B Y T E :

I am growing up so quickly!
Now that I am mature enough to
give you a reactive NST, I should do
this well or even better every time you test me! If not,
beware!

There are variations in the parameters used to define the NST and its results. Both the period of time in which the NST is performed and the number of accelerations required during this period to deem the test reactive differ among institutions. Another variation of the NST includes the definition of a qualifying acceleration. Although the standard definition is that the accelerations rise above the baseline by ≥15 bpm and last ≥15 seconds, this definition may vary based on gestational age. For a fetus less than 32 weeks' gestation, accelerations of ≥10 bpm that last ≥10 seconds in length may be deemed acceptable (National Institute of Child Health and Human Development, 1997). An additional variation is that some institutions require that accelerations coincide with fetal movement in order to be acceptable. Because these discrepancies exist, it is necessary to be aware of and follow institutional policy (Fig. 4–1).

When the result of the NST is reactive, the patient will most likely be scheduled for testing on a weekly or twice-weekly basis, depending on gestational age and the indication for antepartum surveillance. Women who have maternal or obstetric indications that require twice-weekly testing include, but are not limited to, those with a postterm gestation, intrauterine growth restriction, type 1 diabetes mellitus, and pregnancy-induced hypertension. Some high-risk conditions may warrant testing on a more frequent basis. Isolated episodes that occur during a normal-risk pregnancy that warrant performance of an NST (such as complaint of decreased fetal movement) and are subsequently ruled out might not be followed with any regular schedule of testing. A reactive NST has a negative predictive value of 99.8%, meaning that the possibility of stillbirth occurring within 1 week after a reactive NST is extremely low (Freeman, Anderson, & Dorchester, 1982).

If the NST is reactive, but nonreassuring components of the FHR tracing such as variable, late, or prolonged decelerations are present, continued monitoring and further evaluation are indicated. If variable decelerations are brief (<30 seconds in length) and occur infrequently, they do not require intervention (Meis et al., 1986). If repetitive variable decelerations are present, measurement of the amniotic fluid volume by sonographic examination will determine if oligohydramnios is the underlying cause of this pattern. It is well established that oligohydramnios is associated with increased perinatal morbidity and mortality (Casey et al., 2000) and requires immediate attention and possible intervention. Further sonographic examination may reveal structural anomalies of the maternal–fetal unit that may be causing decelerations of the FHR to occur (Fig. 4–2).

If the NST is judged to be nonreactive, meaning that no accelerations or an insufficient number of accelerations are produced during a 40-minute time period (extended length of time to account for fetal sleep cycles), additional testing of the fetus is indicated. Intervention is not based solely on a nonreactive NST, because 80% to 90% of the nonreactive tracings are due to fetal sleep and are not the result of hypoxia (Evertson, Gauthier,

Table 4–1. INDICATIONS FOR ANTEPARTUM FETAL SURVEILLANCE

Preexisting Indications	Obstetric Indications
Type 1 diabetes mellitus	Postterm gestation
Chronic hypertension	Polyhydramnios or oligohydramnios
Previous demise	Decreased fetal movement
Autoimmune disease	Intrauterine growth restriction
Renal disease	Multiple gestation
Endocrine disease	Isoimmunization
Cardiovascular disease	Chronic abruptio placentae
Hemoglobinopathy	Pregnancy-induced hypertension
	Gestational diabetes

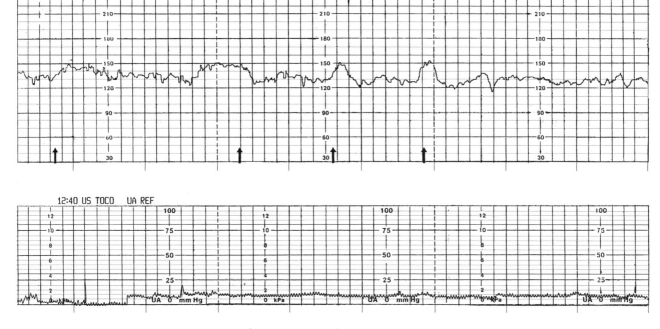

Figure 4–1. Reactive nonstress test.

Schifrin, & Paul, 1979; Evertson & Paul, 1978; Fig. 4–3).

A nonreactive NST that also has nonreassuring components of the FHR, such as variable, late, or prolonged decelerations, is of great concern. Such findings warrant immediate investigation and consideration of the need for delivery.

In summary, whether the tracing is considered reactive or nonreactive, if any part of the tracing is nonreassuring, further evaluation is needed. This may consist of any one or a combination of the tests mentioned in this chapter. It is important to understand that, although the NST is an effective screening tool for the evaluation of fetal

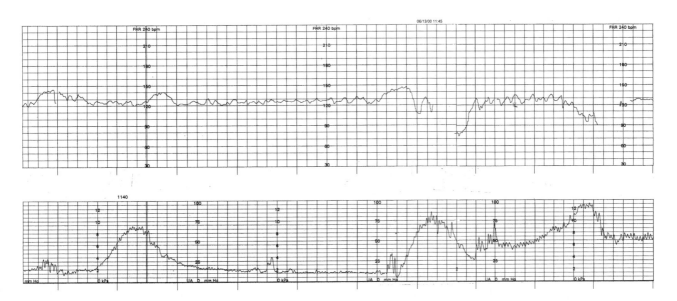

Figure 4–2. Reactive nonstress test with variable decelerations.

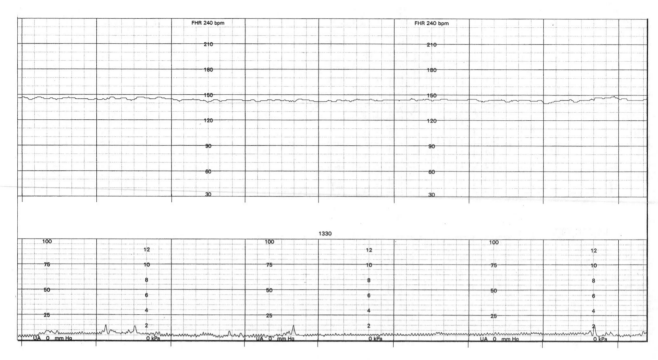

Figure 4–3. Nonreactive nonstress test.

well-being and is often used as the primary method of testing, it has poor positive predictive value for determining fetal hypoxia/acidosis (Salamalekis et al., 1997). Adjunct methods of assessment should be employed any time fetal status is in question.

Fetal Acoustic Stimulation Test (FAST)/Vibra-acoustic Stimulation (VAS)

A combination of vibratory and acoustic stimulation can be used to elicit acceleration(s) of the FHR and safely reduce the testing time of the NST (Smith, Phelan, Platt, Broussard, & Paul, 1986; AAP & ACOG, 2002; ACOG, 1999). The FHR tracing is then judged to be either reactive or nonreactive, based on the same criteria explained previously in regard to the NST. A prolonged acceleration(s) is frequently observed in response to fetal acoustic stimulation (Miller-Slade et al., 1991) and is interpreted as a reactive test (Fig. 4–4). For this reason, it is important to have established the baseline FHR before applying vibra-acoustic stimulation. A fetus that shows no response to the applied stimulus needs further

evaluation. The concern is that a fetus who does not have the ability to produce accelerations may be neurologically compromised or acidotic.

STORK BYTE:

Let me reassure you. . .
If I can raise my heart rate at least
15 beats above my FHR baseline for
at least 15 seconds, then I am likely getting enough oxygen and am not acidotic.

The fetal acoustic stimulator is attached by a connector to the EFM and annotates directly on the FHR tracing when stimulation is given. The patient end of the fetal acoustic stimulator is placed on the maternal abdomen in the area of the fetal head and up to a 3-second stimulus is given. If no reaction occurs, stimulation may be repeated after 1 minute. A total of three attempts at fetal acoustic stimulation may be made, each at a minimum of 1-minute intervals. Some advantages to using fetal acoustic stimulation are that the procedure is noninvasive, easy to perform, and may decrease both testing time and the incidence of nonreactive NSTs (Marden, McDuffie, Allen, & Abitz, 1997; Saracoglu,

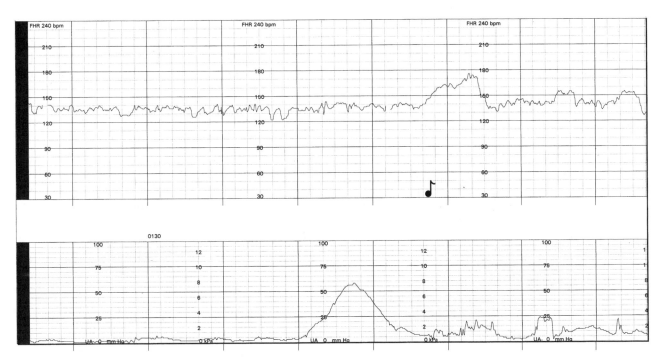

Figure 4–4. Acceleration in response to fetal acoustic stimulation (musical note).

Gol, Sahin, Turkkani, & Oztopcu, 1999). If fetal hypoxia/acidosis is suspected, an alternative method to assess fetal status should be used.

Some limitations to the use of fetal acoustic stimulation include the possibility of variable decelerations or tachycardia in response to the stimulus. The occurrence of either result prompts further monitoring and investigation. If the fetus fails to respond to acoustic stimulation by producing a reactive NST, further testing is indicated, such as with a contraction stress test or biophysical profile. It is also important to note that, when magnesium sulfate is being administered to the patient, FHR accelerations may be blunted and fetal movements reduced in response to vibro-acoustic stimulation (Scherer, 1994). If fetal hypoxia/acidosis is suspected, an alternative method to assess fetal status should be used.

Contraction Stress Test (CST)

The contraction stress test (CST) is another screening test that involves observing the FHR response to three palpable contractions (≥40 seconds' duration) that occur within a 10-minute period. The

FHR pattern is assessed for the presence of late decelerations, which represent possible evidence of uteroplacental insufficiency. The advantage of using the CST is that, in progressive fetal compromise, late decelerations may appear before the disappearance of accelerations. As such, the CST may be an earlier predictor of declining fetal status than the NST (Freeman, 1985). Additionally, if performed as an adjunct assessment after a nonreactive NST, the CST can assist in determining whether the nonreactive result is indicative of hypoxia/acidosis.

There are variations as to how the contraction pattern for the performance of the CST is initiated. These include assessing the patient who is experiencing spontaneous contractions, having the patient perform nipple stimulation to elicit contractions, or by administering oxytocin intravenously (also referred to as an oxytocin challenge test). Nipple stimulation is the most efficient means of eliciting a contraction pattern for the purposes of the CST. This can be accomplished by having the patient rub one nipple through her clothing until contractions occur. If this activity does not prompt an adequate contraction pattern within 2 minutes, the patient is instructed to stop performing stimulation. She may attempt this technique again after 5 minutes (AAP & ACOG, 2002; ACOG, 1999; Huddleston, Sutliff, & Robinson, 1984).

If nipple stimulation is not successful in generating an adequate contraction pattern, administration of oxytocin may produce the desired results. Oxytocin is administered intravenously with the aid of an infusion pump, starting at a rate of 0.5 mU/min. The dosage may be doubled at a frequency of 20-minute intervals until an adequate contraction pattern is initiated (ACOG, 1999).

Some limitations to performing the CST include that it is not always possible to elicit enough contractions or, of greater concern, it is possible to cause too many contractions (hyperstimulation). Also, administration of oxytocin requires the placement of an intravenous catheter, an invasive procedure that carries risk and may cause maternal discomfort. Additionally, the CST is often time consuming and carries a high false-positive rate of 35% to 50% (Schifrin, Lapidus, & Doctor, 1975; Staisch, Westlake & Bashore, 1980) (ie, late decelerations are present during testing, but the fetus is tolerant of subsequent labor induction). Finally, care must be taken not to perform this test in cases

where the presence of contractions would present risk to the patient or fetus, such as when preterm labor, uterine rupture, or bleeding might ensue. Interpretation of the results of the CST are as follows:

Negative—No late decelerations observed during testing (Fig. 4–5)

Positive—Late decelerations occurring in response to 50% or more of the contractions (Fig. 4–6)

Suspicious (equivocal)—Intermittent late decelerations or late decelerations related to uterine hyperstimulation (Fig 4–7)

Unsatisfactory—Inability to achieve the three required contractions within the 10-minute time frame or the tracing is of poor quality (Fig. 4–8)

In most instances, a negative CST will be followed with weekly repeat testing. This may be prescribed in addition to more frequent performance of NSTs or biophysical profiles (discussed later in this chapter). Any result other than a negative CST requires immediate follow-up investigation. If the fetus is mature, the patient with a nonreactive NST and a positive CST should be

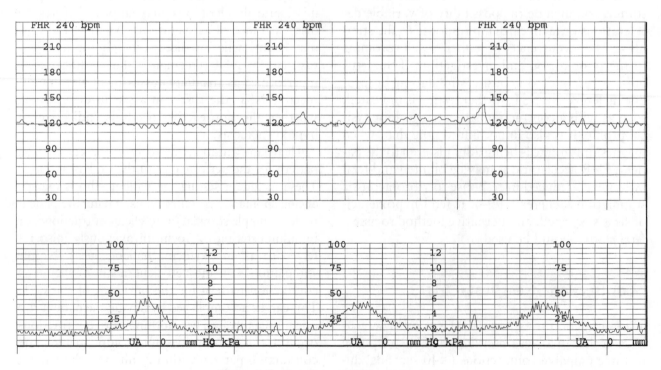

Figure 4–5. Negative contraction stress test.

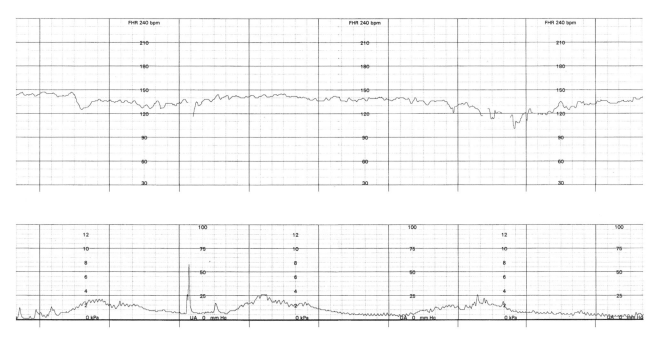

Figure 4–6. Positive contraction stress test.

immediately followed with a sonographic examination to rule out anomalies and, barring their existence, considered for delivery. These test results indicate that the fetus may not be adequately oxygenated by way of the placenta and there is no re-

assurance that the fetus is in a supportive intrauterine environment. A preterm fetus may be either further evaluated by adjunct methods and repeat testing in a timely manner, or it may be decided that extrauterine life would be more

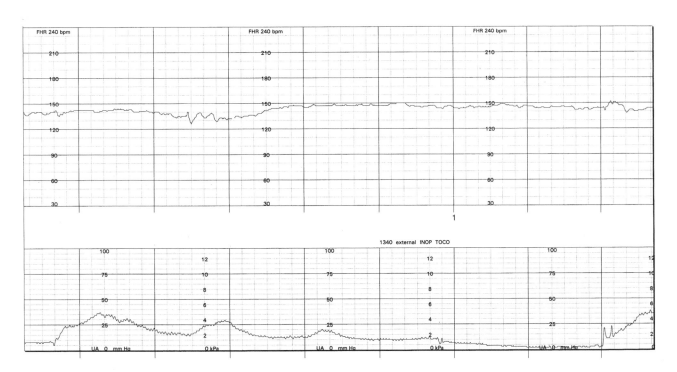

Figure 4–7. Suspicious or equivocal contraction stress test.

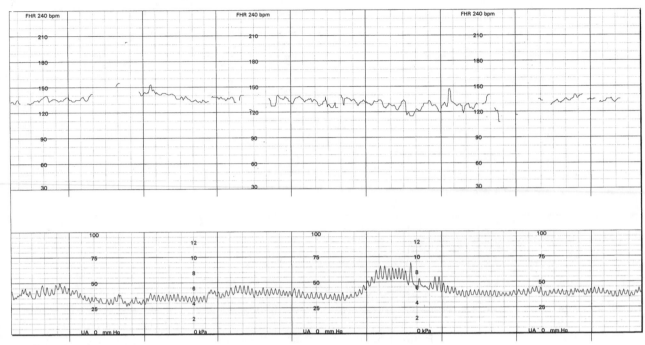

FHR Baseline = Indeterminate

Figure 4–8. Unsatisfactory contraction stress test.

beneficial. This decision requires the evaluation of test results within the context of the entire clinical situation.

A suspicious or unsatisfactory test result presents a more challenging situation. Repeating the CST within 24 hours (Schifrin, Lapidus, & Doctor, 1975) or performing immediate evaluation with a biophysical profile is warranted.

Biophysical Profile (BPP)

The biophysical profile (BPP) involves evaluating the fetus with the use of both EFM and real-time sonography. The fetus is assessed on five separate criteria: The presence or absence of a reactive NST, the presence or absence of fetal breathing movements, the presence or absence of fetal movement and visualization of fetal tone as evidenced by flexion and extension, and the measurement of amniotic fluid volume (Manning, Baskett, Morrison, & Lange, 1981; Vintzileos, Campbell, Ingardia, & Nochimson, 1983). A possible score of 2 points is awarded for the satisfaction of each parameter, whereas a score of 0 is assigned to each criterion that is not met.

The highest and most reassuring BPP test result, therefore, is a score of 10 (Table 4–2).

Interpretation of the BPP is as follows:

10/10, 8/10—Reassuring
6/10—Equivocal
4/10, 2/10, 0/10—Nonreassuring

Two variations in biophysical testing have evolved since its inception. The first variation of the BPP includes the addition of a sixth component, placental grading. If the placenta is observed to be appropriate for gestational age, 2 points are assigned. This raises the total possible score for the BPP to 12 (Vintzileos, Campbell, Ingardia, & Nochimson, 1983). The second variation is the "modified BPP." This involves first performing the NST and then measuring the amniotic fluid index by sonography. If both parameters are reassuring, it can be assumed that the result is equivalent to a BPP of 8/10. This conclusion is derived from the assumption that, if the NST is reactive, fetal movement and fetal tone are likely to be present (Miller, Rabello, & Paul, 1996). More recently, it has been shown that using fetal acoustic stimulation early in the BPP testing can shorten

Table 4-2. BIOPHYSICAL PROFILE (BPP)

Criteria for Evaluation	Nonreassuring Results	Reassuring Results
NST	Nonreactive = 0	Reactive = 2
Fetal breathing movements	Absent or ↓ = 0	Present (one or more episodes sustained for ≥30 seconds occurring within 30 minutes of observation) = 2
Fetal movement	Absent or ↓ = 0	Present (≥3 episodes of body or limb movements occurring within 30 minutes of observation) = 2
Fetal tone	− Flexion / − episode(s) of extension/flexion = 0	Present (≥1 episode of extension of an extremity with return to flexion or opening and closing of a hand) = 2
Amniotic fluid volume	↓ Fluid = 0	Adequate fluid (>2 cm vertical pocket) = 2

the testing time and reduce the number of nonreassuring test results by 5% (Pinette, Blackstone, Wax, & Cartin, 2005).

Any fetus with a score of less than 8/10 on the BPP requires further observation and possible intervention. The equivocal score is managed the same as that of an equivocal CST; the test is to be repeated within 24 hours, preferably sooner. Gestational age is also taken into consideration when determining management strategies. Manning and associates found that there was a significantly lower incidence of cerebral palsy in fetuses at risk who were tested with BPP than in untested patients (Manning et al., 1997; 1998). Any fetus found to have oligohydramnios, regardless of the result of the BPP, requires further evaluation.

The specific antepartum screening test selected may vary depending on resources, location, or practitioner preference (see Appendix B). Regardless of the type of test(s) chosen or the order of their performance, antepartum testing is a highly predictive indicator of fetal well-being.

REFERENCES

American Academy of Pediatrics and American College of Obstetricians and Gynecologists. (2002). *Guidelines for perinatal care* (5th ed.). Washington, DC: ACOG.

American College of Obstetrics and Gynecology (ACOG). (1999). *Antepartum fetal surveillance.* Practice Bulletin #9 (Replaces Technical Bulletin #188). Washington, DC: Author.

Bishop, E. H. (1981). Fetal acceleration test. *American Journal of Obstetrics and Gynecology, 141,* 905–909.

Casey, B. M., McIntire, D. D., Bloom, S. L., Lucas, M. J., Santos, R., Twickler, D. M., Ramus, R. M., & Levveno, K. (2000). Pregnancy outcomes after antepartum diagnosis of oligohydramnios at or beyond 34 weeks' gestation. *American Journal of Obstetrics and Gynecology, 182,* 909–912.

Clark, S. L., Gimovsky, M. L., & Miller, F. C. (1984). The scalp stimulation test: A clinical alternative to fetal scalp blood sampling. *American Journal of Obstetrics & Gynecology, 148*(3), 274–277.

Druzin, M. L., Fox, A., Kogut, E., & Carlson, C. (1985). The relationship of the nonstress test to gestational age. *American Journal of Obstetrics and Gynecology, 153,* 386–389.

Evertson, L., & Paul, R. (1978). Antepartum fetal heart rate testing: The nonstress test. *American Journal of Obstetrics and Gynecology, 132,* 895–900.

Evertson, L. R., Gauthier, R. J., Schifrin, B. S., Paul, R. H. (1979). Antepartum fetal heart rate testing. I. Evolution of the nonstress test. *American Journal of Obstetrics and Gynecology, 133,* 29–33.

Freeman, R. K. (1985). Early indications of placental insufficiency. *Contemporary OB/GYN, 28*(47), 145–161.

Freeman, R. K., Anderson, G., & Dorchester, W. (1982). A prospective multi-institutional study of antepartum fetal heart rate monitoring. I. Risk of perinatal mortality and morbidity according to antepartum fetal heart rate test results. *American Journal of Obstetrics and Gynecology, 143,* 771–777.

Huddleston, J. F., Sutliff, G., & Robinson, D. (1984). Contraction stress test by intermittent nipple stimulation. *Obstetrics and Gynecology, 63,* 669–673.

Lavin, J. P., Miodovnik, M., & Barden, T. P. (1984). Relationship of nonstress test reactivity and gestational age. *Obstetrics and Gynecology, 63,* 338–344.

Manning, F. A., Baskett, T. F., Morrison, I., & Lange, I. (1981). Fetal biophysical scoring: A prospective study in 1,184 high risk patients. *American Journal of Obstetrics and Gynecology, 140*(3), 289–294.

Manning, F. A., Bondagji, N., Harman, C. R., Casiro, O., Menticoglou, S., & Morrison, I. (1998). Fetal assessment based on biophysical profile scoring. VIII. The incidence of cerebral palsy in tested and untested perinates. *American Journal of Obstetrics and Gynecology, 178*(4), 696– 706.

———. (1997). Fetal assessment based on the fetal biophysical profile score: Relationship of last BPS result to subsequent cerebral palsy. *Journal de Gynecologie, Obstetrique et Biologie de la Reproduction, 26*(7), 720–729.

Marden, D., McDuffie, R. S., Allen, R. & Abitz, D. (1997). A randomized controlled trial of a new fetal acoustic stimulation test for fetal well-being. *American Journal of Obstetrics and Gynecology, 176*(6), 1386–1388.

Meis, P. J., Ureda, J. R., Swaim, M., Kelly, R. T., Perry, M., & Sharp, P. (1986). Variable decelerations during testing are not a sign of fetal compromise. *American Journal of Obstetrics and Gynecology, 154,* 586–590.

Miller, D. A., Rabello, Y. A., & Paul, R. H. (1996). The modified biophysical profile: Antepartum testing in the 1990s. *American Journal of Obstetrics and Gynecology, 174,* 812–817.

Miller-Slade, D., Gloeb, D. J., Bailey, S., Bendell, A., Interlandi, E., Kline-Kaye, V., & Kroesen, J. (1991). Acoustic stimulation induced fetal response compared to traditional nonstress testing. *Journal of Obstetric, Gynecologic, and Neonatal Nursing, 20*(2), 160–167.

National Institute of Child Health and Human Development Research Planning Workshop. (1997). Electronic fetal heart monitoring: Research guidelines for interpretation. *Journal of Obstetric, Gynecologic, and Neonatal Nursing, 26*(6), 635–640.

Pinette, M. G., Blackstone, J., Wax, J. R., & Cartin, A. (2005). Using fetal acoustic stimulation to shorten the biophysical profile. *Journal of Clinical Ultrasound, 33*(5), 223–225.

Salamalekis, E., Loghis, C., Panayotopoulos, N., Vitoratos, N., Giannaki, G., & Christodoulacos, G. (1997). Nonstress test: A fifteen-year clinical appraisal. *Clinical and Experimental Obstetrics and Gynecology, 24*(2), 79–81.

Saracoglu, F., Gol, K., Sahin, I., Turkkani, B., & Oztopcu, C. (1999). The predictive value of fetal acoustic stimulation. *Journal of Perinatology, 19*(2), 103–105.

Schifrin, B., Lapidus, M., & Doctor, G. S. (1975). Contraction stress test for antepartum evaluation. *Obstetrics and Gynecology, 45,* 433–438.

Sherer, D. M. (1994). Blunted response to vibroacoustic stimulation associated with maternal IV magnesium sulfate therapy. *American Journal of Perinatology, 11*(6), 401–403.

Smith, C. V., Davis, S. R., Rayburn, W. F., & Nelson, R. M. (1991). Fetal habituation to vibroacoustic stimulation in uncomplicated term pregnancies. *American Journal of Perinatology, 8*(6), 380–382.

Smith, C. V., Phelan, J. P., Platt, L. D., Broussard, P., & Paul, R. H. FAST.II. (1986). A randomized clinical comparison with the nonstress test. *American Journal of Obstetrics and Gynecology, 155,* 131–134.

Staisch, K. J., Westlake, J. R., & Bashore, R. A. (1980). Blind oxytocin challenge test and perinatal outcome. *American Journal of Obstetrics and Gynecology, 138* (4), 399–403.

Vintzileos, A. M., Campbell, W. A., Ingardia, C. J., & Nochimson, D. (1983). The biophysical profile and its predictive value. *Obstetrics and Gynecology, 62*(2), 271–278.

5 | Exercises in Electronic Fetal Monitoring

The exercises presented in this chapter are meant to facilitate the integration of the didactic information contained within the text of this book into the processes of critical thinking necessary for practicing the skill of electronic fetal monitoring (EFM). In each of the following case studies, select portions of the fetal strip chart are presented along with the contemporaneous nurse's notes. When gaps in the data occur, the passage of time is denoted at the start of the subsequent portion of the fetal strip chart.

Proper completion of the exercises includes comparison of one's interpretation of the fetal strip with the Guide to Interpretation that is located at the end of this chapter. It is necessary to recognize that the information presented within the case studies has been preserved for the purpose of being as accurately reflective of actual circumstances as is possible without breaching confidentiality. Therefore, the interpretations and interventions presented within each case study are not necessarily reflective of the current standard of care. Comparison with the Guide to Interpretation and with current, evidence-based practice is essential in promoting appropriate clinical decision-making. It must be kept in mind that minor variations in interpretation are expected to occur as a result of multiple factors (as discussed in Chapters 3, 7, and 8). The Guide to Interpretation is, therefore, based upon the reasoning and parameters for evaluating EFM data as have been explained throughout the preceding chapters.

For purposes of confidentiality, all proper pronouns have been removed from the case studies. All other identifying data has been altered to protect the privacy of the patient. Only the clinical designation of the person mentioned (eg, RN, CNM, MD, etc.) is presented. When multiple persons of the same title are involved in the case, such circumstances are denoted numerically, in order of their entrée into the scenario (eg, MD #1, MD #2, etc.).

The commentary appearing above the strip chart corresponds with the numerical annotations located in the center margin of the paper strip chart. Abbreviations and nomenclature may vary from case to case, based upon regional or individual differences in expression (eg, use of the terms UC or CTX to express *uterine contraction*).

For the purposes of clarity and consistency, the Guide to Interpretation at the end of this chapter utilizes the terminology suggested by the National Institute of Child Health and Human Development Research Planning Workshop (see Chapter 3). When the case studies present monitoring of uterine activity through use of an intrauterine pressure catheter (IUPC), the strength of contractions is expressed in a peak-minus-baseline format. It is necessary to recognize that the selected methods for expressing interpretation of the strip chart employed in the Guide to Interpretation may not be reflective of individual institutional standards or culture. Additionally, minor inter-observer variations in interpretation are likely to occur. Such differences should be viewed objectively and utilized as a catalyst for discussion and continued learning.

The case studies are presented on strip charts that are printed with 30–240 bpm paper scaling. As the examples are presented at 3cm/min paper speed, each regularly ocurring vertical marker represents the passage of 10 seconds of time. Every sixth vertical line is emphasized to represent the passage of one minute of time (six 10-second segments).

Case Examples

HX OF PATIENT A: 22 YO, G_2P_1, 40+ WKS, AWAKENED BY SPONTANEOUS LABOR AT 0400.

1) 05/22/98 07:48
   VE BY MD = 5 CMS. AROM WITH SPIRAL ELECTRODE APPLICATION - NO FLUID SEEN.

2) 05/22/98 07:54
   COMMENTS: PT TO LT SIDE. SPIRAL ELECTRODE NOT WORKING CORRECTLY. REPLACED BY MD.

Strip Chart A-1

1) 05/22/98 08:08
   COMMENTS: POSITION CHANGE TO RIGHT SIDE.

2) 05/22/98 08:19
   BASELINE OFFSCALE.

3) 05/22/98 08:22
   COMMENTS: IUPC INSERTED BY MD, 6 CM, AMNIOINFUSION ORDERED.

Strip Chart A-2

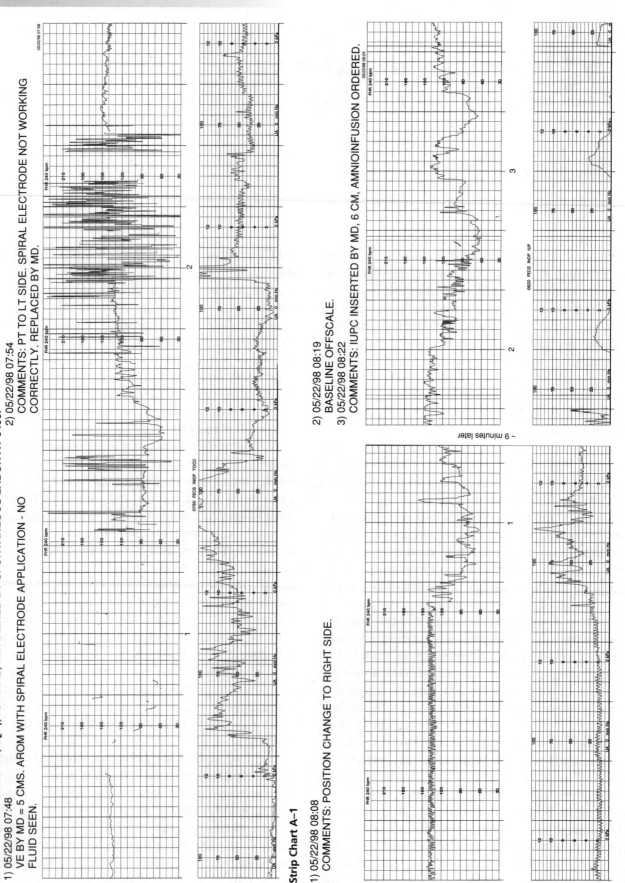

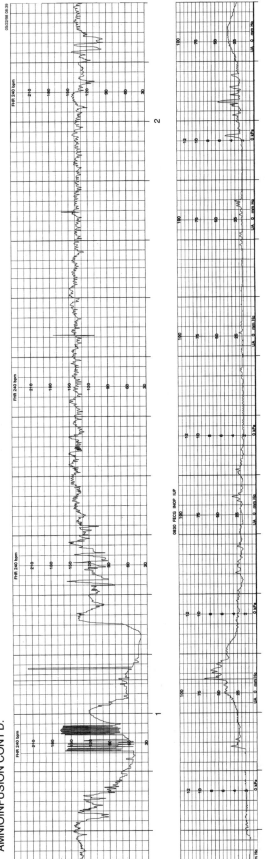

Strip Chart A-3

1) 05/22/98 09:00 COMMENTS: PT TO RT SIDE PER ANES. SM AMT OF FLUID SEEN. LOOKS LIKE MEC. + PINK SHOW. O2 IN PLACE VIA FACEMASK AT 10 L, IV LR INF WIDE 05/22/98 09:01

2) 05/22/98 09:01 BP 137/78 M 93 P 103 COMMENTS: PT BACK TO LEFT SIDE. MORE FLUID SEEN. PINKISH TINGED. MEC SEEN. PERI CARE. PAD PLACED.

1) 05/22/98 08:28
COMMENTS: MD AT BEDSIDE TALKING TO PT ABOUT POSSIBILITY OF C/S. TERB .25 MG IV GIVEN. O2 CONT VIA MASK, IV OPEN, PT ON L SIDE, AMNIOINFUSION CONT'D.

2) 05/22/98 08:37
COMMENTS: FOLEY PLACED. DRAINING TO GRAV/CL YELLOW URINE. SHAVE. AMNIO INF., IV LR INF WIDE. PT REQUESTING EPI/ANES PAGED.

3) 05/22/98 09:04 COMMENTS: REPORT TO ONCOMING RN. PATIENT RESTING ON LEFT SIDE. ? LT MEC FLUID.

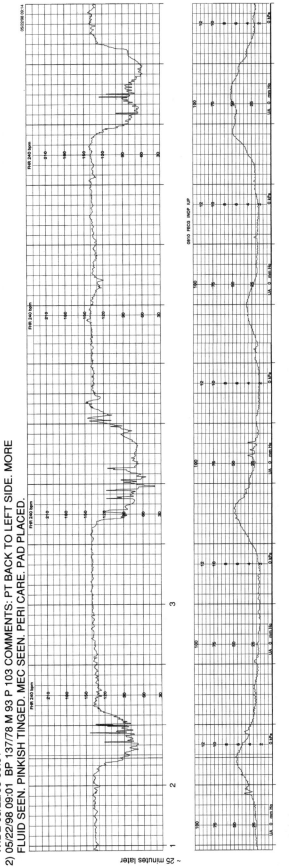

Strip Chart A-4

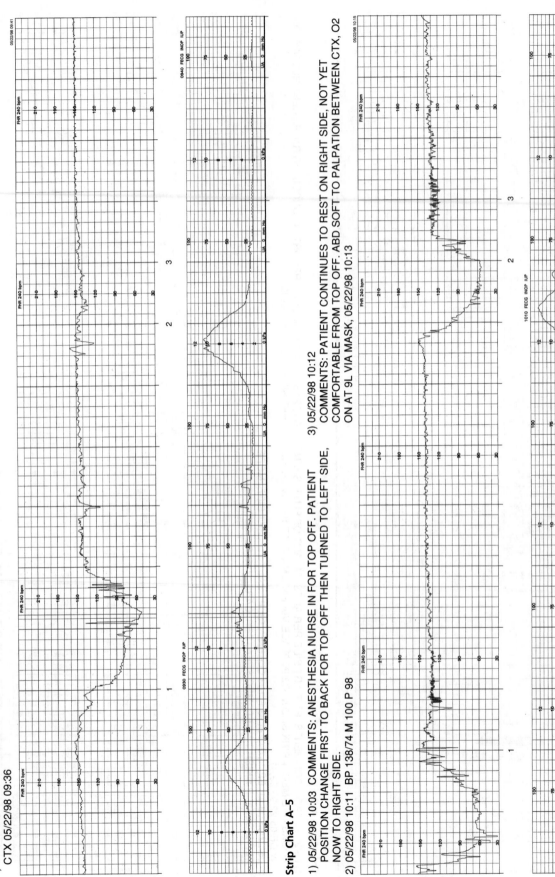

1) 05/22/98 09:30   COMMENTS: POSITION CHANGE AT MARK TO RIGHT SIDE. CNM IN ROOM TRACING VIEWED.

2) 05/22/98 09:36   COMMENTS: PATIENT STATES FEELING SOME PRESSURE WITH CTX 05/22/98 09:36

3) 05/22/98 09:37   COMMENTS: ABD SOFT TO PALPATION BETWEEN CTX NO FLUID SEEN OUT, REPORTED TO CNM WHEN LAST IN ROOM.

Strip Chart A–5

1) 05/22/98 10:03   COMMENTS: ANESTHESIA NURSE IN FOR TOP OFF. PATIENT POSITION CHANGE FIRST TO BACK FOR TOP OFF THEN TURNED TO LEFT SIDE, NOW TO RIGHT SIDE.

2) 05/22/98 10:11   BP 138/74 M 100 P 98

3) 05/22/98 10:12   COMMENTS: PATIENT CONTINUES TO REST ON RIGHT SIDE, NOT YET COMFORTABLE FROM TOP OFF. ABD SOFT TO PALPATION BETWEEN CTX, O2 ON AT 9L VIA MASK, 05/22/98 10:13

Strip Chart A–6

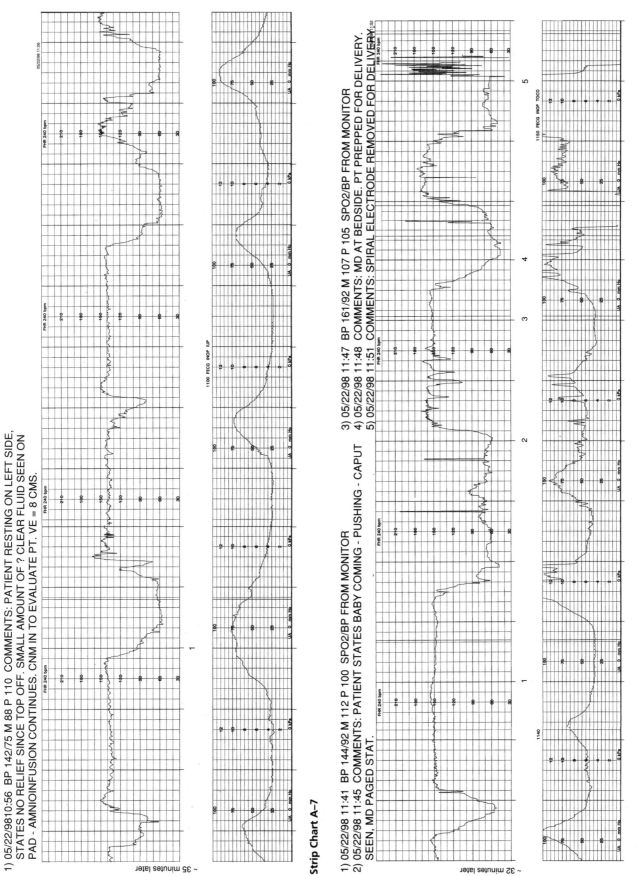

1) 05/22/98 10:56 BP 142/75 M 88 P 110 COMMENTS: PATIENT RESTING ON LEFT SIDE, STATES NO RELIEF SINCE TOP OFF. SMALL AMOUNT OF ? CLEAR FLUID SEEN ON PAD - AMNIOINFUSION CONTINUES. CNM IN TO EVALUATE PT. VE = 8 CMS.

Strip Chart A-7

1) 05/22/98 11:41 BP 144/92 M 112 P 100 SPO2/BP FROM MONITOR
2) 05/22/98 11:45 COMMENTS: PATIENT STATES BABY COMING - PUSHING - CAPUT SEEN, MD PAGED STAT.
3) 05/22/98 11:47 BP 161/92 M 107 P 105 SPO2/BP FROM MONITOR
4) 05/22/98 11:48 COMMENTS: MD AT BEDSIDE. PT PREPPED FOR DELIVERY.
5) 05/22/98 11:51 COMMENTS: SPIRAL ELECTRODE REMOVED FOR DELIVERY.

Strip Chart A-8

HX OF PATIENT B: 32 YO, G₂P₀, 39 WKS. FULLY DILATED AND ENCOURAGED TO PUSH SINCE 1600. EPIDURAL IN PLACE.

1) 04/19/99 16:18
   COMMENTS: CNM IN TO EXAMINE PT, CAPUT SEEN FETUS CONTINUES ROP.
   BP 103/53 M 72 P94

Strip Chart B–1

1) 04/19/99 16:33
   BP 106/53 M 77 P82.

2) 04/19/99 16:39
   COMMENTS: PT PUSHING WITH GOOD EFFORT W/ CONTRACTIONS, FEELS "PRESSURE" WITH SOME CONTRACTIONS BUT EPIDURAL STILL VERY EFFECTIVE. NO COMPLAINT OF PAIN.

Strip Chart B–2

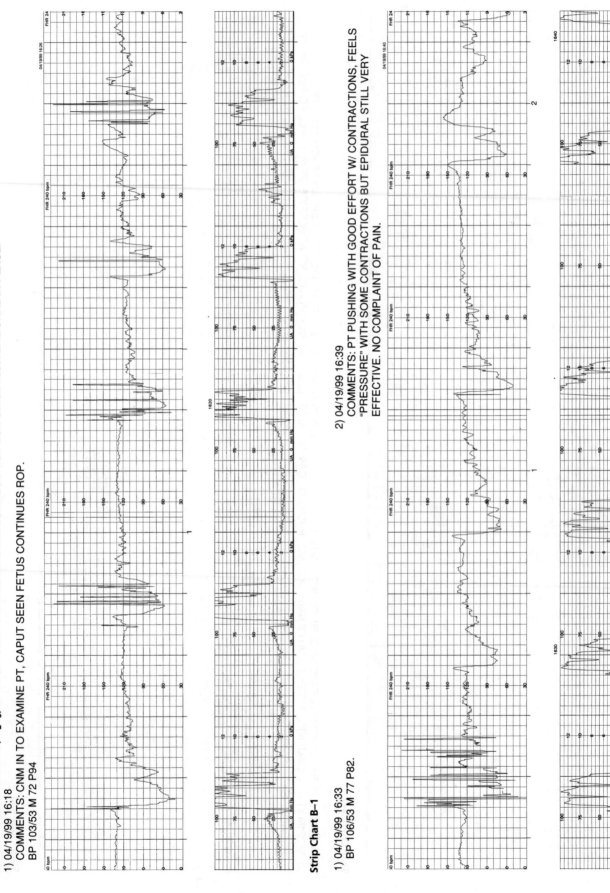

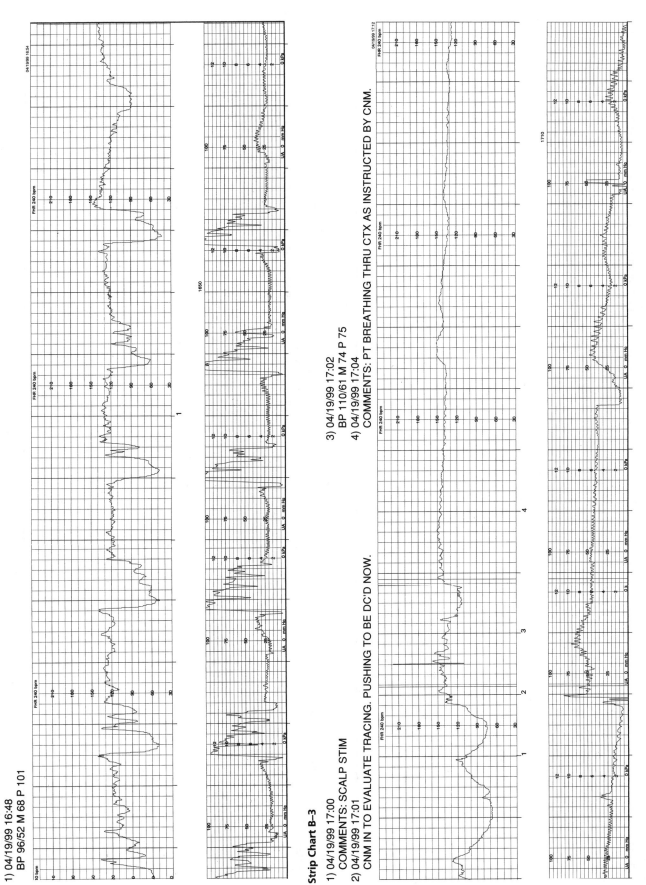

1) 04/19/99 16:48
   BP 96/52 M 68 P 101

Strip Chart B-3

1) 04/19/99 17:00
   COMMENTS: SCALP STIM
2) 04/19/99 17:01
   CNM IN TO EVALUATE TRACING. PUSHING TO BE DC'D NOW.

3) 04/19/99 17:02
   BP 110/61 M 74 P 75
4) 04/19/99 17:04
   COMMENTS: PT BREATHING THRU CTX AS INSTRUCTED BY CNM.

Strip Chart B-4

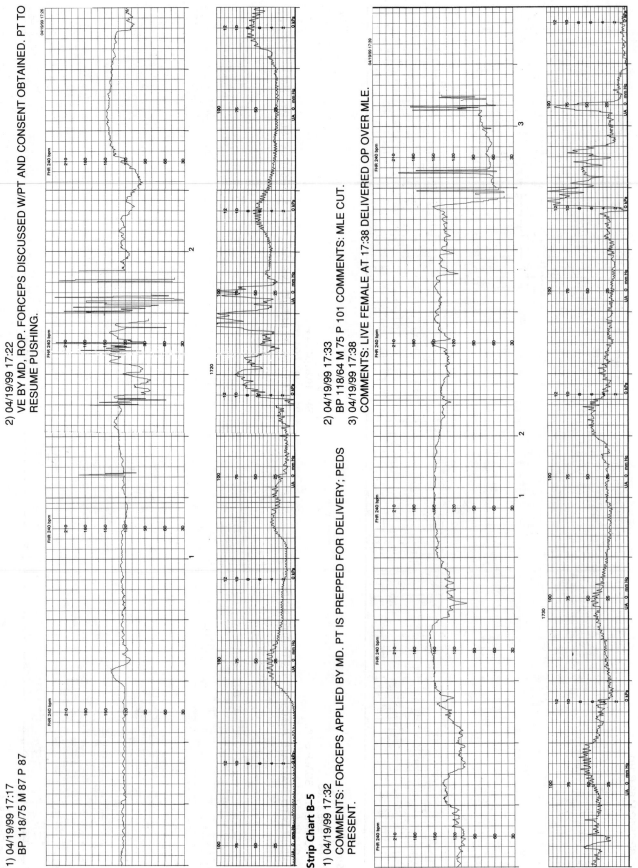

1) 04/19/99 17:17
BP 118/75 M 87 P 87

2) 04/19/99 17:22
VE BY MD, ROP. FORCEPS DISCUSSED W/PT AND CONSENT OBTAINED. PT TO RESUME PUSHING.

Strip Chart B-5

1) 04/19/99 17:32
COMMENTS: FORCEPS APPLIED BY MD. PT IS PREPPED FOR DELIVERY; PEDS PRESENT.

2) 04/19/99 17:33
BP 118/64 M 75 P 101 COMMENTS: MLE CUT.

3) 04/19/99 17:38
COMMENTS: LIVE FEMALE AT 17:38 DELIVERED OP OVER MLE.

Strip Chart B-6

HX OF PATIENT C: 34 YO, G₂P₁, 28+ WKS, CHRONIC HYPERTENSIVE ADMITTED FOR TREATMENT OF FETAL SVT. FHR AUSCULTATED 200-240 BPM IN MD OFFICE, CONFIRMED BY SONOGRAPHIC EVALUATION.

1) 09/26/00 16:52
BP 147/97 M 113 P 87

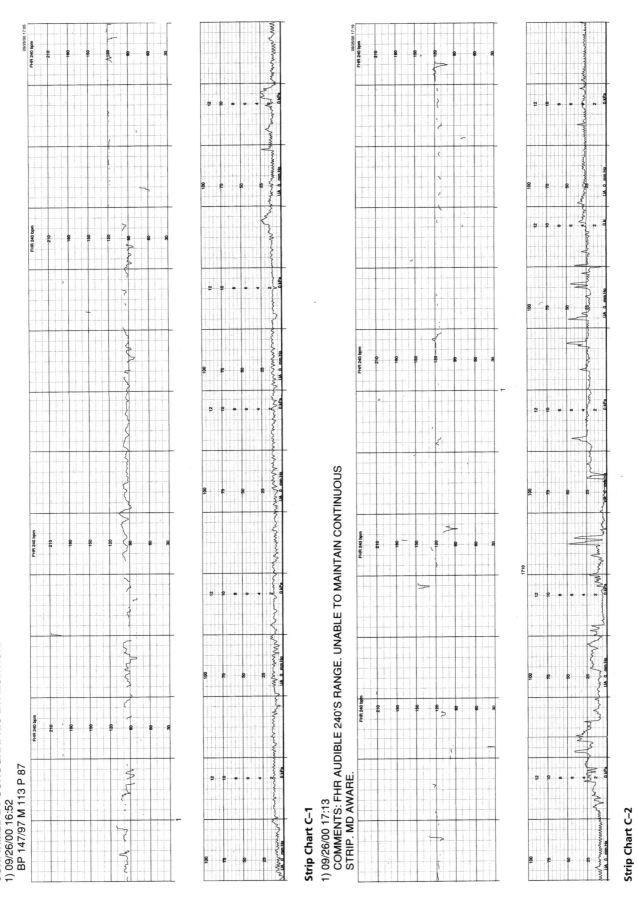

Strip Chart C-1

1) 09/26/00 17:13
COMMENTS: FHR AUDIBLE 240'S RANGE. UNABLE TO MAINTAIN CONTINUOUS STRIP. MD AWARE.

Strip Chart C-2

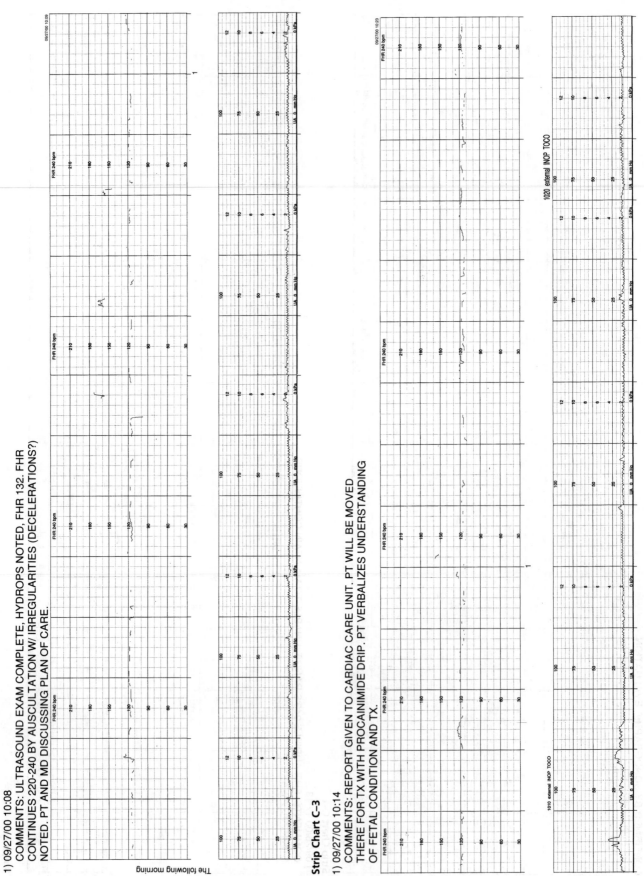

1) 09/27/00 10:08

COMMENTS: ULTRASOUND EXAM COMPLETE, HYDROPS NOTED, FHR 132. FHR CONTINUES 220-240 BY AUSCULTATION W/ IRREGULARITIES (DECELERATIONS?) NOTED. PT AND MD DISCUSSING PLAN OF CARE.

The following morning

Strip Chart C-3

1) 09/27/00 10:14

COMMENTS: REPORT GIVEN TO CARDIAC CARE UNIT. PT WILL BE MOVED THERE FOR TX WITH PROCAINIMIDE DRIP. PT VERBALIZES UNDERSTANDING OF FETAL CONDITION AND TX.

Strip Chart C-4

HX OF PATIENT D: 29 YO, G₁P₀, 35+ WKS, INDUCTION FOR PIH

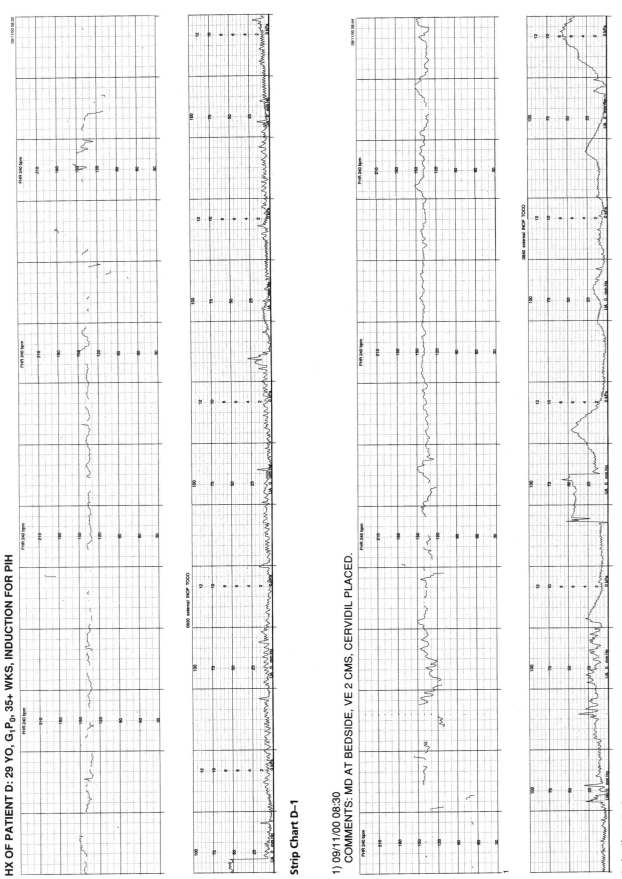

Strip Chart D–1

1) 09/11/00 08:30
COMMENTS: MD AT BEDSIDE, VE 2 CMS, CERVIDIL PLACED.

Strip Chart D–2

1) 09/11/00 08:56

COMMENTS: PT TO LEFT SIDE FOR COMFORT. UCS PALPATE MODERATE.
BP 138/84, P 80 R 18. ENCOURAGED WITH BREATHING TECHNIQUES.

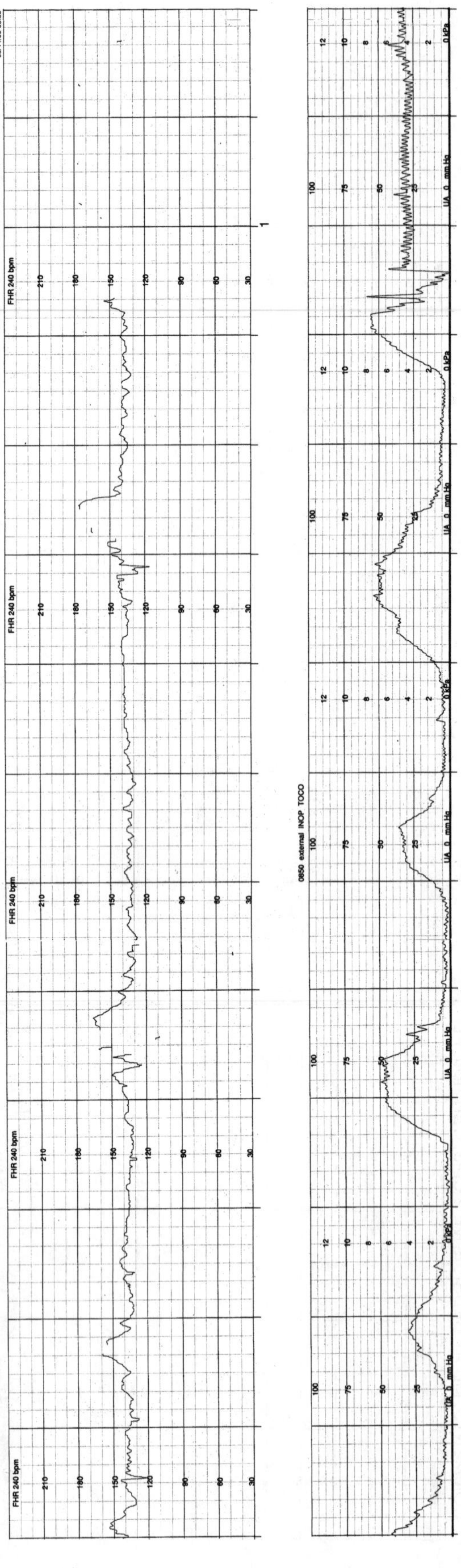

Strip Chart D-3

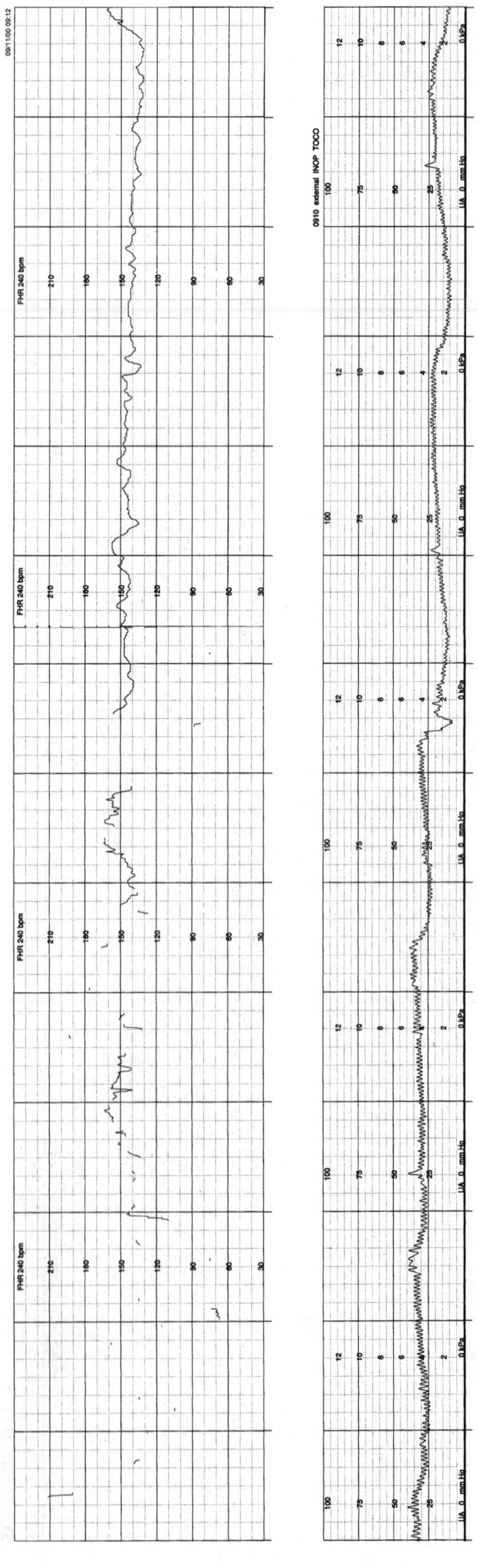

Strip Chart D-4

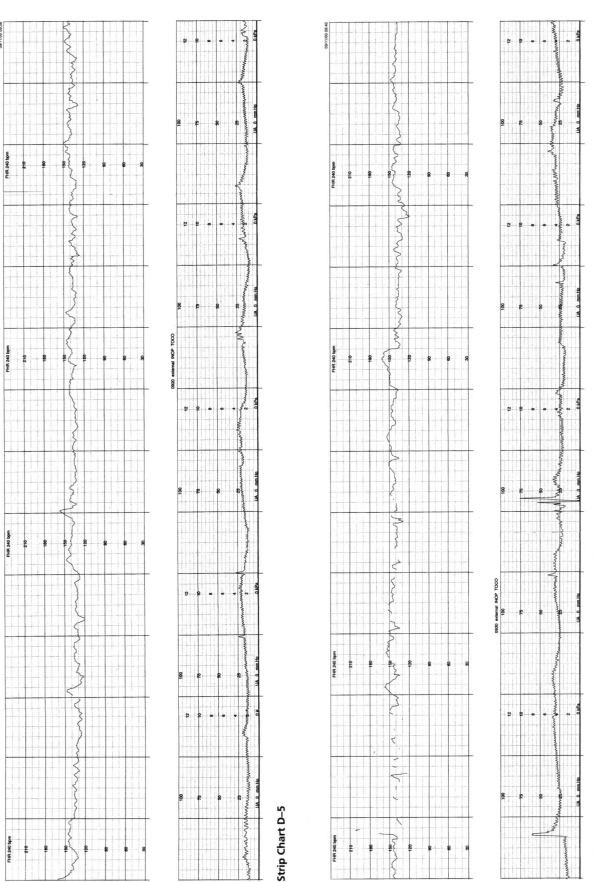

Strip Chart D–5

Strip Chart D–6

1) 09/11/00 09:50

COMMENTS: PT ONTO HER BACK, TO SEMI-FOWLERS. COPING WELL WITH UCS. CERVIDIL REMAINS IN PLACE. UCS MODERATE BY PALPATION. UTERUS SOFT BETWEEN.

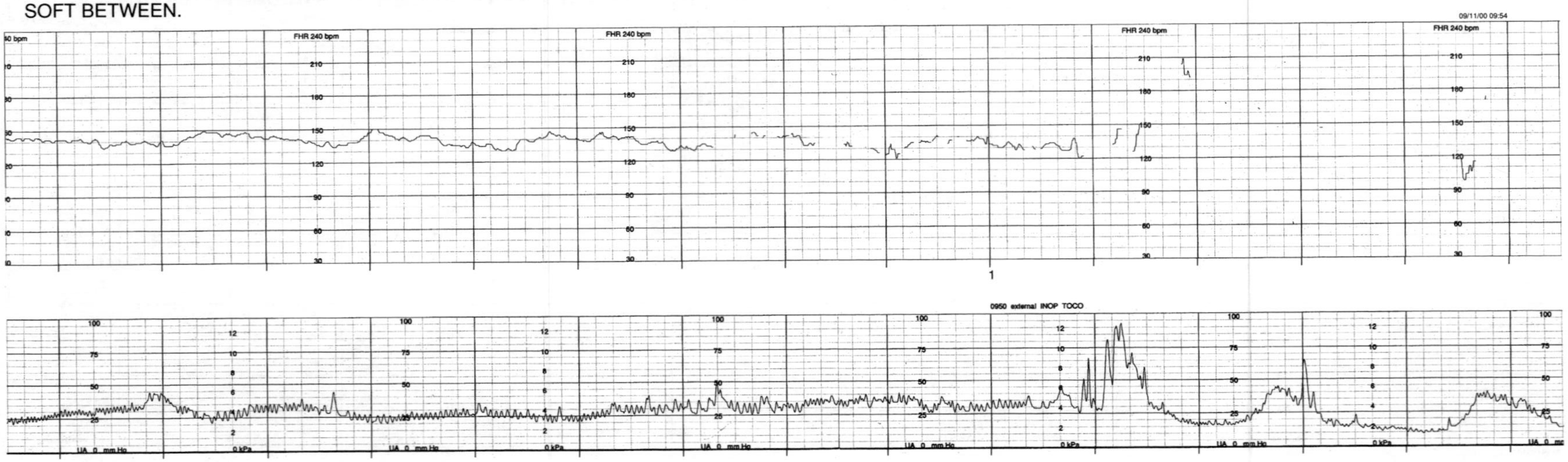

Strip Chart D-7

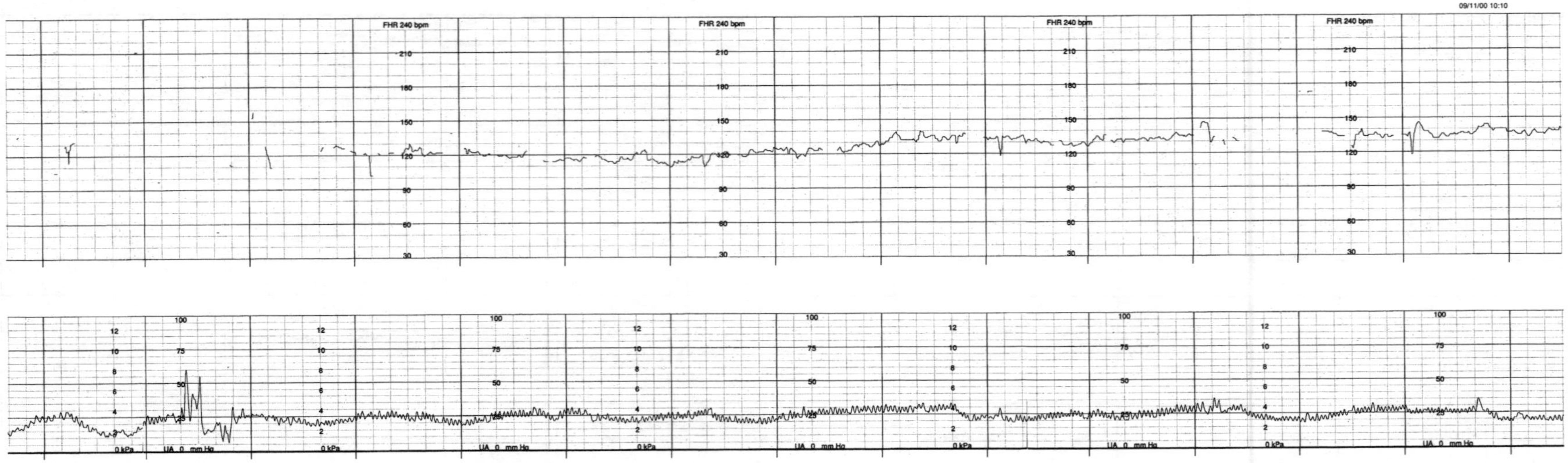

Strip Chart D-8

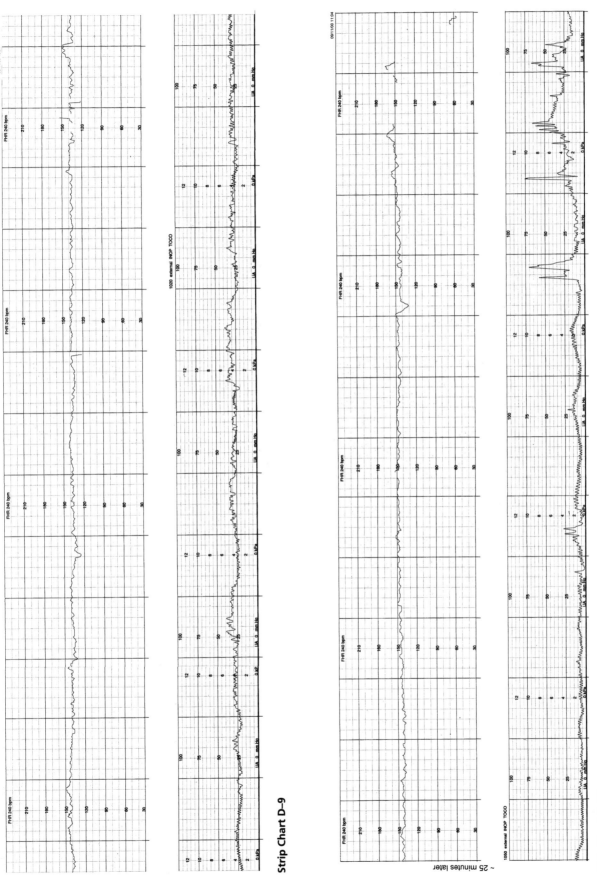

Strip Chart D-9

~ 25 minutes later

Strip Chart D-10

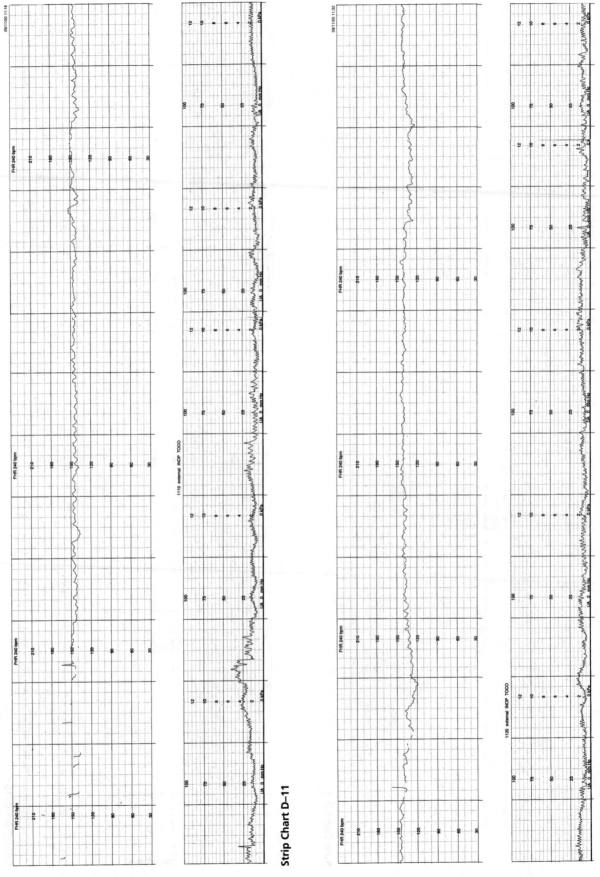

Strip Chart D-11

Strip Chart D-12

1) 09/11/00 11:35
COMMENTS: PT TO R SIDE; C/O UC PAIN, CONTINUES USING BREATHING
TECHNIQUES. COMFORT MEASURES GIVEN.

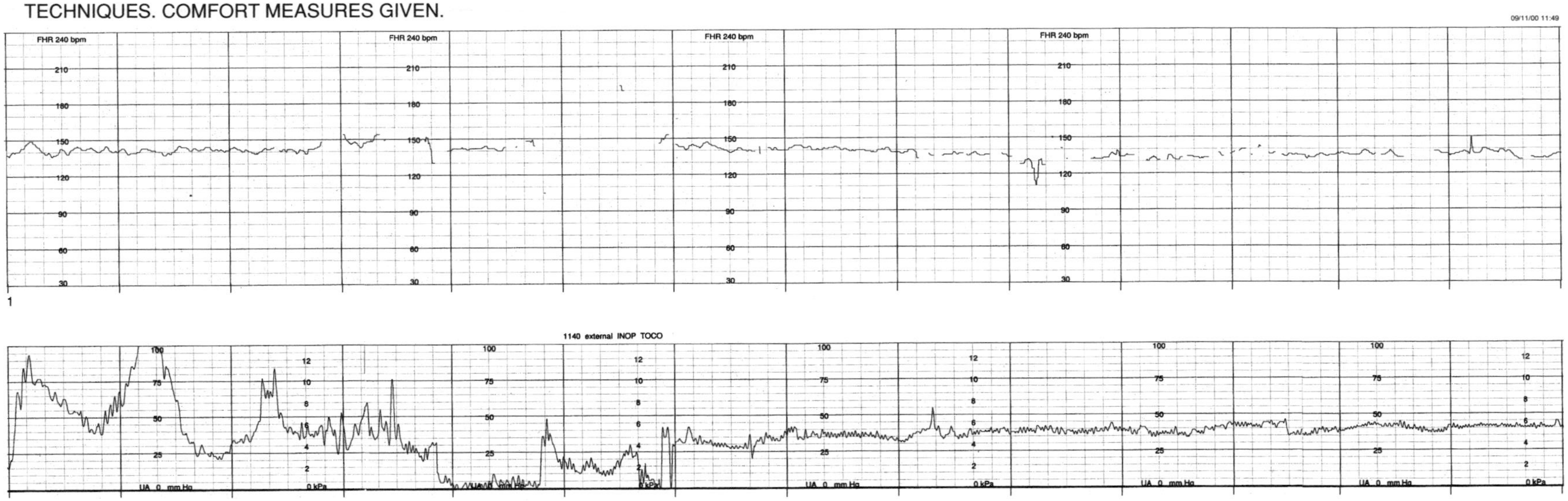

Strip Chart D–13

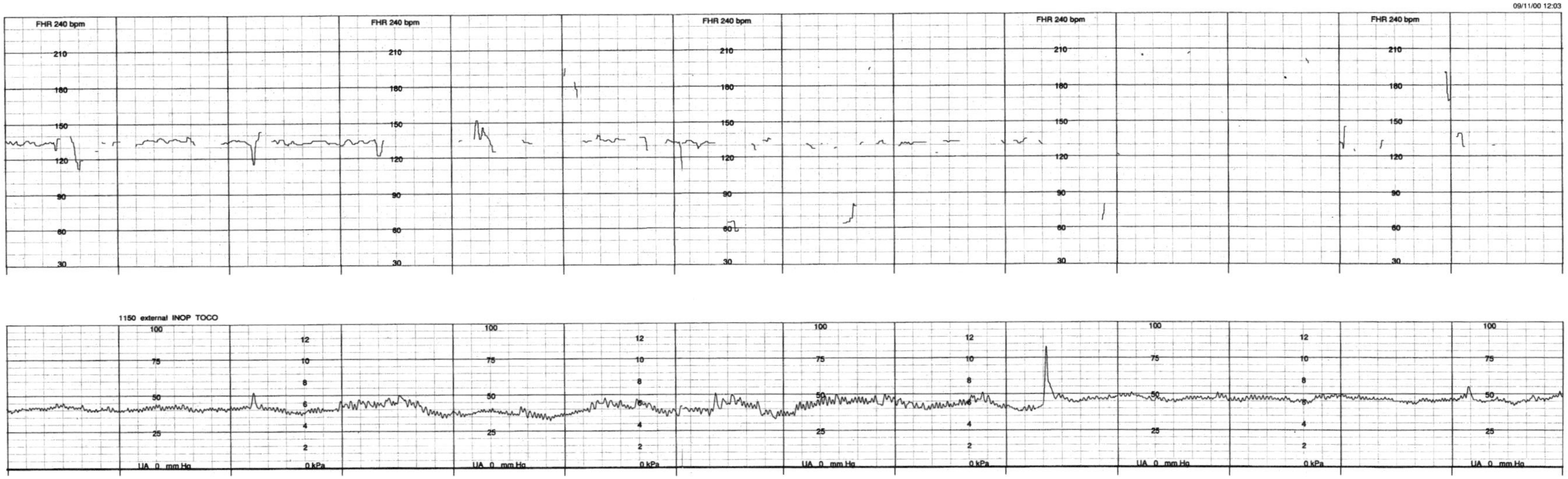

Strip Chart D–14

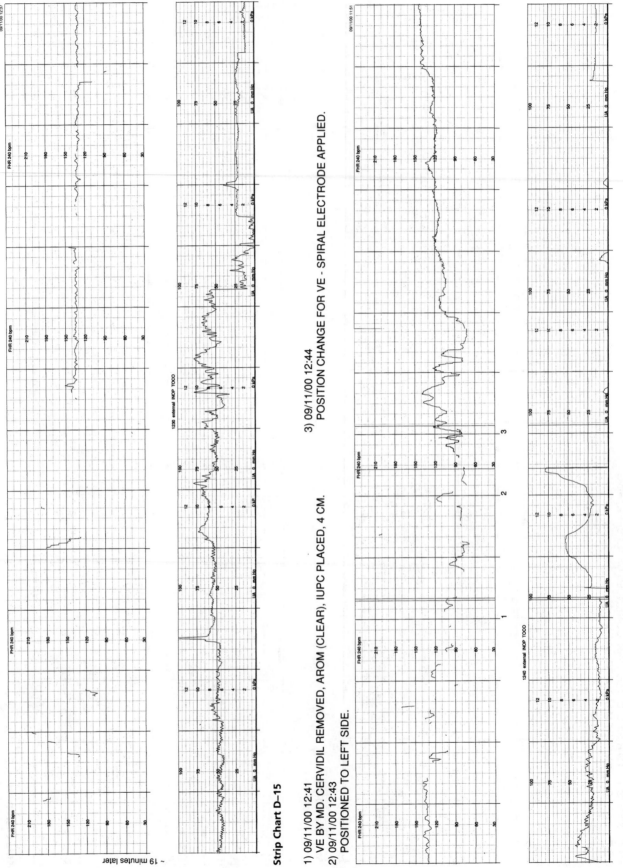

Strip Chart D–15

1) 09/11/00 12:41
   VE BY MD. CERVIDIL REMOVED, AROM (CLEAR), IUPC PLACED, 4 CM.
2) 09/11/00 12:43
   POSITIONED TO LEFT SIDE.

3) 09/11/00 12:44
   POSITION CHANGE FOR VE - SPIRAL ELECTRODE APPLIED.

~ 19 minutes later

Strip Chart D–16

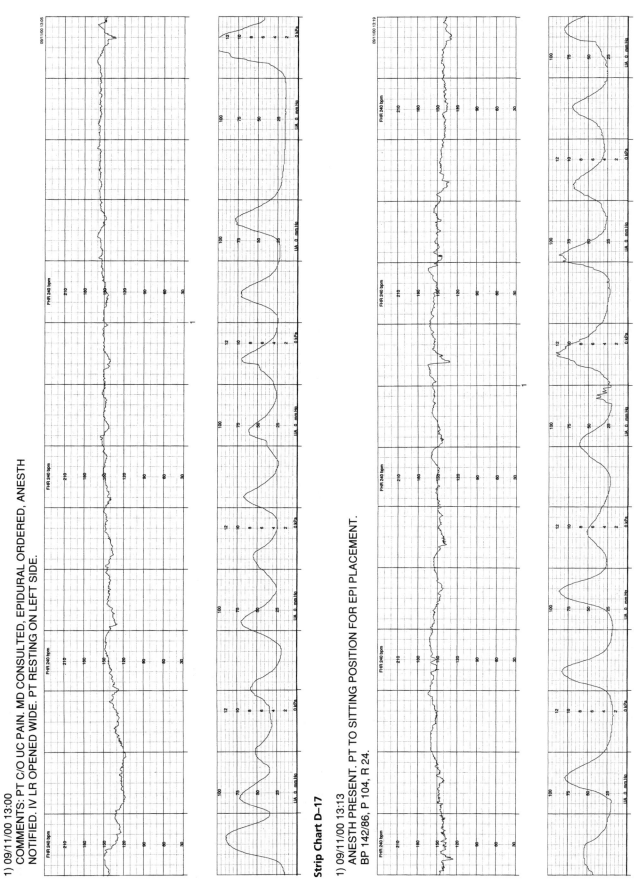

1) 09/11/00 13:00
COMMENTS: PT C/O UC PAIN. MD CONSULTED, EPIDURAL ORDERED, ANESTH
NOTIFIED. IV LR OPENED WIDE. PT RESTING ON LEFT SIDE.

Strip Chart D-17

1) 09/11/00 13:13
ANESTH PRESENT. PT TO SITTING POSITION FOR EPI PLACEMENT.
BP 142/86, P 104, R 24.

Strip Chart D-18

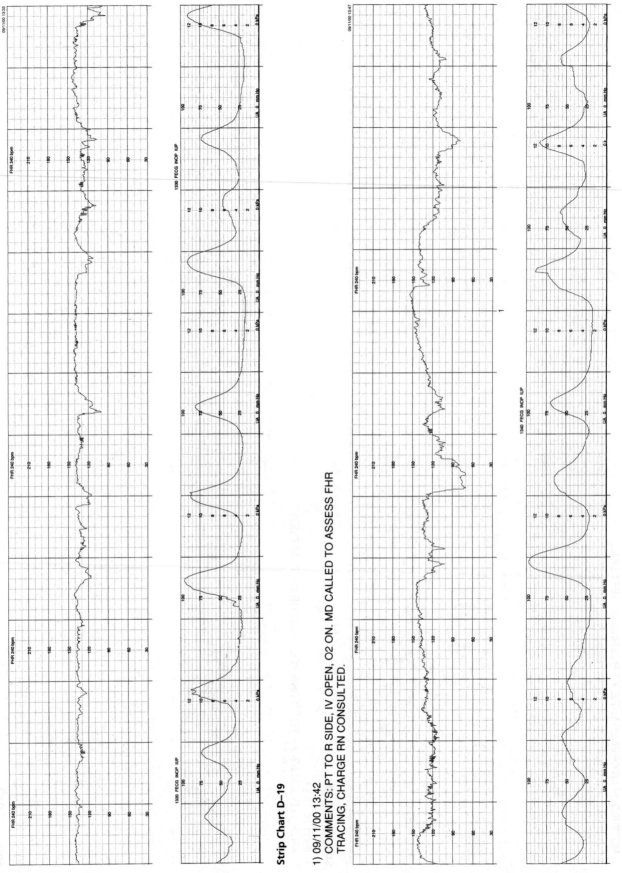

Strip Chart D-19

1) 09/11/00 13:42
COMMENTS: PT TO R SIDE, IV OPEN, O2 ON. MD CALLED TO ASSESS FHR
TRACING, CHARGE RN CONSULTED.

Strip Chart D-20

1) 09/11/00 14:00
COMMENTS: PT C/O FEELING "PRESSURE". VE- FULLY. MD CALLED- PT NOT TO
PUSH AT THIS TIME.

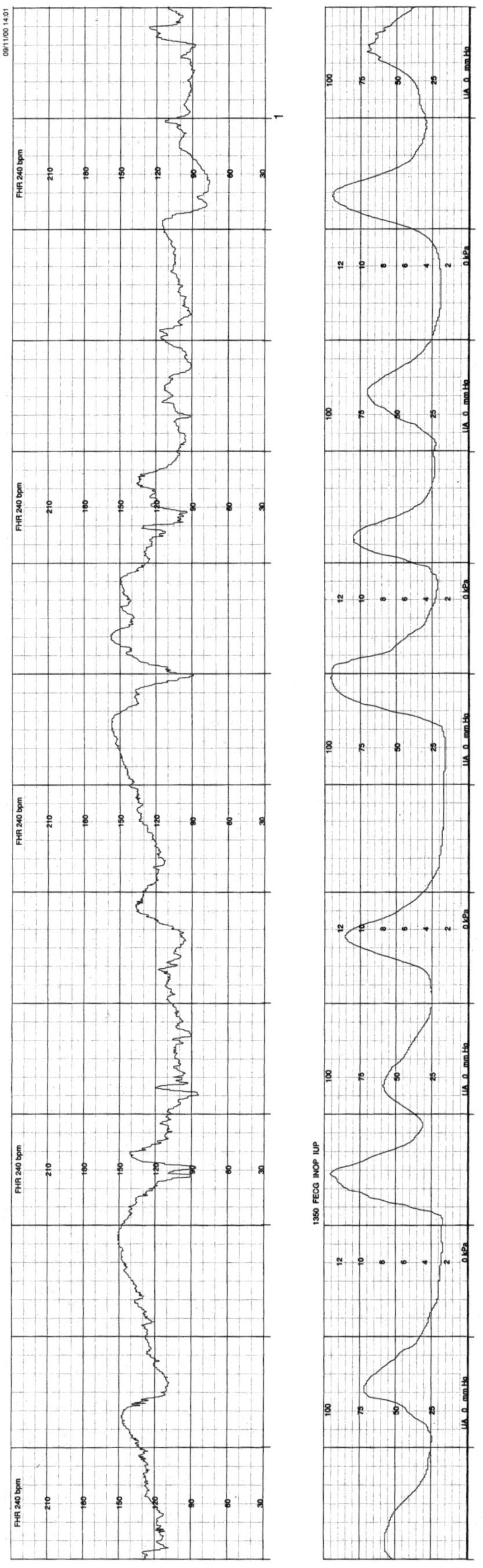

Strip Chart D–21

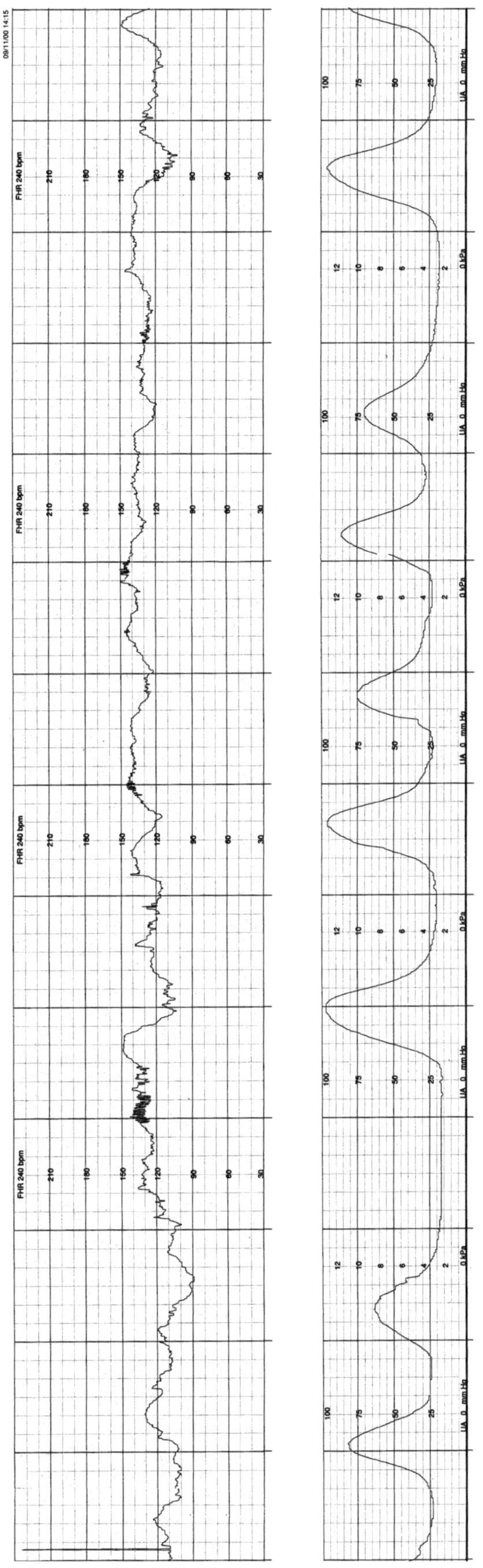

Strip Chart D–22

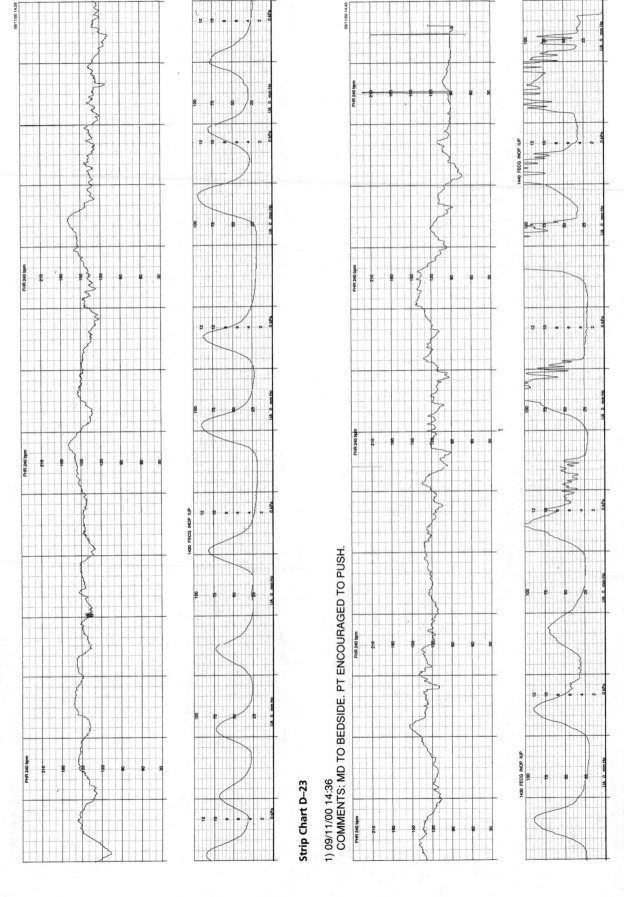

Strip Chart D–23

1) 09/11/00 14:36
COMMENTS: MD TO BEDSIDE. PT ENCOURAGED TO PUSH.

Strip Chart D–24

HX OF PATIENT E: 17 YO, G$_1$P$_0$, 42 WKS, 1/2 PPD SMOKER. INDUCTION BEGUN AT 1030 WITH PGE$_1$ FOLLOWING ANTEPARTUM TEST RESULTS OF NONREACTIVE NST AND BPP 6/10. EPIDURAL IN PLACE SINCE 1815.

1) 04/16/99 22:18 BP 104/59 M 71 P 76
2) 04/16/99 22:21 BP 108/63 M 76 P 72
3) 04/16/99 22:22 COMMENTS: PIT INCREASED TO 8 MU/MIN VIA INF PUMP.
4) 04/16/99 22:31 COMMENTS: MD IN ROOM, TRACING VIEWED, VE- NO CERVICAL CHANGE; 5 CM 90% - 1

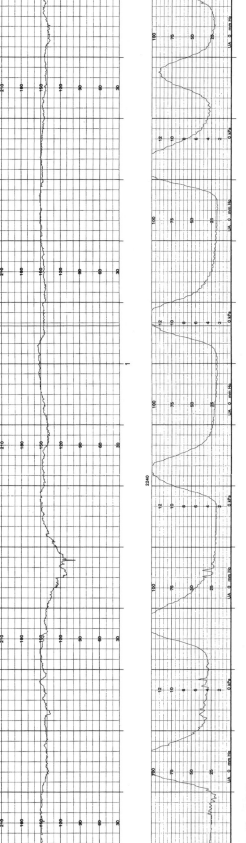

Strip Chart E-1

1) 04/16/99 22:42
BP 119/83 M 93 P 76

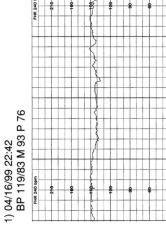

Strip Chart E-2

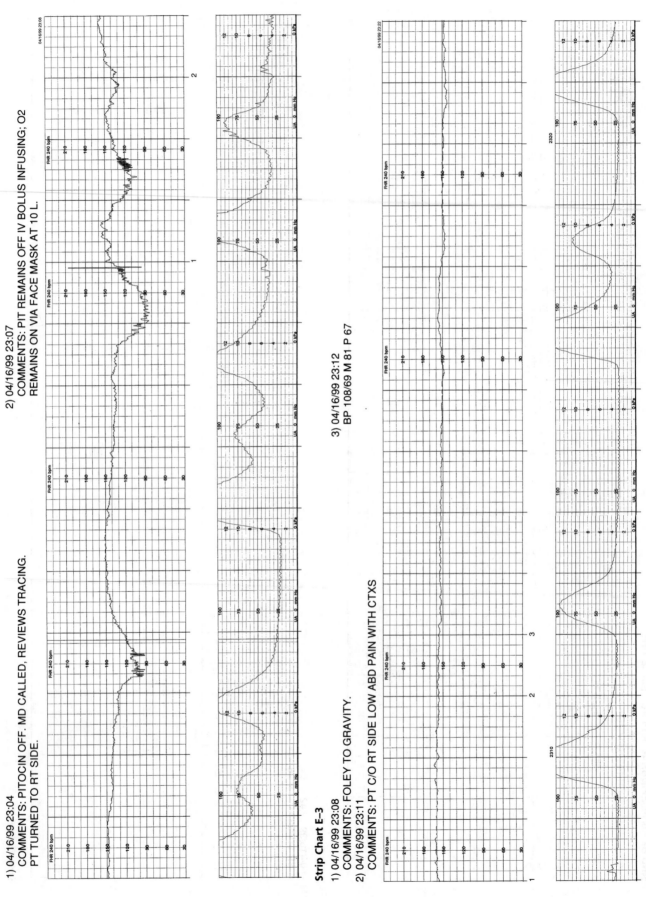

1) 04/16/99 23:04
COMMENTS: PITOCIN OFF. MD CALLED, REVIEWS TRACING.
PT TURNED TO RT SIDE.

2) 04/16/99 23:07
COMMENTS: PIT REMAINS OFF IV BOLUS INFUSING; O2
REMAINS ON VIA FACE MASK AT 10 L.

Strip Chart E-3

1) 04/16/99 23:08
COMMENTS: FOLEY TO GRAVITY.

2) 04/16/99 23:11
COMMENTS: PT C/O RT SIDE LOW ABD PAIN WITH CTXS

3) 04/16/99 23:12
BP 108/69 M 81 P 67

Strip Chart E-4

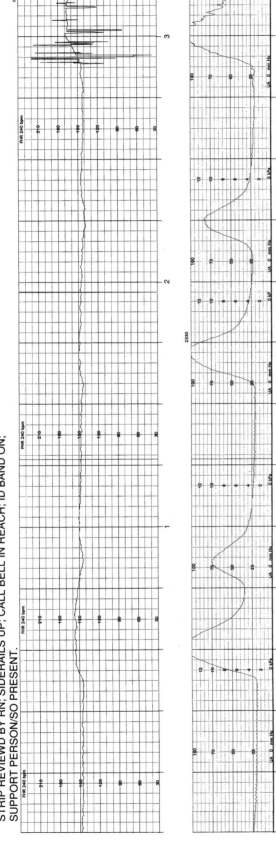

2) 04/16/99 23:31 COMMENTS: CONTRACTIONS MODERATE TO PALPATION; PIT OFF, IV LR INFUSING WELL, O2 ON @ 8 L VIA MASK, PT SLEEPING ON LT SIDE. STRIP REVIEWD BY RN; SIDERAILS UP; CALL BELL IN REACH; ID BAND ON; SUPPORT PERSON/SO PRESENT.

VE BY MD, DILATION: 6.
COMMENTS: SCALP STIMULATION GIVEN

Strip Chart E–5

1) 04/16/99 23:37
COMMENTS: PERICARE GIVEN, PT REPOSITIONED TO RT SIDE.

2) 04/16/99 23:40
COMMENTS: TEMP 96.4 AX

3) 04/16/99 23:42
COMMENTS: PT C/O PAIN ON RT SIDE

4) 04/16/99 23:43
COMMENTS: PIT RESTARTED @ 1 MU/MIN PER MD ORDER. BP 122/82 M 97 P 71.

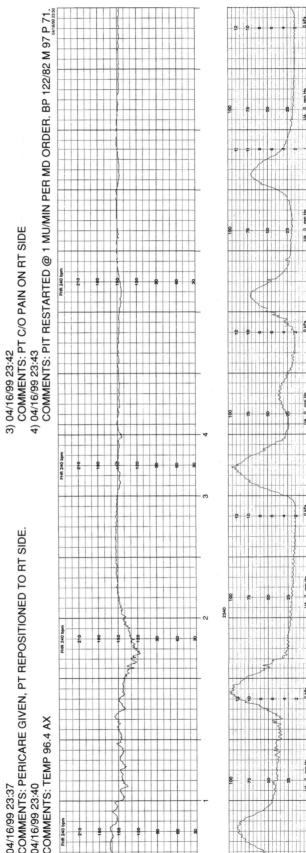

Strip Chart E–6

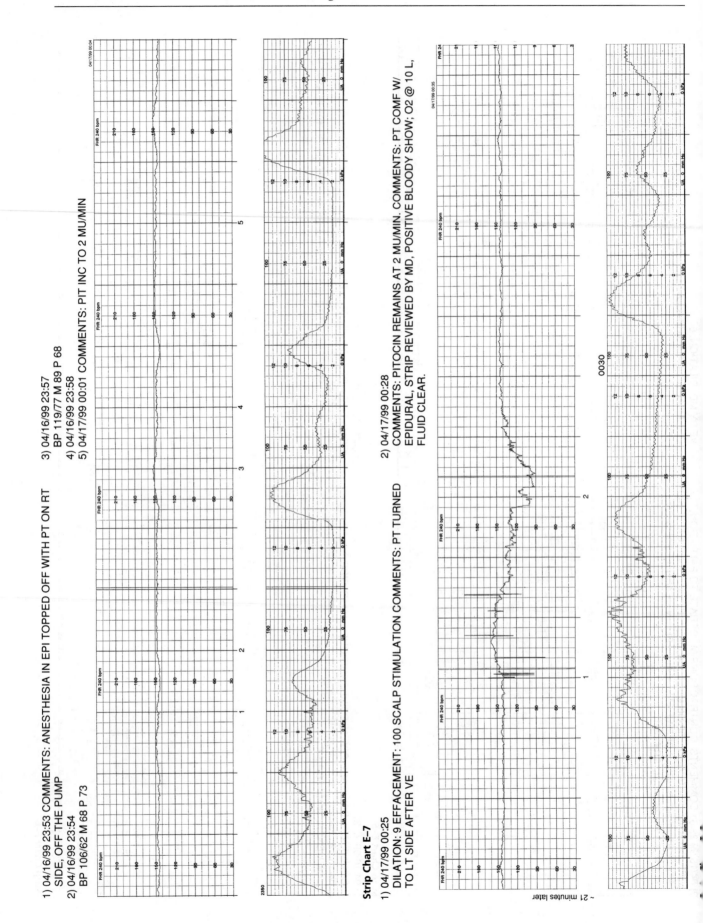

1) 04/16/99 23:53 COMMENTS: ANESTHESIA IN EPI TOPPED OFF WITH PT ON RT SIDE, OFF THE PUMP

2) 04/16/99 23:54
BP 106/62 M 68 P 73

3) 04/16/99 23:57
BP 119/77 M 89 P 68

4) 04/16/99 23:58

5) 04/17/99 00:01 COMMENTS: PIT INC TO 2 MU/MIN

Strip Chart E–7

1) 04/17/99 00:25
DILATION: 9 EFFACEMENT: 100 SCALP STIMULATION COMMENTS: PT TURNED TO LT SIDE AFTER VE

2) 04/17/99 00:28
COMMENTS: PITOCIN REMAINS AT 2 MU/MIN. COMMENTS: PT COMF W/ EPIDURAL, STRIP REVIEWED BY MD, POSITIVE BLOODY SHOW; O2 @ 10 L, FLUID CLEAR.

~ 21 minutes later

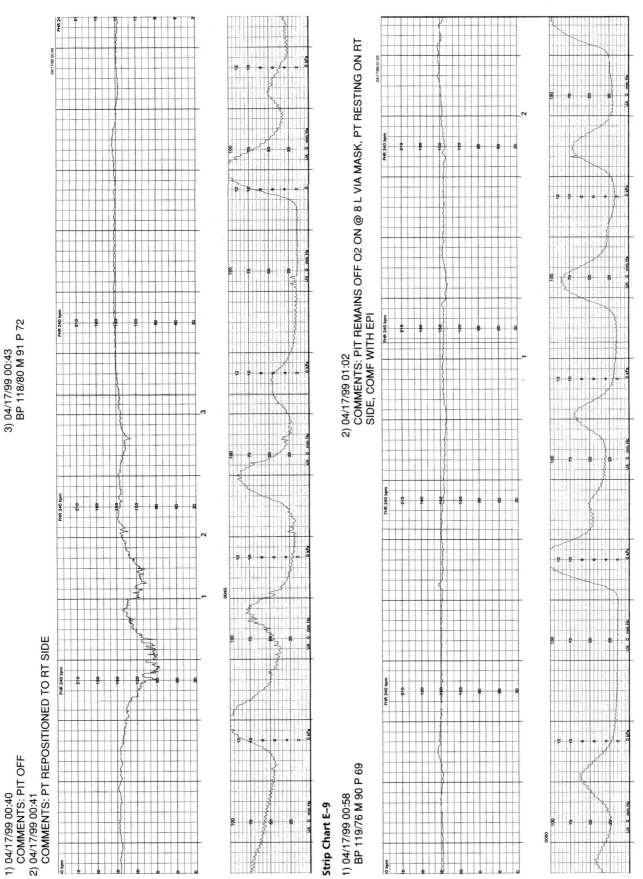

1) 04/17/99 00:40
COMMENTS: PIT OFF

2) 04/17/99 00:41
COMMENTS: PT REPOSITIONED TO RT SIDE

3) 04/17/99 00:43
BP 118/80 M 91 P 72

Strip Chart E-9

1) 04/17/99 00:58
BP 119/76 M 90 P 69

2) 04/17/99 01:02
COMMENTS: PIT REMAINS OFF O2 ON @ 8 L VIA MASK, PT RESTING ON RT SIDE, COMF WITH EPI

Strip Chart E-10

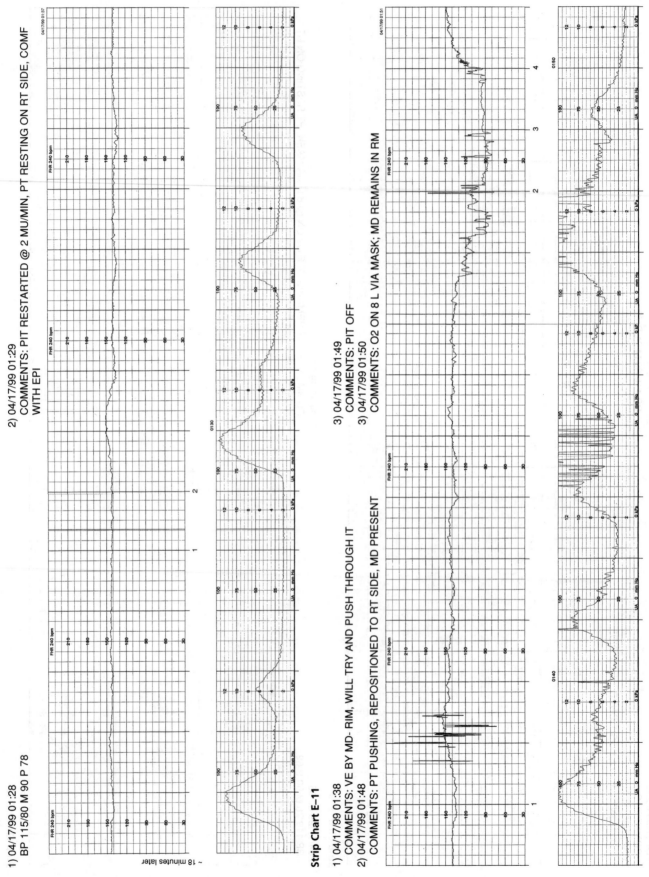

1) 04/17/99 01:28
BP 115/80 M 90 P 78

2) 04/17/99 01:29
COMMENTS: PIT RESTARTED @ 2 MU/MIN, PT RESTING ON RT SIDE, COMF
WITH EPI

~ 18 minutes later

Strip Chart E-11

1) 04/17/99 01:38
COMMENTS: VE BY MD- RIM, WILL TRY AND PUSH THROUGH IT
2) 04/17/99 01:48
COMMENTS: PT PUSHING, REPOSITIONED TO RT SIDE, MD PRESENT
3) 04/17/99 01:49
COMMENTS: PIT OFF
3) 04/17/99 01:50
COMMENTS: O2 ON 8 L VIA MASK; MD REMAINS IN RM

Strip Chart E-12

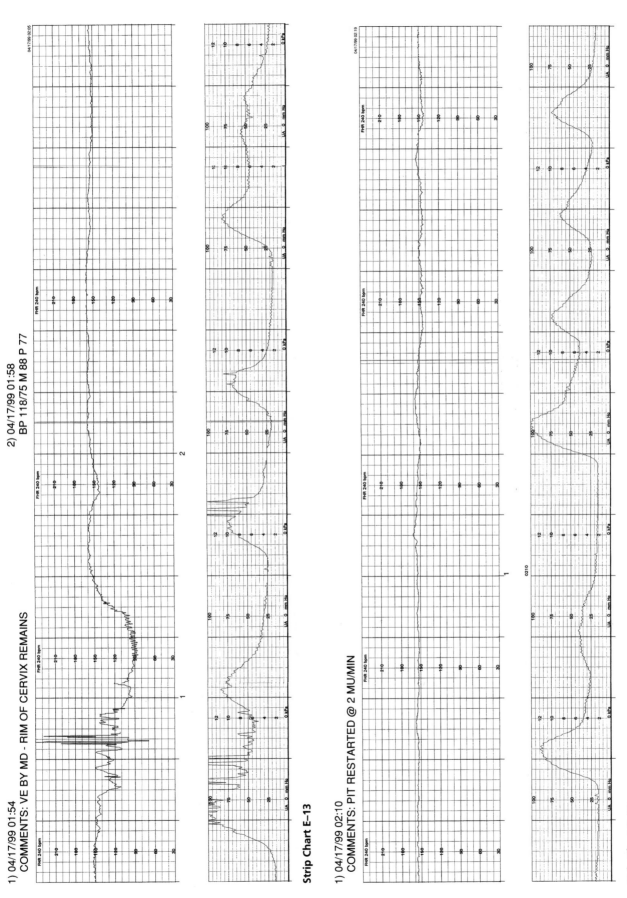

1) 04/17/99 01:54
COMMENTS: VE BY MD - RIM OF CERVIX REMAINS

2) 04/17/99 01:58
BP 118/75 M 88 P 77

Strip Chart E-13

1) 04/17/99 02:10
COMMENTS: PIT RESTARTED @ 2 MU/MIN

Strip Chart E-14

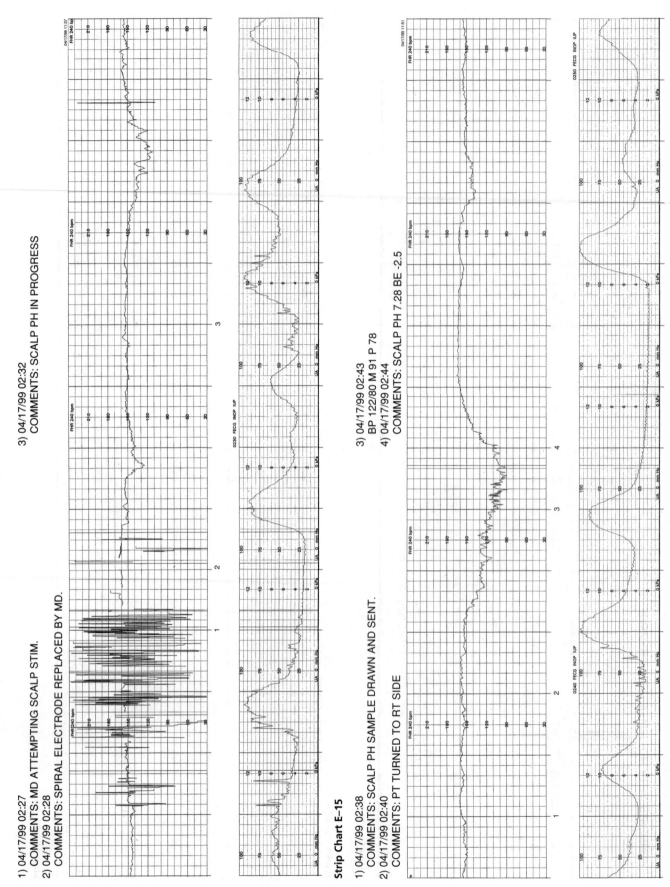

1) 04/17/99 02:27
   COMMENTS: MD ATTEMPTING SCALP STIM.
2) 04/17/99 02:28
   COMMENTS: SPIRAL ELECTRODE REPLACED BY MD.

3) 04/17/99 02:32
   COMMENTS: SCALP PH IN PROGRESS

Strip Chart E-15

1) 04/17/99 02:38
   COMMENTS: SCALP PH SAMPLE DRAWN AND SENT.
2) 04/17/99 02:40
   COMMENTS: PT TURNED TO RT SIDE

3) 04/17/99 02:43
   BP 122/80 M 91 P 78
4) 04/17/99 02:44
   COMMENTS: SCALP PH 7.28 BE -2.5

Strip Chart E-16

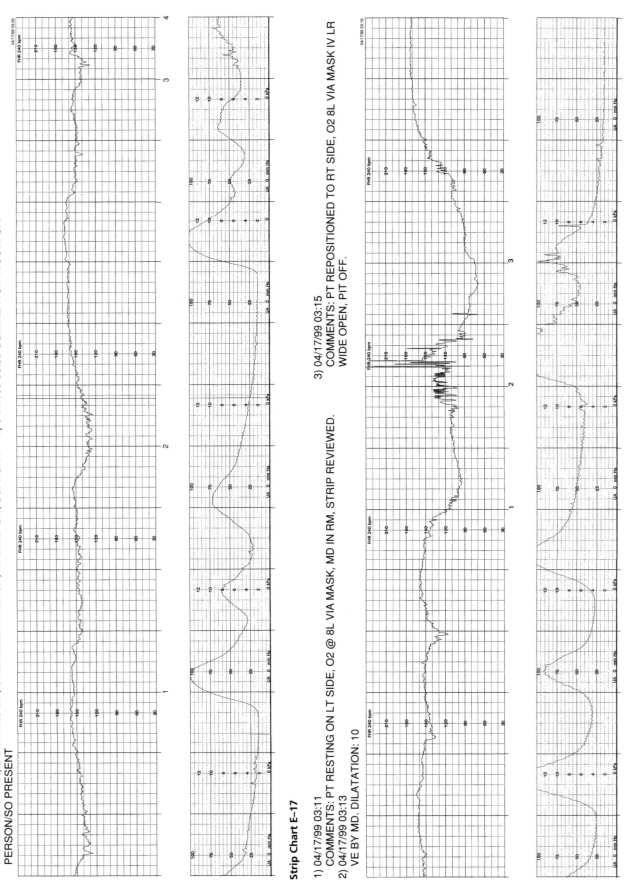

1) 04/17/99 02:59 CONTRACTIONS MODERATE TO MUDERATE TOTAL, COMMENTS. 11
RESTING ON RT SIDE, O2 ON @ 8 L VIA MASK, PITOCIN @ 3 MU/MIN, STRIP
REVIEWED BY RN; SIDERAILS UP; CALL BELL IN REACH; ID BAND ON; SUPPORT
PERSON/SO PRESENT

2) 04/11/99 02:59 07:59 BY 11970 M 07:10
3) 04/17/99 03:04 COMMENTS: PT REPOSITIONED TO LT SIDE
4) 04/17/99 03:05 COMMENTS: PITOCIN OFF

Strip Chart E–17

1) 04/17/99 03:11
   COMMENTS: PT RESTING ON LT SIDE, O2 @ 8L VIA MASK, MD IN RM, STRIP REVIEWED.
2) 04/17/99 03:13
   VE BY MD. DILATATION: 10

3) 04/17/99 03:15
   COMMENTS: PT REPOSITIONED TO RT SIDE, O2 8L VIA MASK IV LR
   WIDE OPEN, PIT OFF.

Strip Chart E–18

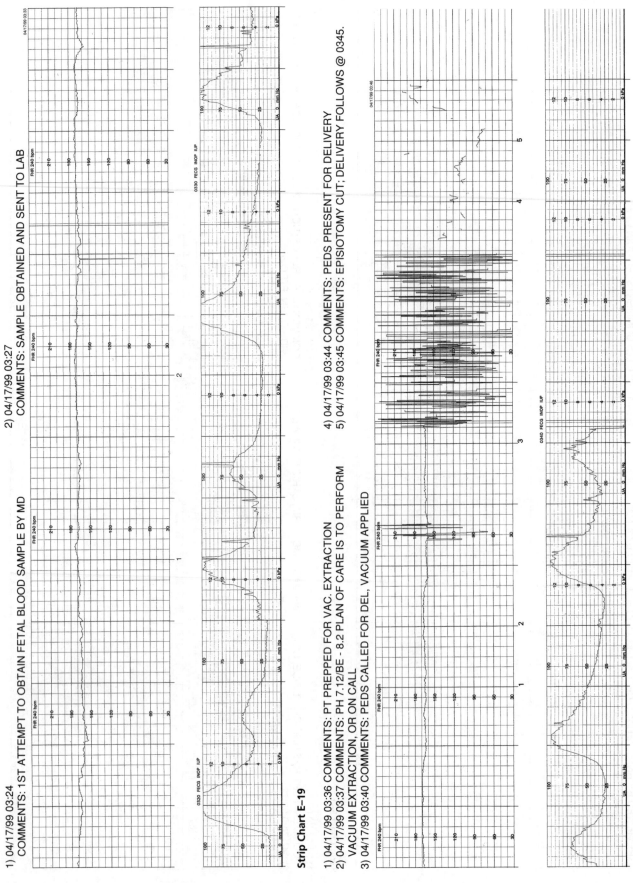

1) 04/17/99 03:24
   COMMENTS: 1ST ATTEMPT TO OBTAIN FETAL BLOOD SAMPLE BY MD

2) 04/17/99 03:27
   COMMENTS: SAMPLE OBTAINED AND SENT TO LAB

Strip Chart E-19

1) 04/17/99 03:36 COMMENTS: PT PREPPED FOR VAC. EXTRACTION
2) 04/17/99 03:37 COMMENTS: PH 7.12/BE - 8.2 PLAN OF CARE IS TO PERFORM
   VACUUM EXTRACTION, OR ON CALL
3) 04/17/99 03:40 COMMENTS: PEDS CALLED FOR DEL, VACUUM APPLIED

4) 04/17/99 03:44 COMMENTS: PEDS PRESENT FOR DELIVERY
5) 04/17/99 03:45 COMMENTS: EPISIOTOMY CUT; DELIVERY FOLLOWS @ 0345.

Strip Chart E-20

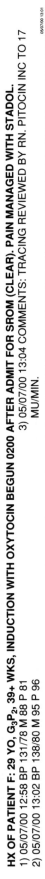

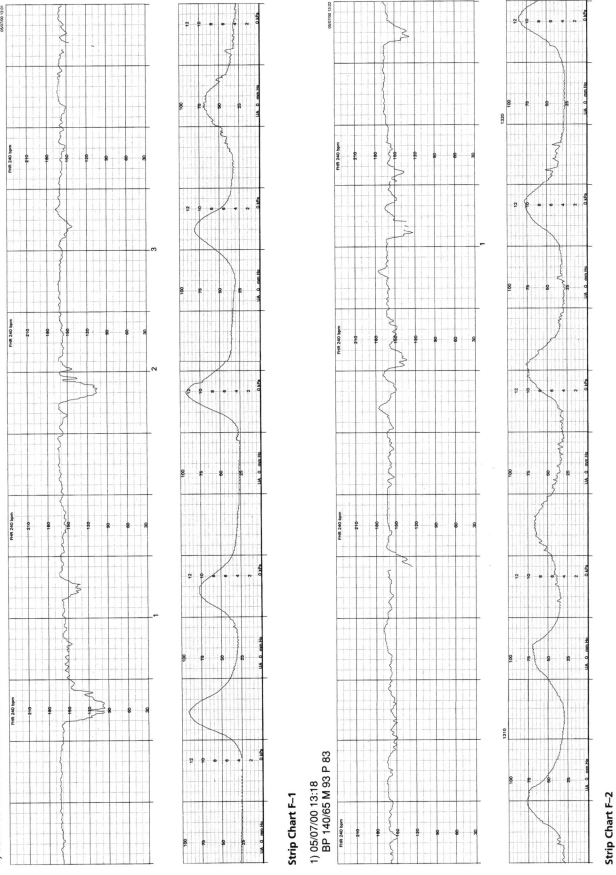

HX OF PATIENT F: 29 YO, G₃P₂, 39+ WKS, INDUCTION WITH OXYTOCIN BEGUN 0200 AFTER ADMIT FOR SROM (CLEAR). PAIN MANAGED WITH STADOL.
1) 05/07/00 12:58 BP 131/78 M 88 P 81
2) 05/07/00 13:02 BP 138/80 M 95 P 96
3) 05/07/00 13:04 COMMENTS: TRACING REVIEWED BY RN. PITOCIN INC TO 17 MU/MIN.

Strip Chart F-1

1) 05/07/00 13:18
BP 140/65 M 93 P 83

Strip Chart F-2

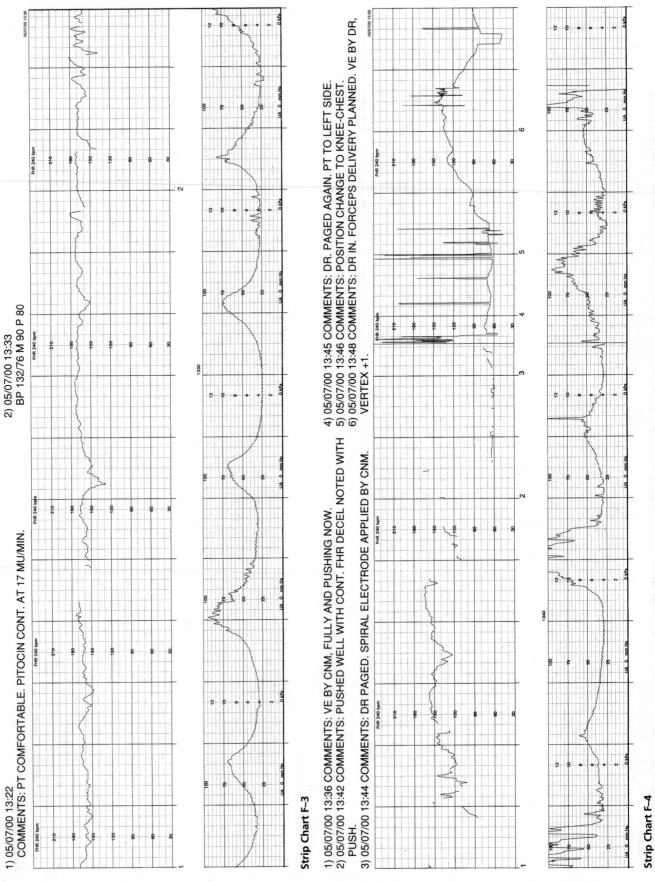

1) 05/07/00 13:22
COMMENTS: PT COMFORTABLE. PITOCIN CONT. AT 17 MU/MIN.

2) 05/07/00 13:33
BP 132/76 M 90 P 80

Strip Chart F-3

1) 05/07/00 13:36 COMMENTS: VE BY CNM, FULLY AND PUSHING NOW.
2) 05/07/00 13:42 COMMENTS: PUSHED WELL WITH CONT. FHR DECEL NOTED WITH PUSH.
3) 05/07/00 13:44 COMMENTS: DR PAGED. SPIRAL ELECTRODE APPLIED BY CNM.

4) 05/07/00 13:45 COMMENTS: DR. PAGED AGAIN. PT TO LEFT SIDE.
5) 05/07/00 13:46 COMMENTS: POSITION CHANGE TO KNEE-CHEST.
6) 05/07/00 13:48 COMMENTS: DR IN. FORCEPS DELIVERY PLANNED. VE BY DR, VERTEX +1.

Strip Chart F-4

1) 05/07/00 13:50 COMMENTS: REMOVED IUPC BY DR
2) 05/07/00 13:51 COMMENTS: SPIRAL ELECTRODE OFF BY MD
3) 05/07/00 13:52 COMMENTS: FORCEPS APPLIED. FHR BY ULTRASOUND TRANSDUCER.
4) 05/07/00 13:53 COMMENTS: REAPPLIED FORCEPS, PITOCIN OFF.

5) 05/07/00 13:54 COMMENTS: FORCEPS REMOVED AND REAPPLIED BY DR. AWARE OF FHR
6) 05/07/00 13:56 COMMENTS: NEO TEAM PRESENT. FHR AUDIBLE 50'S/60'S.
7) 05/07/00 13:57 BP 145/85 M 96 P 128
8) 05/07/00 14:03 COMMENTS: BP 144/110 M 117 P 107 COMMENTS: FETUS DEL'D AND TO PEDS.

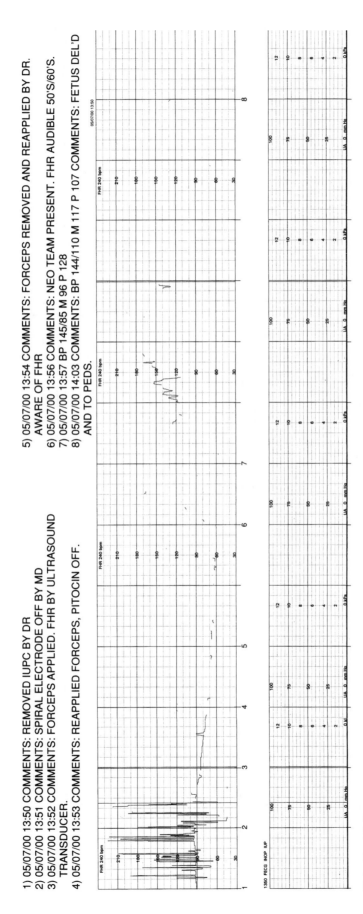

Strip Chart F–5

HX OF PATIENT G: 33 YO, G2P0, 38+ WKS, SROM (CLEAR) 0900. SPONTANEOUS CONTRACTIONS SINCE 1300, REGULAR SINCE 1530. 3-4 CM/60%/-2 BY MD EXAM AT 1955.

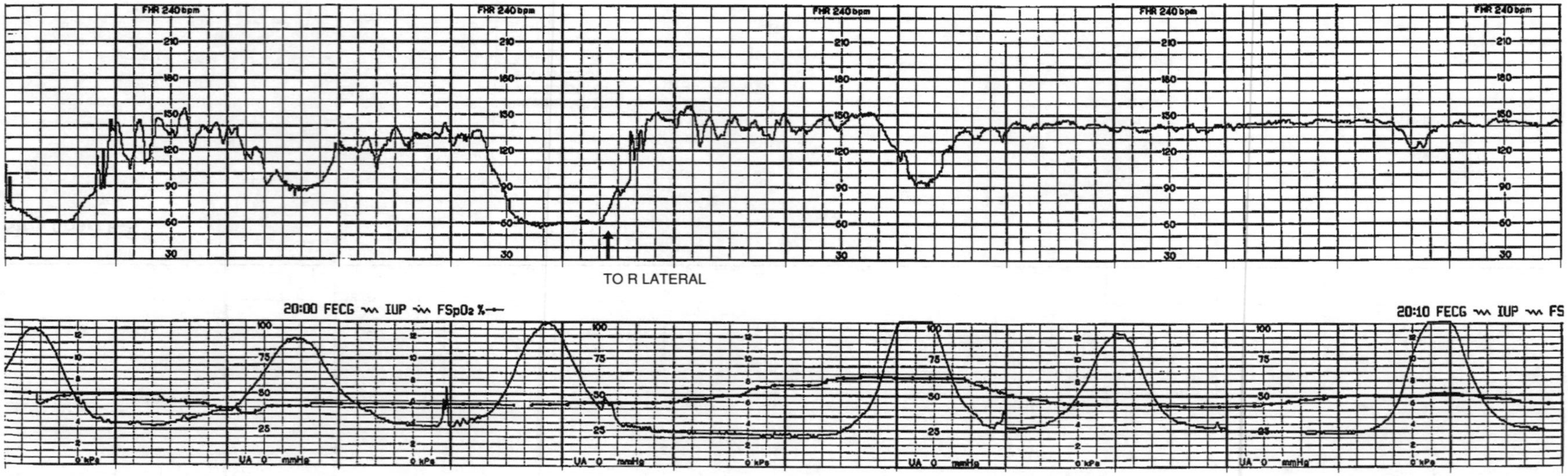

TO R LATERAL

Strip Chart G-1

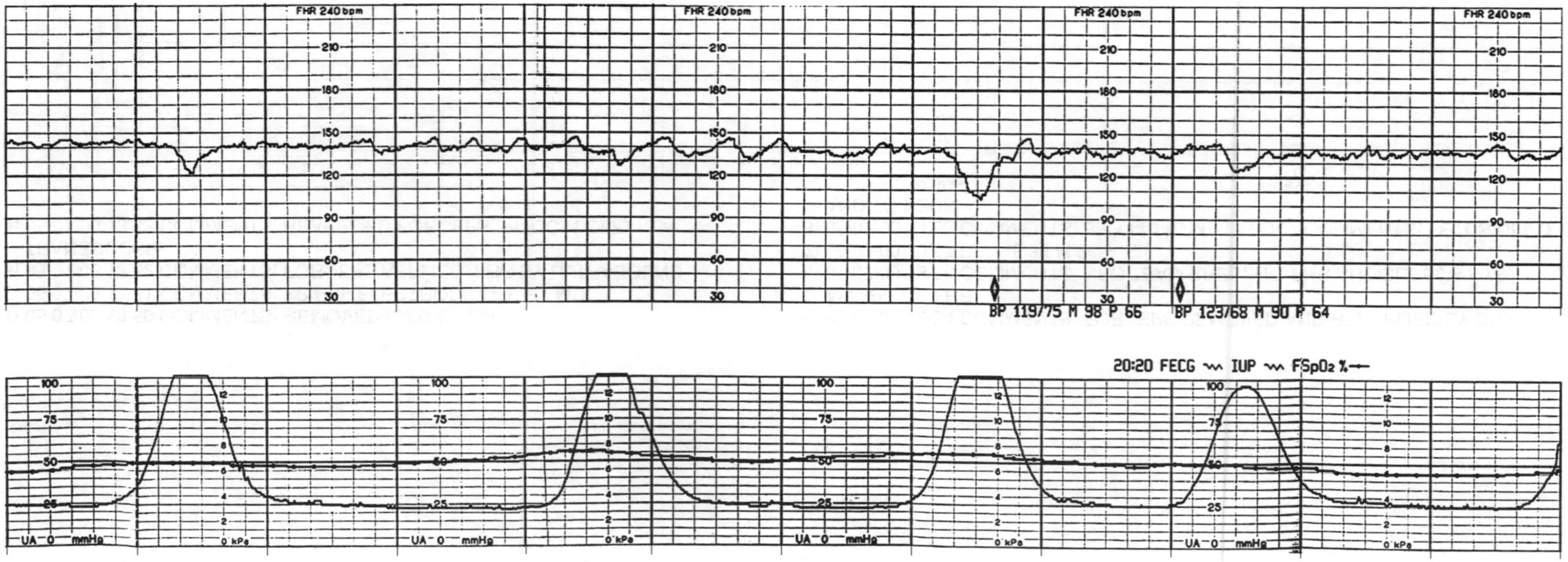

Strip Chart G-2

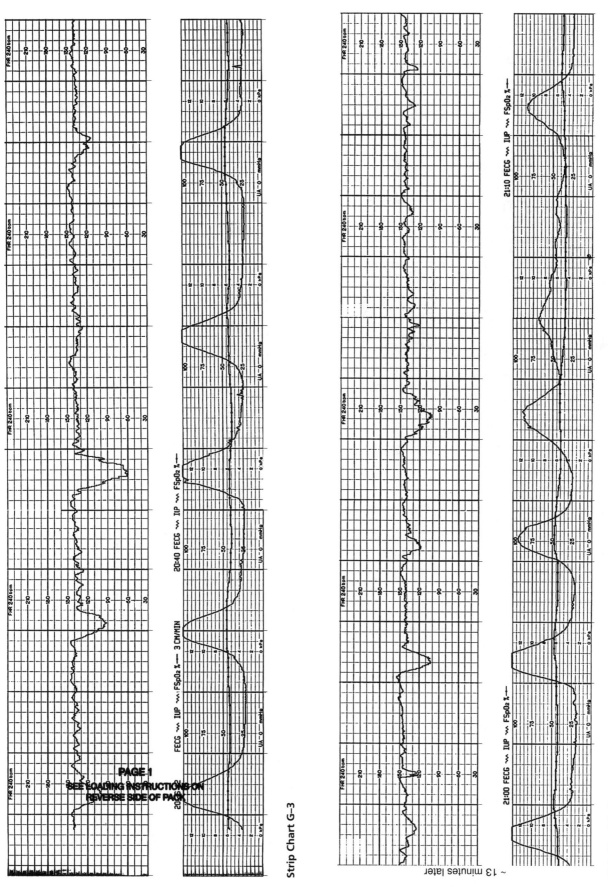

Strip Chart G-3

Strip Chart G-4

~ 13 minutes later

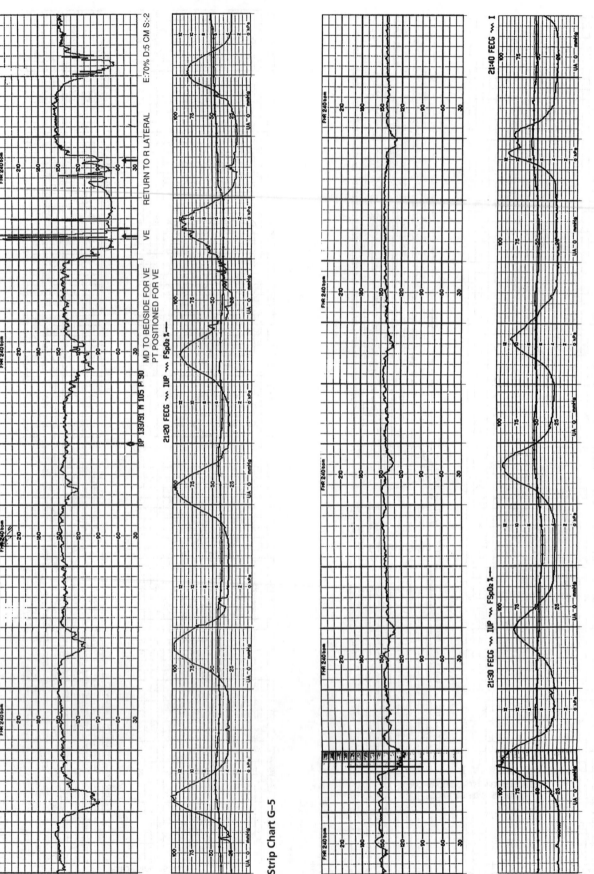

Strip Chart G-5

Strip Chart G-6

HX OF PATIENT H: 18 YO, G₄P₁, 39 WKS, GDM. PRESENTS FOR R/O LABOR.

1) 09/21/00 20:45
COMMENTS: 2 CM/50%/-2

2) 09/21/00 20:47 BP 131/71 M 94 P 72 T 972 COMMENTS: PT.C/O CONTX. DENIES
SROM. CONTX PALPATE MILD, PT TALKING THROUGH THEM.

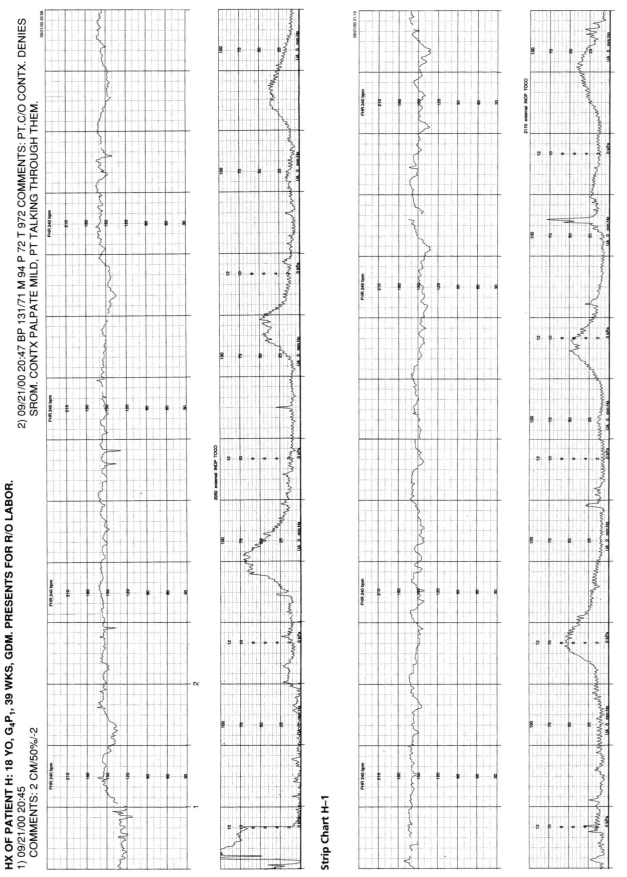

Strip Chart H-1

Strip Chart H-2

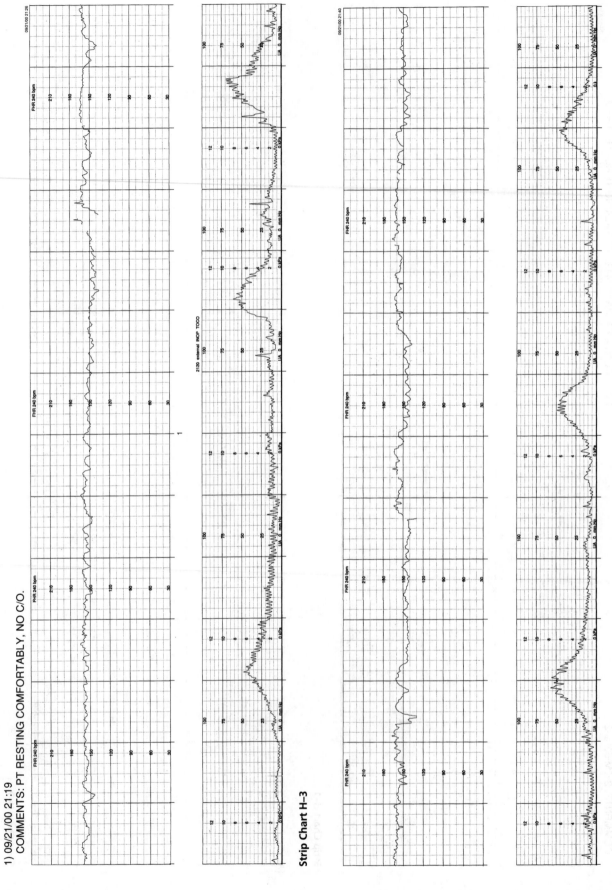

1) 09/21/00 21:19
COMMENTS: PT RESTING COMFORTABLY, NO C/O.

Strip Chart H-3

Strip Chart H-4

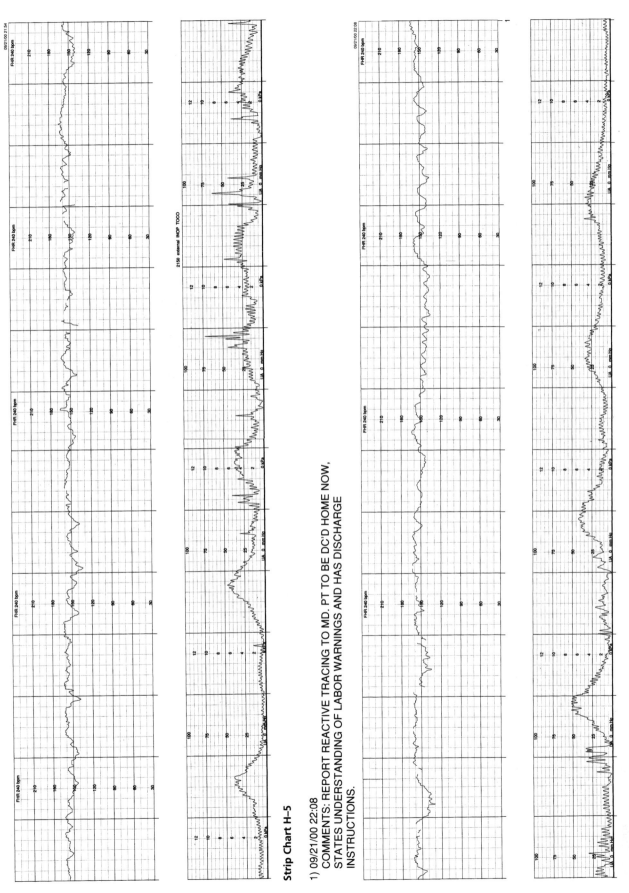

Strip Chart H–5

1) 09/21/00 22:08
COMMENTS: REPORT REACTIVE TRACING TO MD. PT TO BE DC'D HOME NOW, STATES UNDERSTANDING OF LABOR WARNINGS AND HAS DISCHARGE INSTRUCTIONS.

Strip Chart H–6

HX OF PATIENT I: 38 WKS, G₂P₁, GDM (INSULIN DEPENDENT), VBAC (PRIOR C-BIRTH FOR ARREST OF DESCENT AND MACROSOMIA). INDUCTION WITH OXYTOCIN @ 1800, AROM @ 1830 (LIGHT MECONIUM).

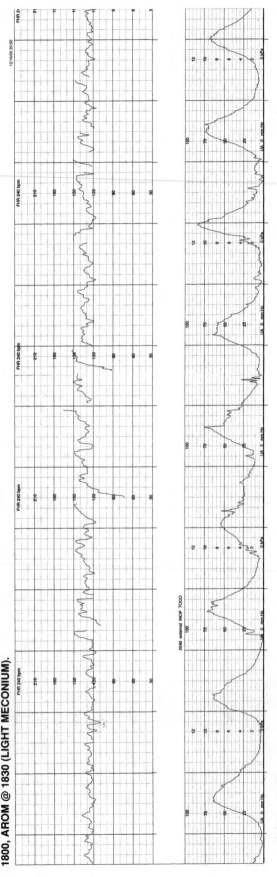

Strip Chart I-1

1) 12/16/00 20:57
COMMENTS: PT C/O UC PAIN. REPOSITIONED, MD CONSULTED. UC'S PALPATE MODERATE.

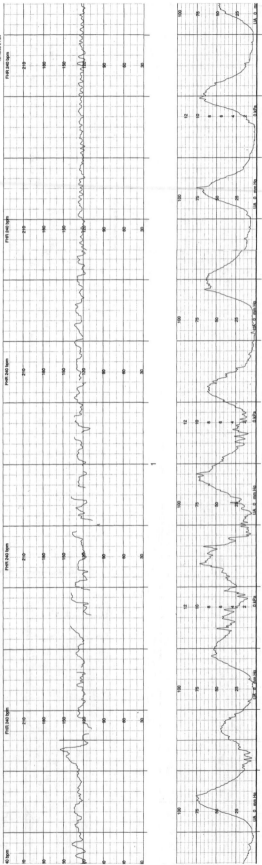

Strip Chart I-2

1) 12/16/00 21:12
FLD AMT LARGE; FLD CLR; FLD ODOR NORMAL; NUBAIN 10 MG; DILATION: 2
EFFACEMENT: 75 STATION: -2

2) 12/16/00 21:20
LOWERED HB, PT TO R SIDE NOW.

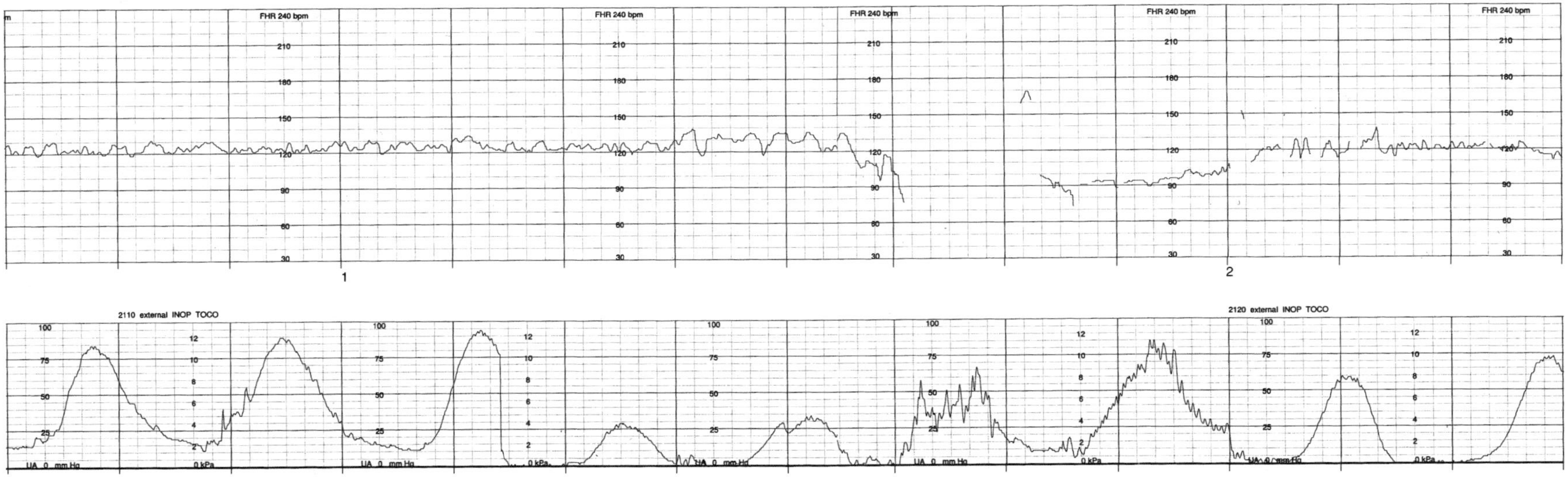

Strip Chart I-3

1) 12/16/00 21:32
PT RESTING R SIDE, NO COMPLAINT, DOZING THRU UCS. UCS PALPATE
MODERATE, UTERUS SOFT BETWEEN UCS

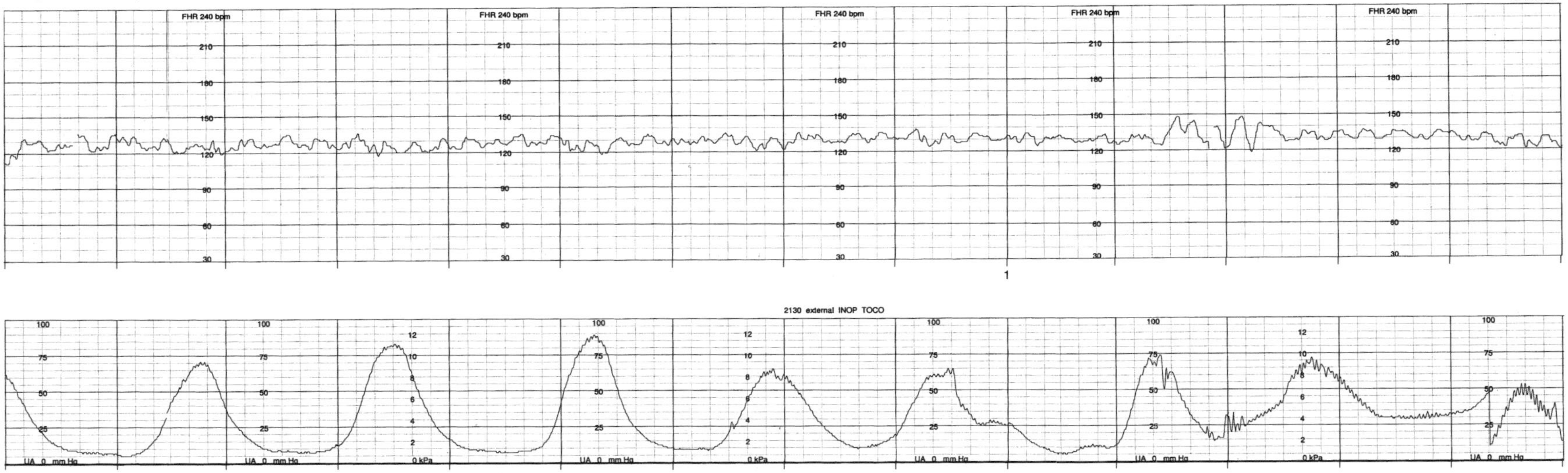

Strip Chart I-4

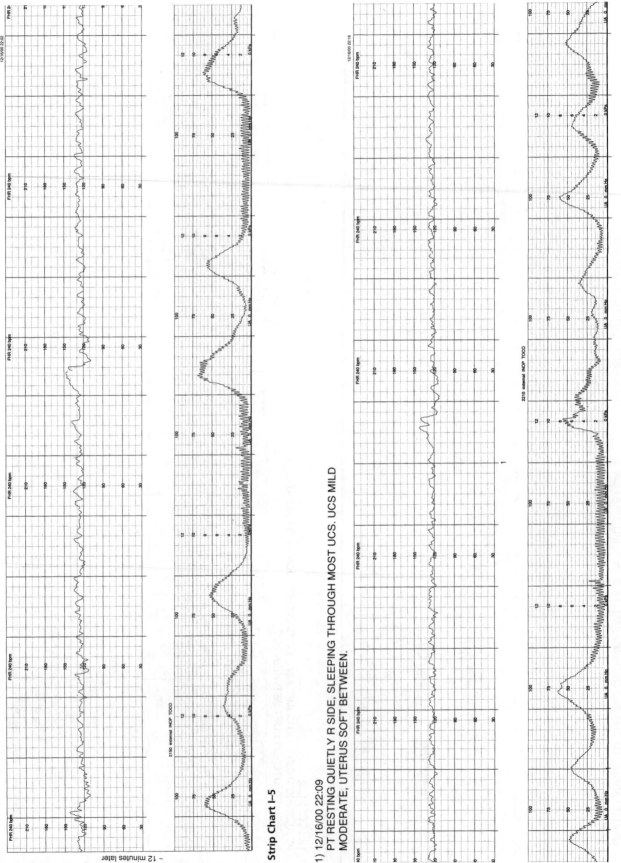

Strip Chart I-5

1) 12/16/00 22:09
PT RESTING QUIETLY R SIDE, SLEEPING THROUGH MOST UCS. UCS MILD
MODERATE, UTERUS SOFT BETWEEN.

Strip Chart I-6

1) 12/17/00 05:50
PITOCIN TO 6 MU. BP 128/82 P88 R 18. MD CONSULTED TO VIEW TRACING.

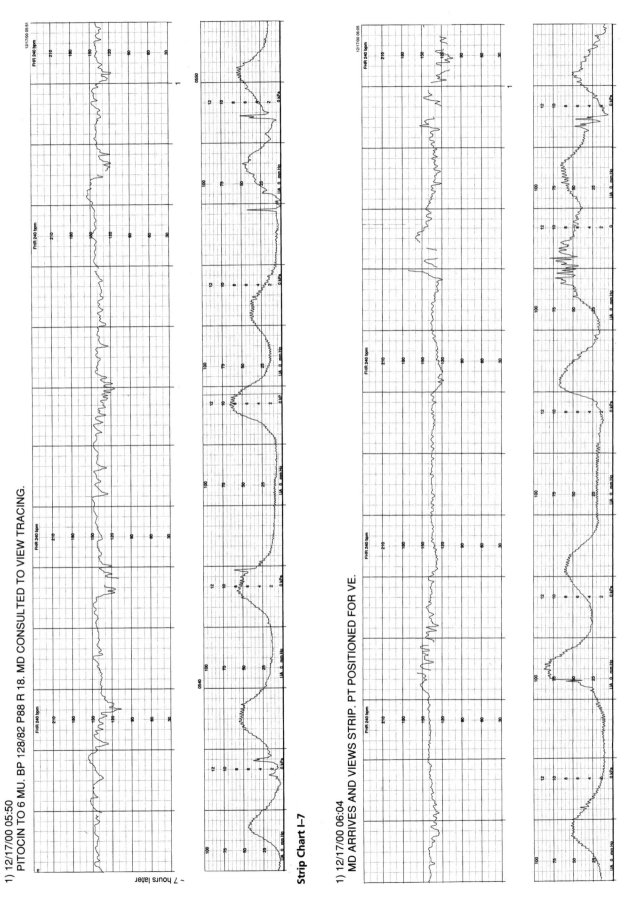

Strip Chart I–7

1) 12/17/00 06:04
MD ARRIVES AND VIEWS STRIP. PT POSITIONED FOR VE.

Strip Chart I–8

1) 12/17/00 06:07
DILATION: 3-4 EFFACEMENT: 80% STATION: -2 PT REQUESTS EPIDURAL, BOLUS
BEGUN.

2) 12/17/00 06:11
TO L SIDE.

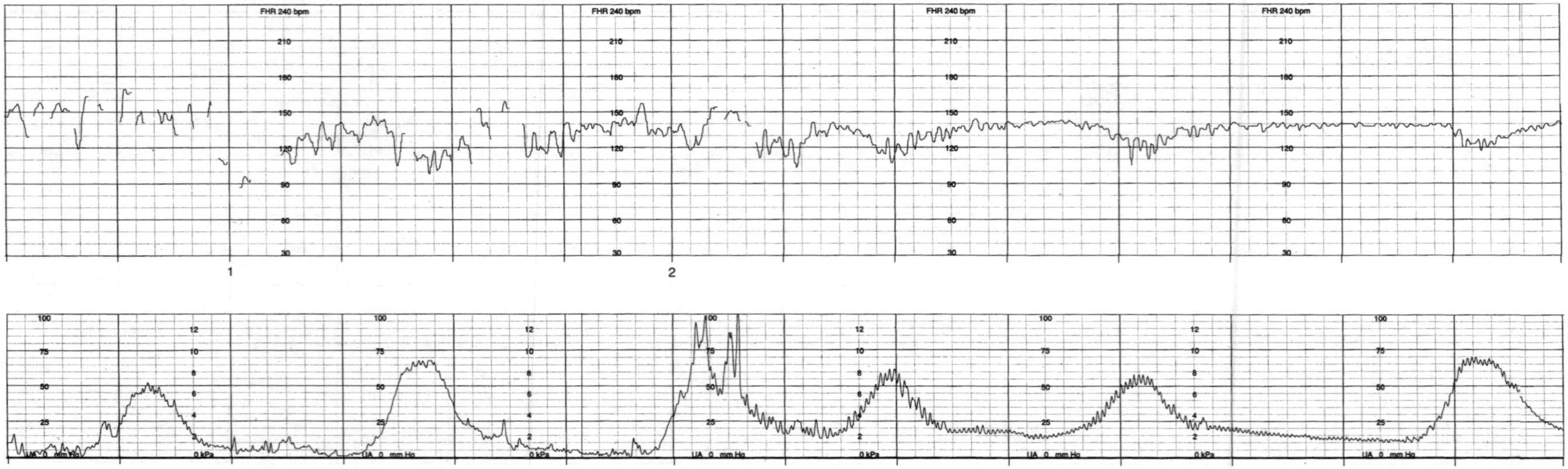

Strip Chart I-9

1) 12/17/00 06:20
PT CONTINUES RESTING ON LT SIDE. PITOCIN TO 8 MU NOW. BP 134/88 P 92 R
24. ANESTHESIA PAGED FOR EPIDURAL. PT COACHED THRU UCS. UCS
PALPATE MODERATE WITH REST BETWEEN.

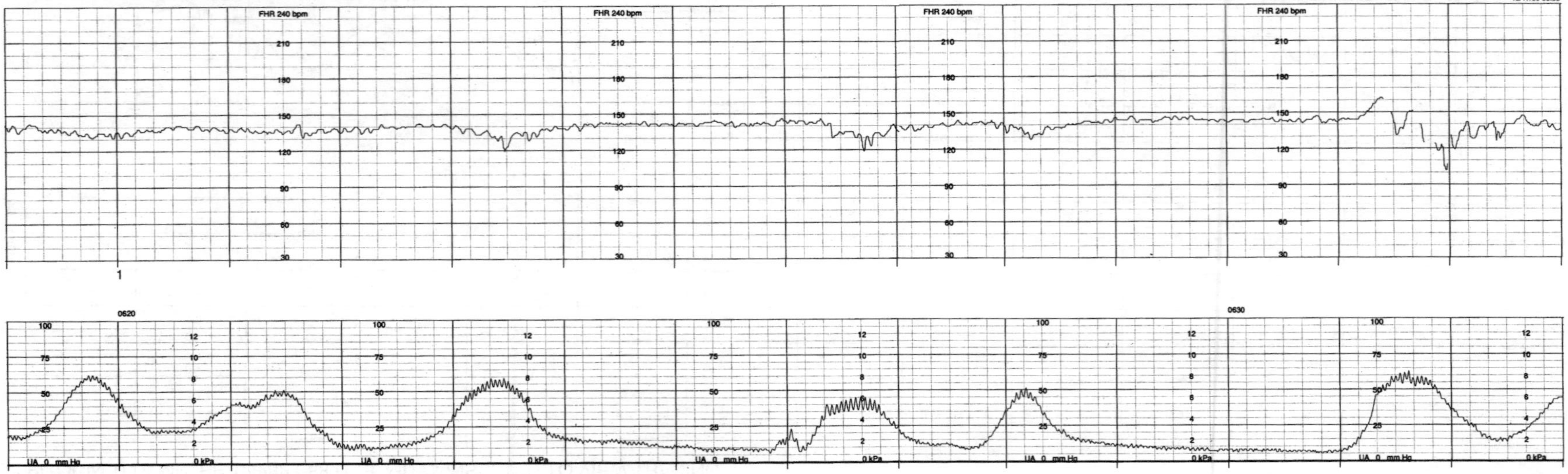

Strip Chart I-10

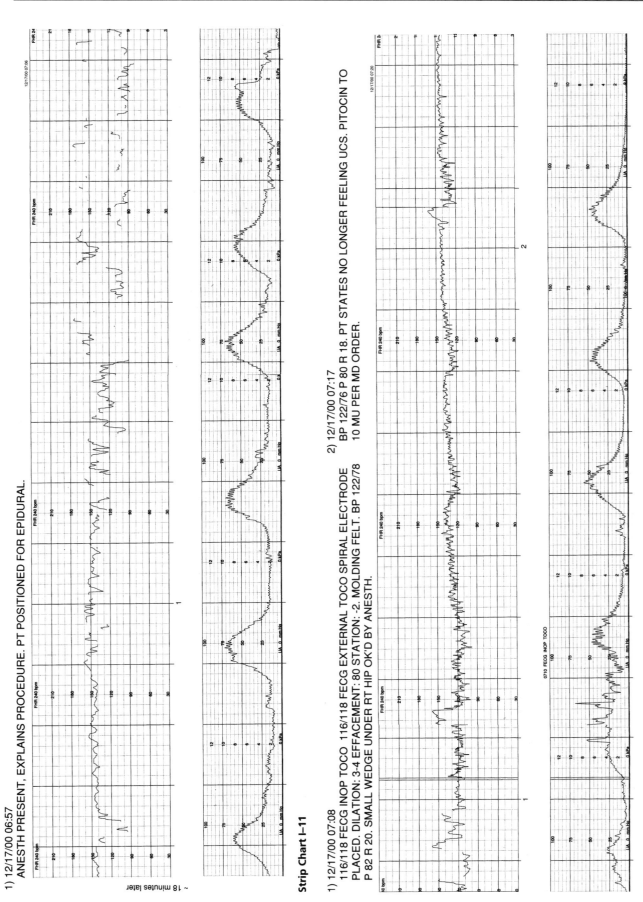

1) 12/17/00 06:57
ANESTH PRESENT, EXPLAINS PROCEDURE. PT POSITIONED FOR EPIDURAL.

~ 18 minutes later

Strip Chart I-11

1) 12/17/00 07:08
116/118 FECG INOP TOCO 116/118 FECG EXTERNAL TOCO SPIRAL ELECTRODE
PLACED. DILATION: 3-4 EFFACEMENT: 80 STATION: -2. MOLDING FELT. BP 122/78
P 82 R 20. SMALL WEDGE UNDER RT HIP OK'D BY ANESTH.

2) 12/17/00 07:17
BP 122/76 P 80 R 18. PT STATES NO LONGER FEELING UCS. PITOCIN TO
10 MU PER MD ORDER.

Strip Chart I-12

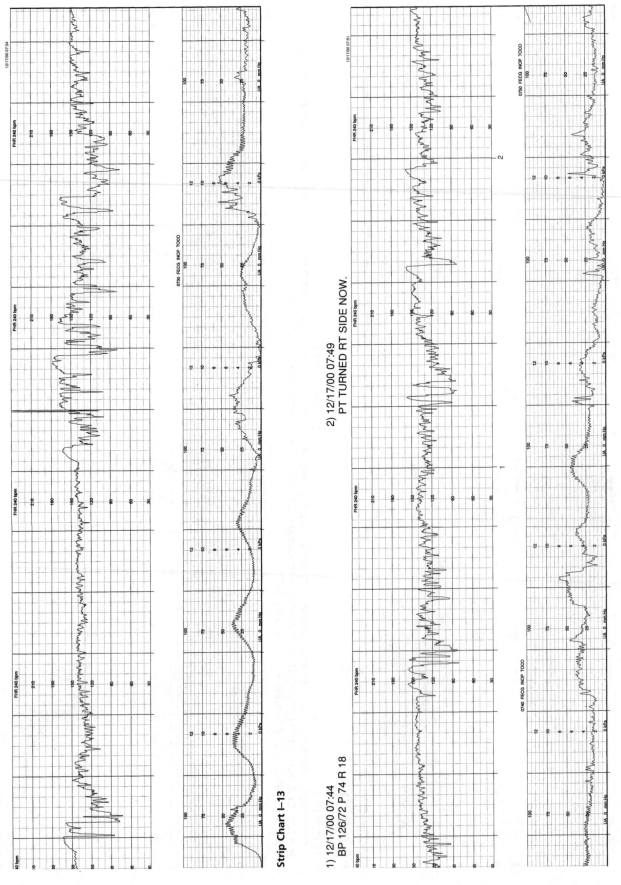

Strip Chart I-13

1) 12/17/00 07:44
   BP 126/72 P 74 R 18

2) 12/17/00 07:49
   PT TURNED RT SIDE NOW.

Strip Chart I-14

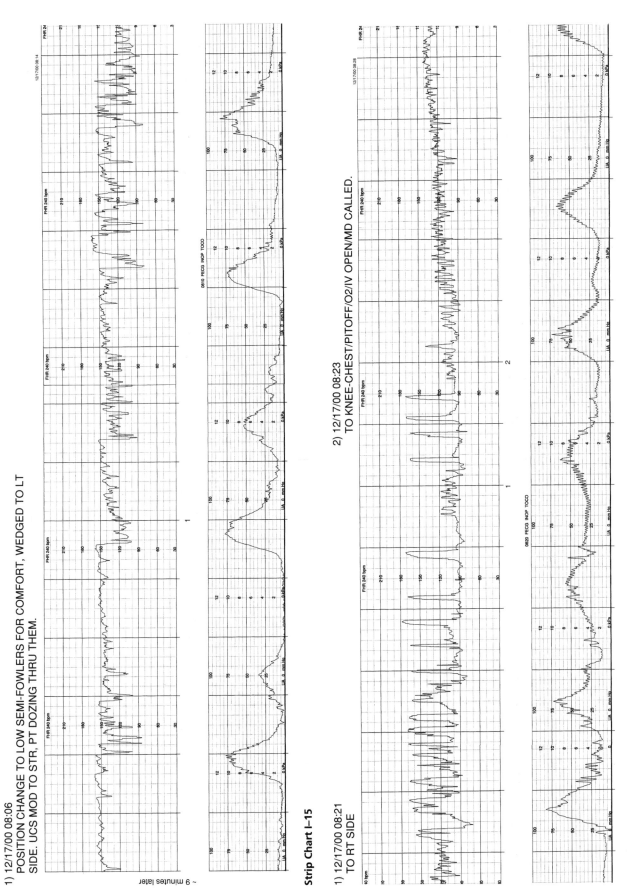

1) 12/17/00 08:06
POSITION CHANGE TO LOW SEMI-FOWLERS FOR COMFORT, WEDGED TO LT
SIDE. UCS MOD TO STR, PT DOZING THRU THEM.

Strip Chart I-15

1) 12/17/00 08:21
TO RT SIDE

2) 12/17/00 08:23
TO KNEE-CHEST/PITOFF/O2/IV OPEN/MD CALLED.

Strip Chart I-16

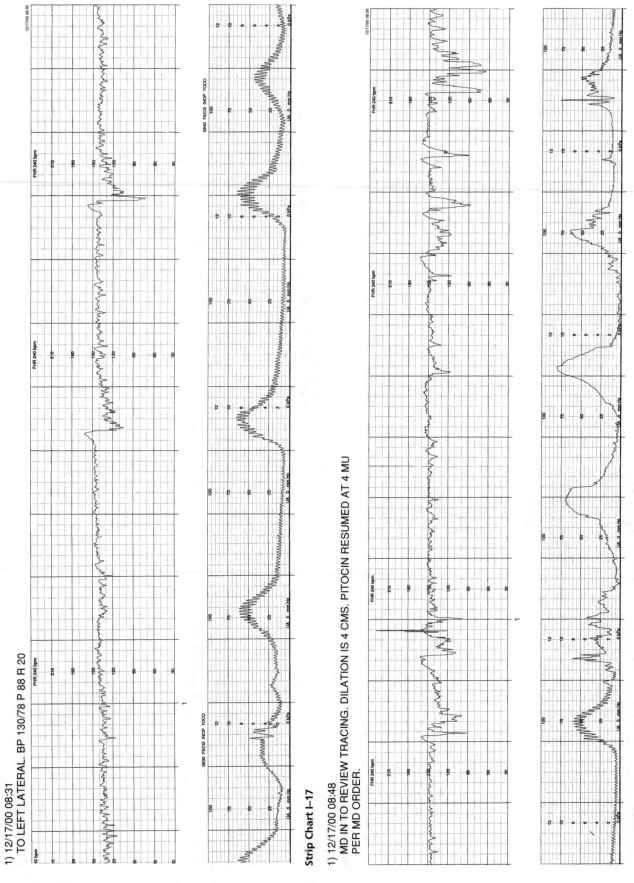

1) 12/17/00 08:31
TO LEFT LATERAL. BP 130/78 P 88 R 20

Strip Chart I-17

1) 12/17/00 08:48
MD IN TO REVIEW TRACING. DILATION IS 4 CMS. PITOCIN RESUMED AT 4 MU PER MD ORDER.

Strip Chart I-18

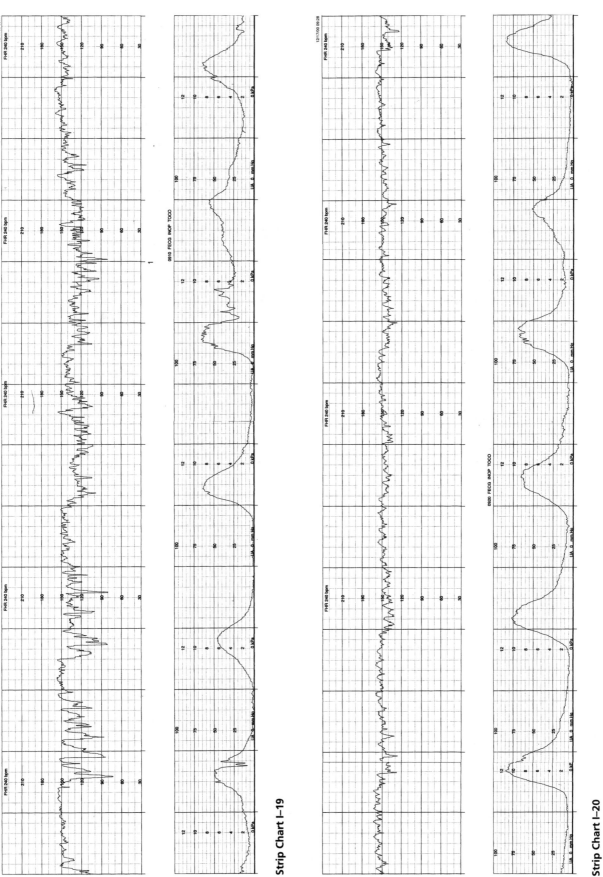

1) 12/17/00 09:10
TO RIGHT SIDE. PITOCIN DC'D. O2 CONTINUES AT 10 L BY MASK. MD NOTIFIED
OF TRACING AND PIT OFF.

Strip Chart I-19

Strip Chart I-20

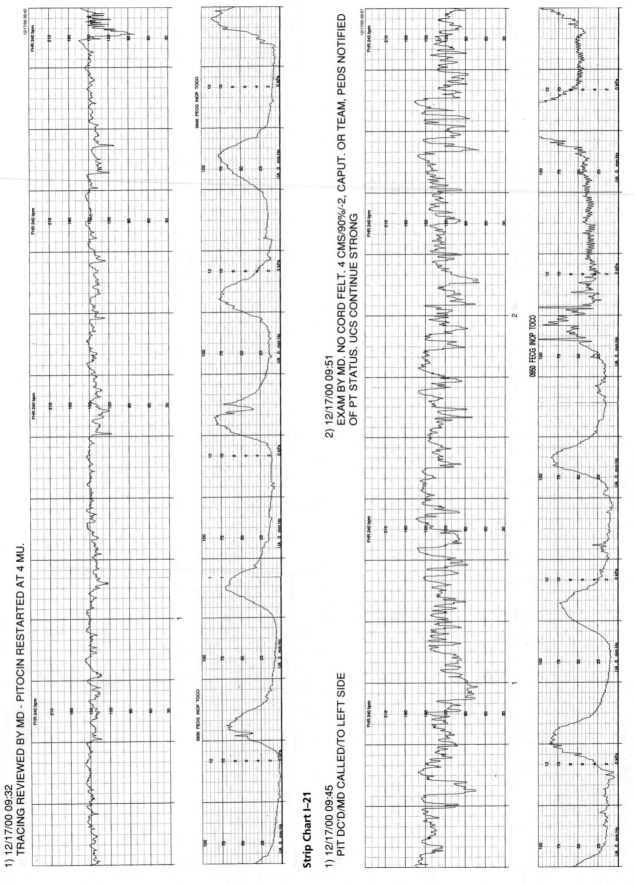

1) 12/17/00 09:32
TRACING REVIEWED BY MD - PITOCIN RESTARTED AT 4 MU.

Strip Chart I-21

1) 12/17/00 09:45
PIT DC'D/MD CALLED/TO LEFT SIDE

2) 12/17/00 09:51
EXAM BY MD. NO CORD FELT. 4 CMS/90%/-2, CAPUT. OR TEAM, PEDS NOTIFIED
OF PT STATUS. UCS CONTINUE STRONG

Strip Chart I-22

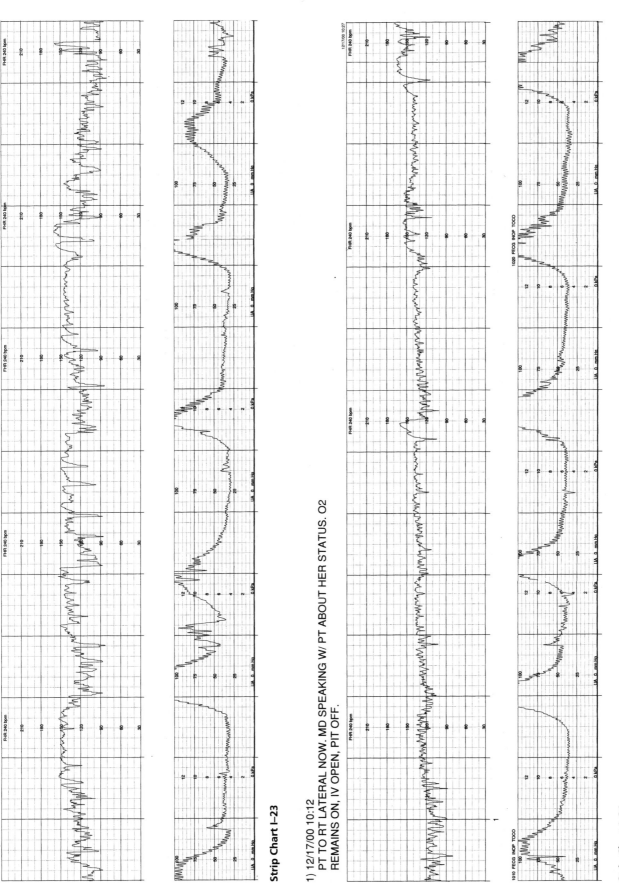

Strip Chart I-23

1) 12/17/00 10:12
PT TO RT LATERAL NOW. MD SPEAKING W/ PT ABOUT HER STATUS. O2
REMAINS ON, IV OPEN, PIT OFF.

Strip Chart I-24

1) 12/17/00 10:27
FOLEY INSERTED, PT RETURNED TO RIGHT SIDE. FOLEY W/ 900 CC CLEAR, PALE RETURN ON INSERTION AND CONTINUING TO DRAIN.

2) 12/17/00 10:34
SCALP STIM BY MD. 4 CMS/90%/-2. EXAM UNCHANGED. RESULTS EXPLAINED TO PT, CONSENT SIGNED.

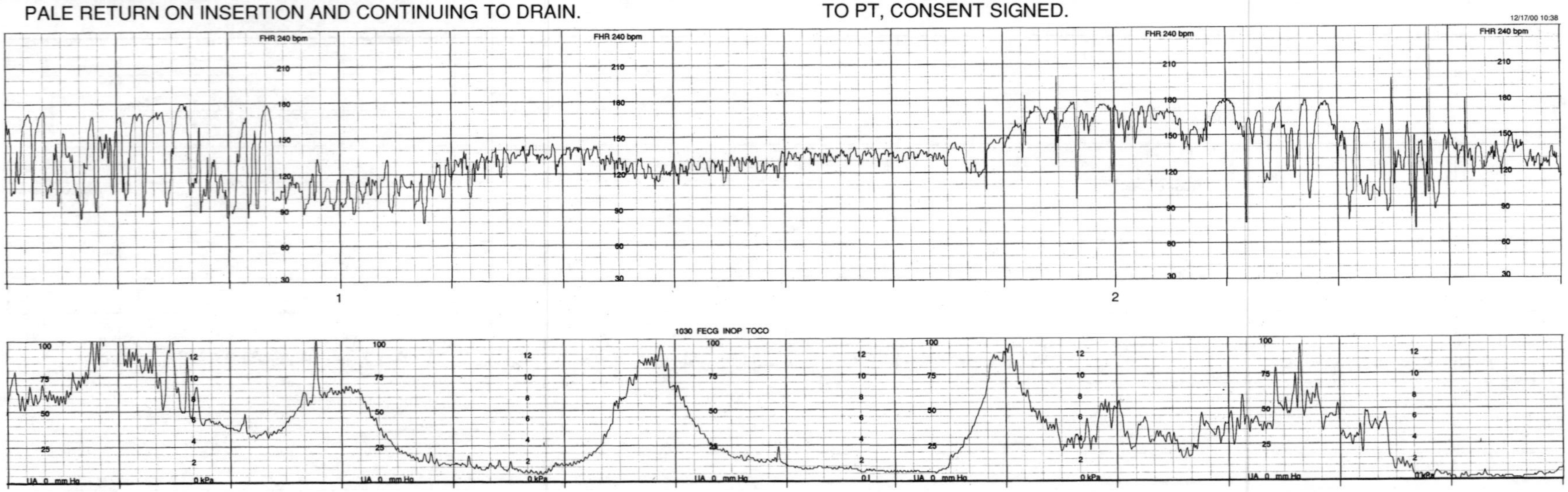

Strip Chart I-25

1) 12/17/00 10:39
PT PREPPED FOR C/S.

2) 12/17/00 10:48
116/118 EXTERNAL INOP TOCO 116/118 INOP INOP TOCO VE- NO PROGRESS. SPIRAL ELECTRODE REMOVED, PT TURNED TO HER SIDE

3) 12/17/00 10:52 TO OR #2.

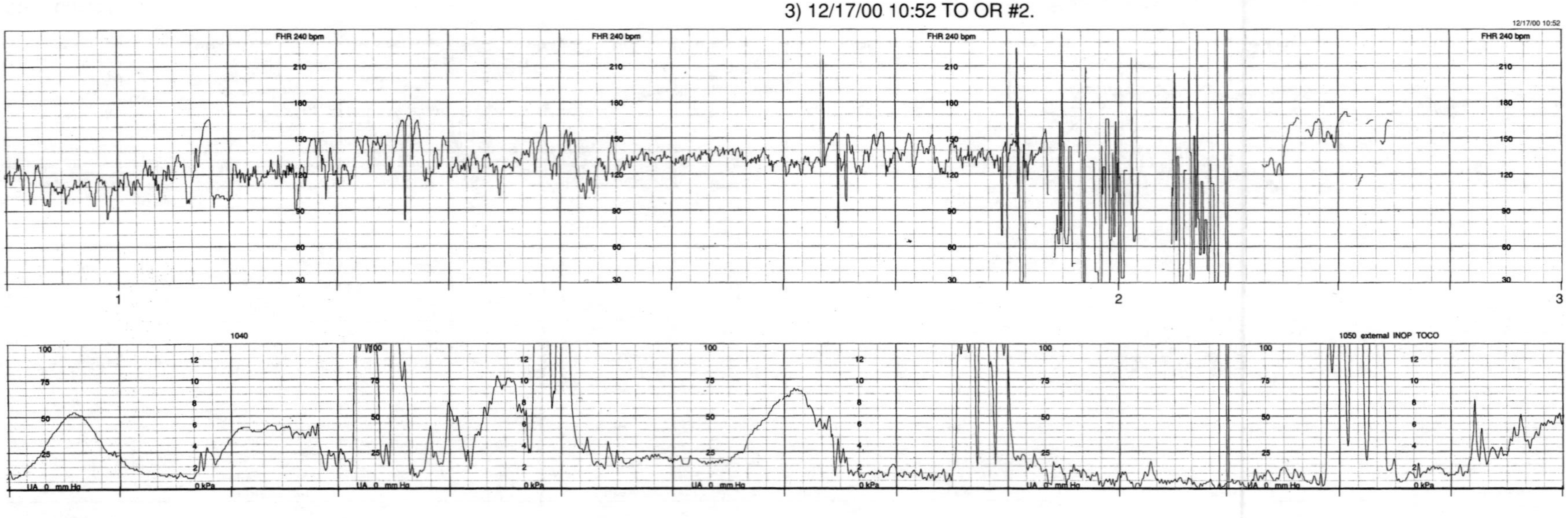

Strip Chart I-26

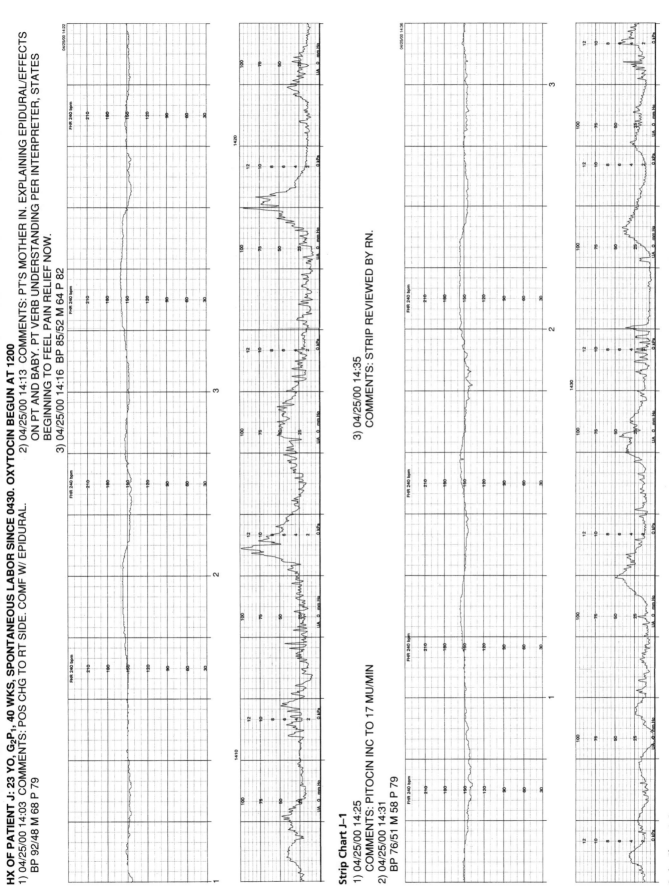

HX OF PATIENT J: 23 YO, G₂P₁, 40 WKS, SPONTANEOUS LABOR SINCE 0430. OXYTOCIN BEGUN AT 1200

1) 04/25/00 14:03 COMMENTS: POS CHG TO RT SIDE. COMF W/ EPIDURAL.
   BP 92/48 M 68 P 79

2) 04/25/00 14:13 COMMENTS: PT'S MOTHER IN. EXPLAINING EPIDURAL/EFFECTS
   ON PT AND BABY. PT VERB UNDERSTANDING PER INTERPRETER, STATES
   BEGINNING TO FEEL PAIN RELIEF NOW.

3) 04/25/00 14:16 BP 85/52 M 64 P 82

Strip Chart J–1

1) 04/25/00 14:25
   COMMENTS: PITOCIN INC TO 17 MU/MIN

2) 04/25/00 14:31
   BP 76/51 M 58 P 79

3) 04/25/00 14:35
   COMMENTS: STRIP REVIEWED BY RN.

Strip Chart J–2

1) 04/25/00 14:42 COMMENTS: REMAINS ON RT SIDE. COMF W/ EPIDURAL. NO C/O
R 18 PITOCIN AT 17 MU/MIN. CTX MODERATE.
2) 04/25/00 14:44 STRIP REVIEWED BY MD 2. BP 95/50 M 65 P 82
3) 04/25/00 14:45 MARK

4) 04/25/00 14:46 COMMENTS: SCALP STIM AT MARK BY DR 2 CX 5/100/0 W/
MOLDING AT +2
5) 04/25/00 14:48 COMMENTS: AROM AND SPIRAL APPLIED BY MD. REPOS TO
LEFT SIDE. LT MEC NOTED. 116/118 FECG EXTERNAL TOCO
6) 04/25/00 14:49 116/118 FECG INOP TOCO

Strip Chart J-3

1) 04/25/00 14:57
COMMENTS: DR REMAINS IN ROOM/ POS CHG TO RT SIDE. UCS STRONG/MOD
2) 04/25/00 15:00
BP 97/57 M 73 P 93

3) 04/25/00 15:01
COMMENTS: PITOCIN OFF PER DR 2 FOR 20 MIN.
4) 04/25/00 15:02
O2 L/MIN @ 8

Strip Chart J-4

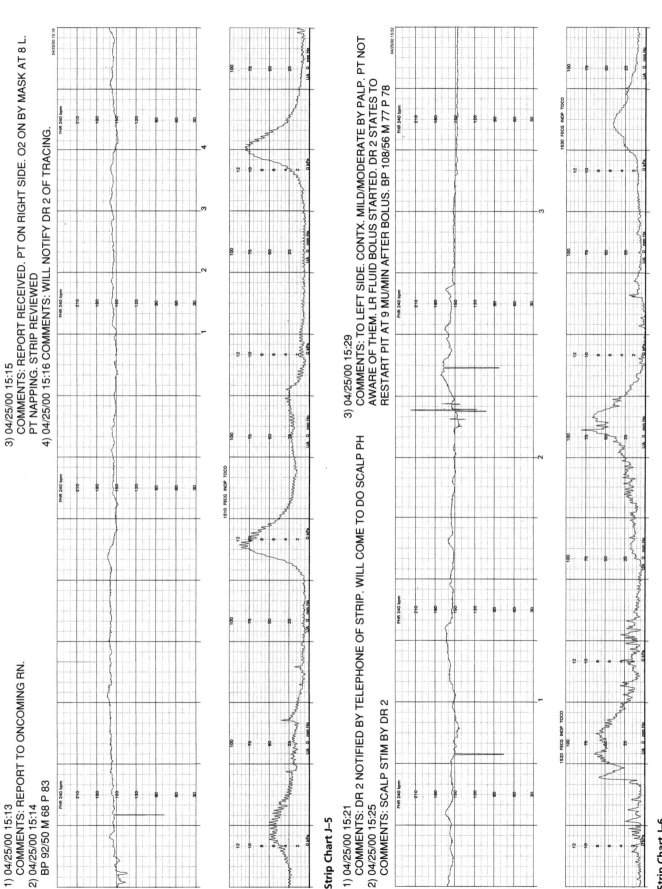

1) 04/25/00 15:13
COMMENTS: REPORT TO ONCOMING RN.
2) 04/25/00 15:14
BP 92/50 M 68 P 83

3) 04/25/00 15:15
COMMENTS: REPORT RECEIVED. PT ON RIGHT SIDE. O2 ON BY MASK AT 8 L.
PT NAPPING. STRIP REVIEWED
4) 04/25/00 15:16 COMMENTS: WILL NOTIFY DR 2 OF TRACING.

Strip Chart J-5

1) 04/25/00 15:21
COMMENTS: DR 2 NOTIFIED BY TELEPHONE OF STRIP. WILL COME TO DO SCALP PH
2) 04/25/00 15:25
COMMENTS: SCALP STIM BY DR 2

3) 04/25/00 15:29
COMMENTS: TO LEFT SIDE. CONTX. MILD/MODERATE BY PALP. PT NOT
AWARE OF THEM. LR FLUID BOLUS STARTED. DR 2 STATES TO
RESTART PIT AT 9 MU/MIN AFTER BOLUS. BP 108/56 M 77 P 78

Strip Chart J-6

1) 04/25/00 15:34
COMMENTS: STRIP REVIEWED BY CHARGE RN. SHE SPOKE WITH MD 1, CHIEF RESIDENT, AND HE AGREES WITH MD 2 TO RESTART PIT. AFTER BOLUS LR BOLUS CONTINUES.

2) 04/25/00 15:44
BP 99/56 M 73 P 80

Strip Chart J-7

1) 04/25/00 15:49
COMMENTS: TEMP. 100.0 PO

2) 04/25/00 15:51
COMMENTS: SCALP STIM BY DR 2.

3) 04/25/00 15:52 COMMENTS: PIT RESTARTED AT 9 MU/MIN PER DR 2.

4) 04/25/00 15:53
COMMENTS: DR 2 AWARE OF PT'S TEMP. MILD/MOD PALP, SOFT BETWEEN CTX.

5) 04/25/00 15:59 BP 107/65 M 82 P 94

Strip Chart J-8

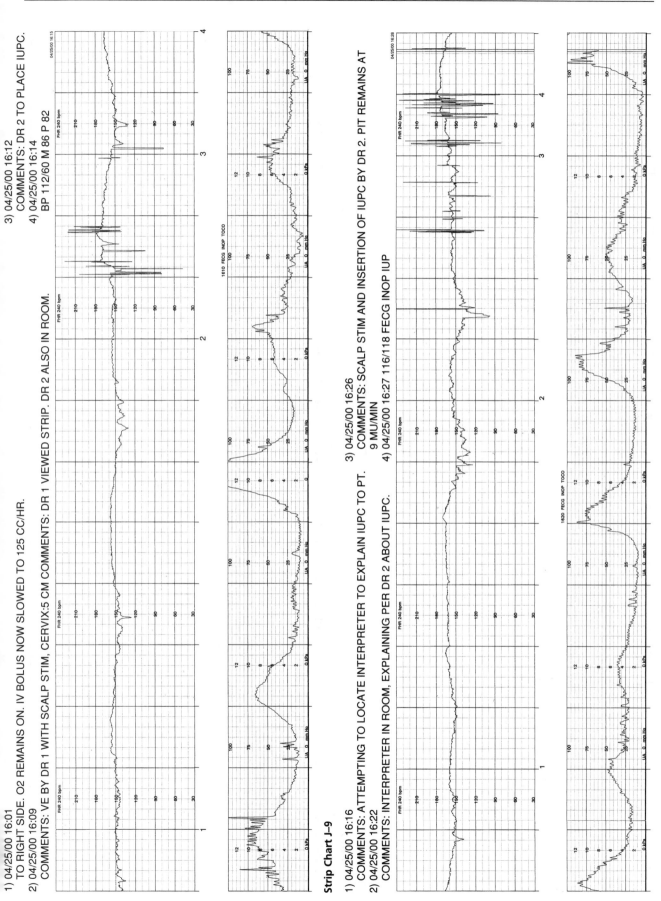

1) 04/25/00 16:01
   TO RIGHT SIDE. O2 REMAINS ON. IV BOLUS NOW SLOWED TO 125 CC/HR.
2) 04/25/00 16:09
   COMMENTS: VE BY DR 1 WITH SCALP STIM, CERVIX:5 CM COMMENTS: DR 1 VIEWED STRIP. DR 2 ALSO IN ROOM.
3) 04/25/00 16:12
   COMMENTS: DR 2 TO PLACE IUPC.
4) 04/25/00 16:14
   BP 112/60 M 86 P 82

Strip Chart J-9

1) 04/25/00 16:16
   COMMENTS: ATTEMPTING TO LOCATE INTERPRETER TO EXPLAIN IUPC TO PT.
2) 04/25/00 16:22
   COMMENTS: INTERPRETER IN ROOM, EXPLAINING PER DR 2 ABOUT IUPC.
3) 04/25/00 16:26
   COMMENTS: SCALP STIM AND INSERTION OF IUPC BY DR 2. PIT REMAINS AT
   9 MU/MIN
4) 04/25/00 16:27 116/118 FECG INOP IUP

Strip Chart J-10

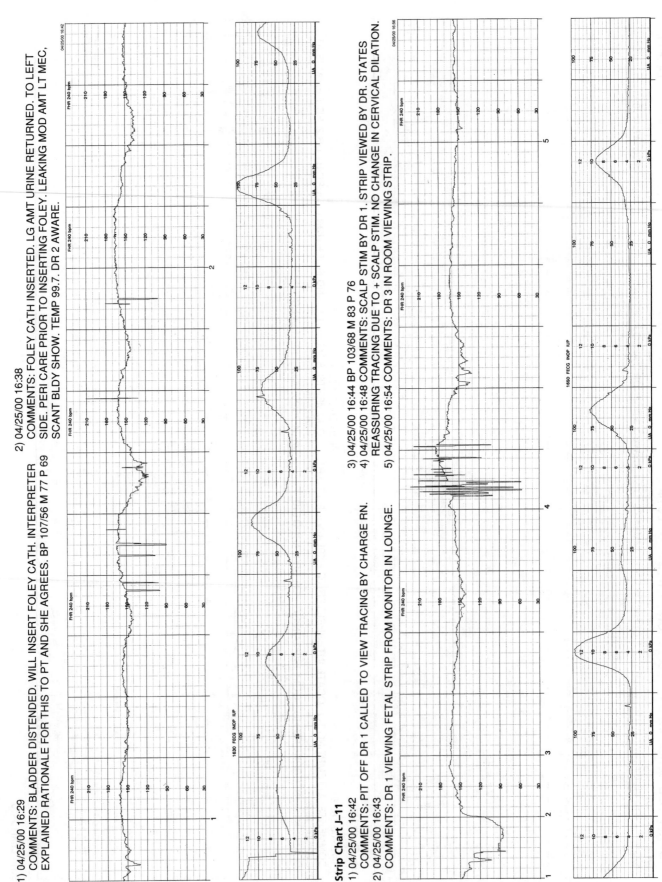

1) 04/25/00 16:29
COMMENTS: BLADDER DISTENDED. WILL INSERT FOLEY CATH. INTERPRETER EXPLAINED RATIONALE FOR THIS TO PT AND SHE AGREES. BP 107/56 M 77 P 69

2) 04/25/00 16:38
COMMENTS: FOLEY CATH INSERTED. LG AMT URINE RETURNED. TO LEFT SIDE. PERI CARE PRIOR TO INSERTING FOLEY. LEAKING MOD AMT LT MEC, SCANT BLDY SHOW. TEMP 99.7. DR 2 AWARE.

Strip Chart J-11

1) 04/25/00 16:42
COMMENTS: PIT OFF DR 1 CALLED TO VIEW TRACING BY CHARGE RN.

2) 04/25/00 16:43
COMMENTS: DR 1 VIEWING FETAL STRIP FROM MONITOR IN LOUNGE.

3) 04/25/00 16:44 BP 103/68 M 83 P 76

4) 04/25/00 16:48 COMMENTS: SCALP STIM BY DR 1. STRIP VIEWED BY DR. DR. STATES REASSURING TRACING DUE TO + SCALP STIM. NO CHANGE IN CERVICAL DILATION.

5) 04/25/00 16:54 COMMENTS: DR 3 IN ROOM VIEWING STRIP.

Strip Chart J-12

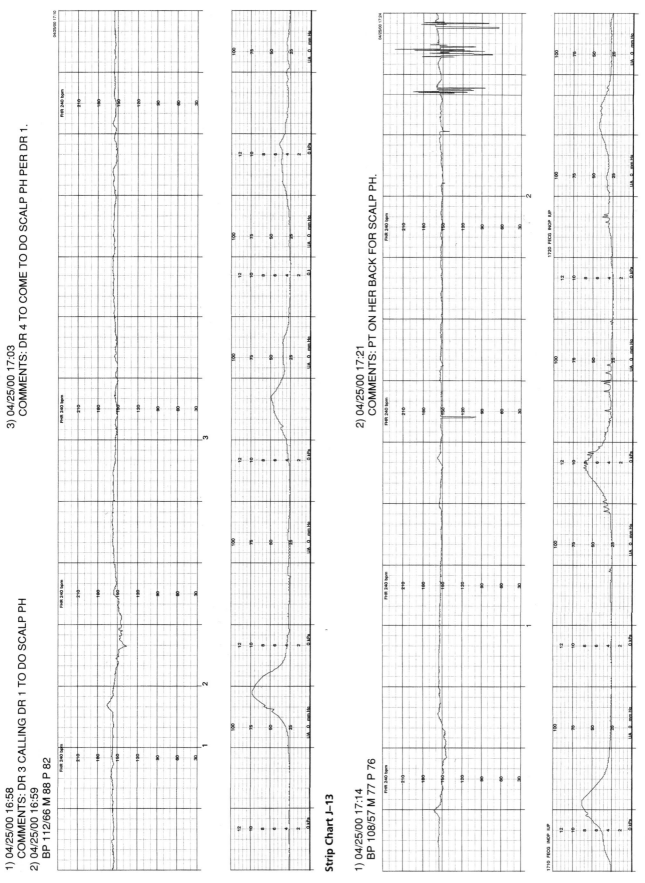

1) 04/25/00 16:58
    COMMENTS: DR 3 CALLING DR 1 TO DO SCALP PH
2) 04/25/00 16:59
    BP 112/66 M 88 P 82

3) 04/25/00 17:03
    COMMENTS: DR 4 TO COME TO DO SCALP PH PER DR 1.

Strip Chart J–13

1) 04/25/00 17:14
    BP 108/57 M 77 P 76

2) 04/25/00 17:21
    COMMENTS: PT ON HER BACK FOR SCALP PH.

Strip Chart J–14

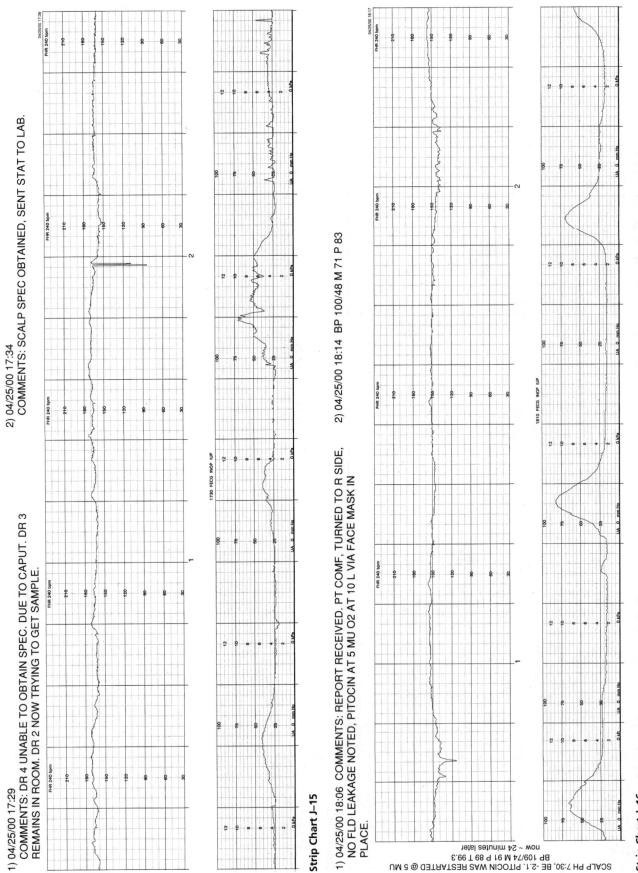

1) 04/25/00 17:29
COMMENTS: DR 4 UNABLE TO OBTAIN SPEC. DUE TO CAPUT. DR 3 REMAINS IN ROOM. DR 2 NOW TRYING TO GET SAMPLE.

2) 04/25/00 17:34
COMMENTS: SCALP SPEC OBTAINED, SENT STAT TO LAB.

Strip Chart J-15

1) 04/25/00 18:06 COMMENTS: REPORT RECEIVED. PT COMF, TURNED TO R SIDE, NO FLD LEAKAGE NOTED, PITOCIN AT 5 MU O2 AT 10 L VIA FACE MASK IN PLACE.

2) 04/25/00 18:14 BP 100/48 M 71 P 83

SCALP PH 7.30, BE -2.1, PITOCIN WAS RESTARTED @ 5 MU
BP 109/74 M 91 P 89 T 99.3
now ~ 24 minutes later

Strip Chart J-16

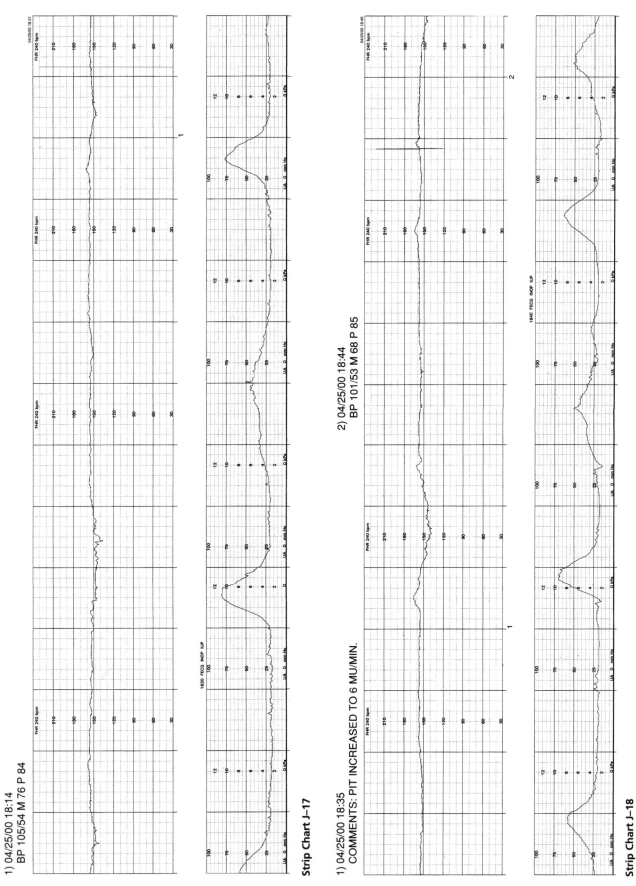

1) 04/25/00 18:14
BP 105/54 M 76 P 84

Strip Chart J-17

1) 04/25/00 18:35
COMMENTS: PIT INCREASED TO 6 MU/MIN.

2) 04/25/00 18:44
BP 101/53 M 68 P 85

Strip Chart J-18

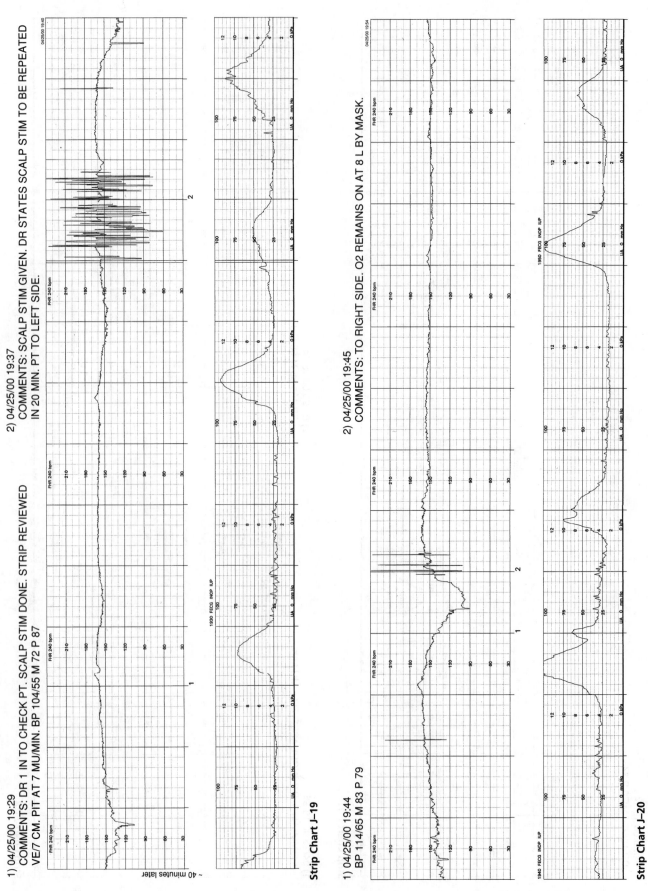

1) 04/25/00 19:29
COMMENTS: DR 1 IN TO CHECK PT. SCALP STIM DONE. STRIP REVIEWED
VE/7 CM. PIT AT 7 MU/MIN. BP 104/55 M 72 P 87

2) 04/25/00 19:37
COMMENTS: SCALP STIM GIVEN. DR STATES SCALP STIM TO BE REPEATED
IN 20 MIN. PT TO LEFT SIDE.

~ 40 minutes later

Strip Chart J-19

1) 04/25/00 19:44
BP 114/65 M 83 P 79

2) 04/25/00 19:45
COMMENTS: TO RIGHT SIDE. O2 REMAINS ON AT 8 L BY MASK.

Strip Chart J-20

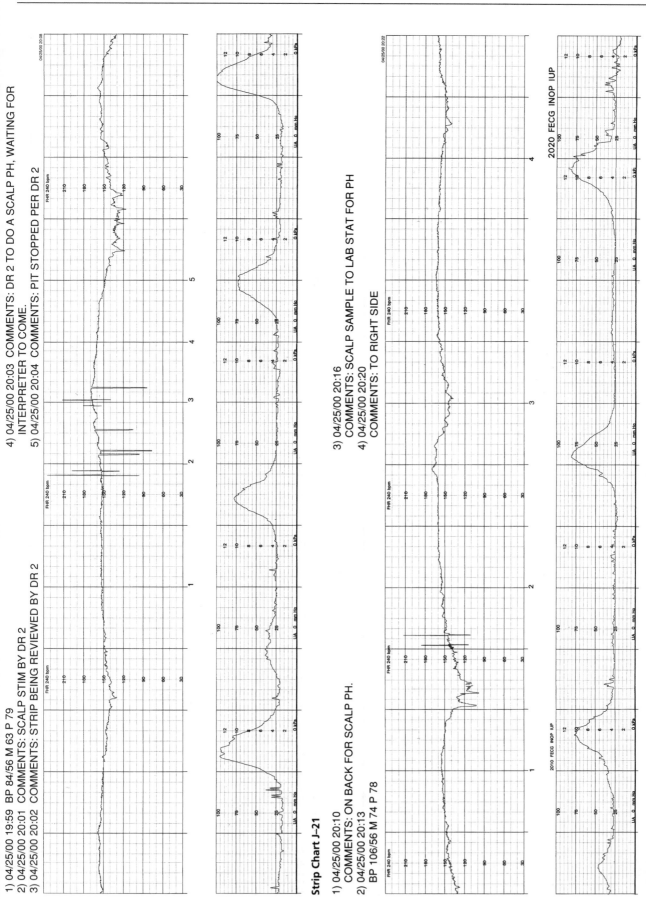

1) 04/25/00 19:59 BP 84/56 M 63 P 79
2) 04/25/00 20:01 COMMENTS: SCALP STIM BY DR 2
3) 04/25/00 20:02 COMMENTS: STRIP BEING REVIEWED BY DR 2

4) 04/25/00 20:03 COMMENTS: DR 2 TO DO A SCALP PH, WAITING FOR
                   INTERPRETER TO COME.
5) 04/25/00 20:04 COMMENTS: PIT STOPPED PER DR 2

Strip Chart J-21

1) 04/25/00 20:10
   COMMENTS: ON BACK FOR SCALP PH.
2) 04/25/00 20:13
   BP 106/56 M 74 P 78

3) 04/25/00 20:16
   COMMENTS: SCALP SAMPLE TO LAB STAT FOR PH
4) 04/25/00 20:20
   COMMENTS: TO RIGHT SIDE

Strip Chart J-22

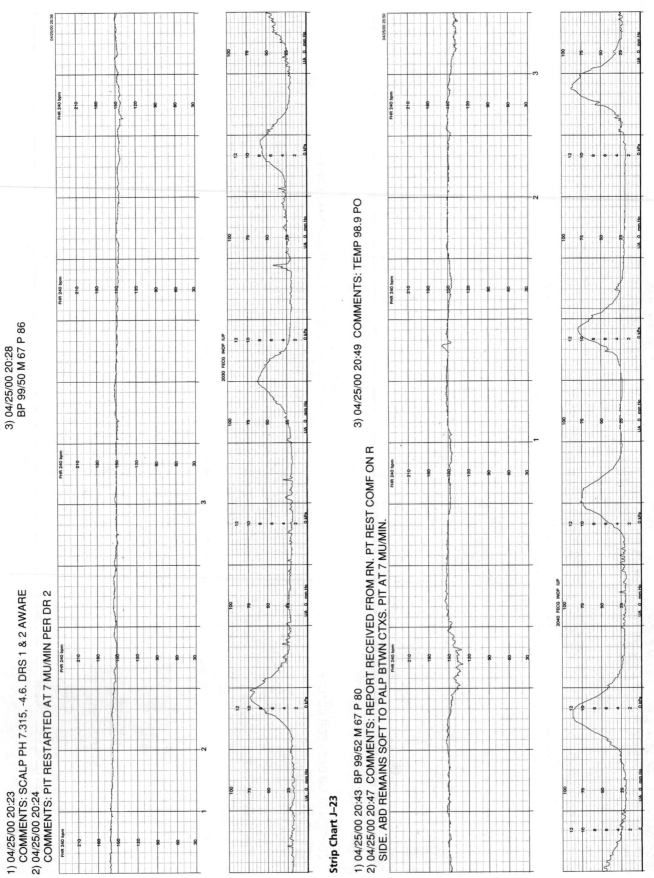

1) 04/25/00 20:23
   COMMENTS: SCALP PH 7.315, -4.6. DRS 1 & 2 AWARE
2) 04/25/00 20:24
   COMMENTS: PIT RESTARTED AT 7 MU/MIN PER DR 2

3) 04/25/00 20:28
   BP 99/50 M 67 P 86

Strip Chart J-23

1) 04/25/00 20:43 BP 99/52 M 67 P 80
2) 04/25/00 20:47 COMMENTS: REPORT RECEIVED FROM RN. PT REST COMF ON R
   SIDE. ABD REMAINS SOFT TO PALP BTWN CTXS. PIT AT 7 MU/MIN.

3) 04/25/00 20:49 COMMENTS: TEMP 98.9 PO

Strip Chart J-24

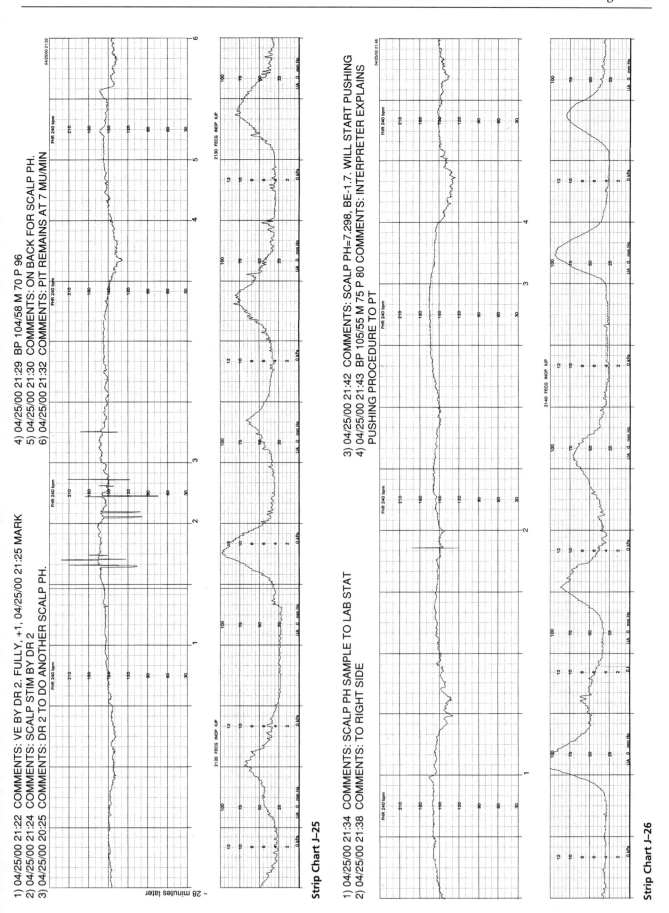

1) 04/25/00 21:22 COMMENTS: VE BY DR 2. FULLY, +1, 04/25/00 21:25 MARK
2) 04/25/00 21:24 COMMENTS: SCALP STIM BY DR 2
3) 04/25/00 20:25 COMMENTS: DR 2 TO DO ANOTHER SCALP PH.

4) 04/25/00 21:29 BP 104/58 M 70 P 96
5) 04/25/00 21:30 COMMENTS: ON BACK FOR SCALP PH.
6) 04/25/00 21:32 COMMENTS: PIT REMAINS AT 7 MU/MIN

Strip Chart J-25

1) 04/25/00 21:34 COMMENTS: SCALP PH SAMPLE TO LAB STAT
2) 04/25/00 21:38 COMMENTS: TO RIGHT SIDE

3) 04/25/00 21:42 COMMENTS: SCALP PH=7.298, BE-1.7. WILL START PUSHING
4) 04/25/00 21:43 BP 105/55 M 75 P 80 COMMENTS: INTERPRETER EXPLAINS
PUSHING PROCEDURE TO PT

Strip Chart J-26

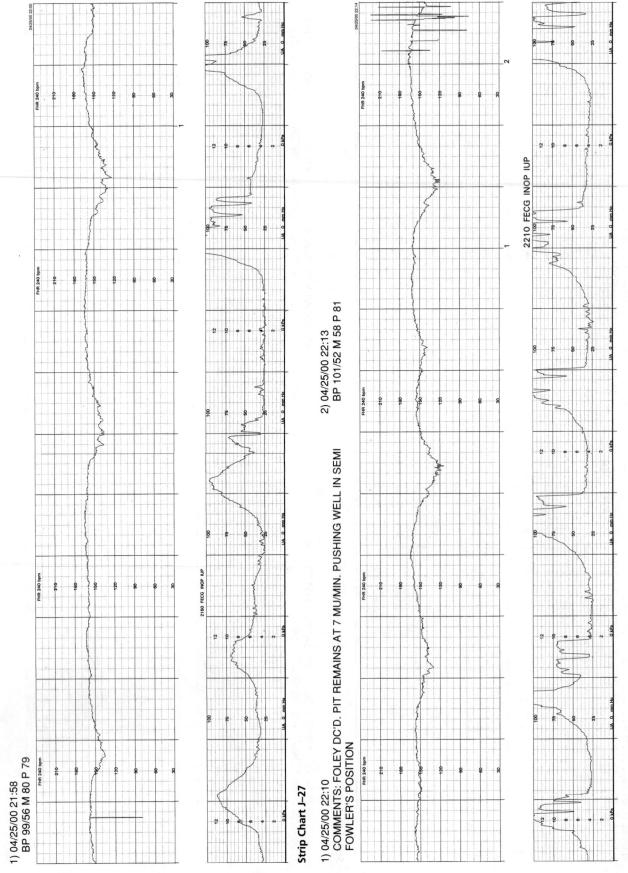

1) 04/25/00 21:58
   BP 99/56 M 80 P 79

Strip Chart J–27

1) 04/25/00 22:10
   COMMENTS: FOLEY DC'D. PIT REMAINS AT 7 MU/MIN. PUSHING WELL IN SEMI
   FOWLER'S POSITION

2) 04/25/00 22:13
   BP 101/52 M 58 P 81

Strip Chart J–28

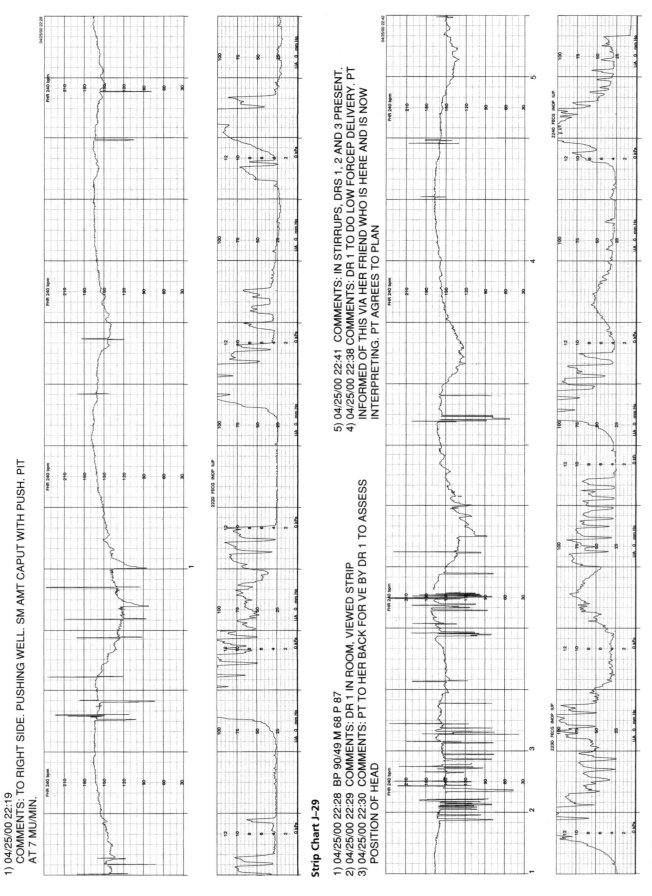

1) 04/25/00 22:19
COMMENTS: TO RIGHT SIDE. PUSHING WELL. SM AMT CAPUT WITH PUSH. PIT
AT 7 MU/MIN.

Strip Chart J-29

1) 04/25/00 22:28   BP 90/49 M 68 P 87
2) 04/25/00 22:29   COMMENTS: DR 1 IN ROOM, VIEWED STRIP
3) 04/25/00 22:30   COMMENTS: PT TO HER BACK FOR VE BY DR 1 TO ASSESS
POSITION OF HEAD

5) 04/25/00 22:41   COMMENTS: IN STIRRUPS, DRS 1, 2 AND 3 PRESENT.
4) 04/25/00 22:38   COMMENTS: DR 1 TO DO LOW FORCEP DELIVERY. PT
INFORMED OF THIS VIA HER FRIEND WHO IS HERE AND IS NOW
INTERPRETING. PT AGREES TO PLAN

Strip Chart J-30

1) 04/25/00 22:44 BP 65/51 M 60 P 88
2) 04/25/00 22:45 COMMENTS: VE BY DR 2. SPIRAL ELECTRODE DC'D.
3) 04/25/00 22:46 COMMENTS: IUPC OUT.
4) 04/25/00 22:48 COMMENTS: FORCEPS ARE BEING APPLIED BY DR 2 AND 1.
   116/118 EXTERNAL INOP TOCO

5) 04/25/00 22:52 COMMENTS: TEMP 100.1 PO
6) 04/25/00 22:54 COMMENTS: FORCEPS OFF. COMMENTS: HEAD OUT. HEAD
   DELIVERED @ 2255 DELEE NOSE & MOUTH.
7) 04/25/00 22:55 PEDS PRESENT FOR DELIVERY; FEMALE

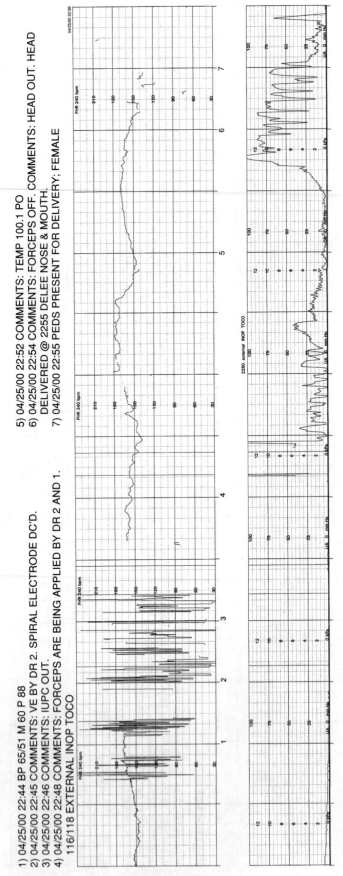

Strip Chart J-31

1) 12/18/99 09:03 COMMENTS: 26 YR OLD G2P0 AT 39 WKS, VTX/VTX TWINS
   PRES FOR INDUCTION. PT WAS 4 CM IN OFFICE ON MONDAY, EXPECTS
   MECHANICAL INDUCTION. DR IN TO SCAN PT, BABIES ARE STILL VTX/VTX
2) 12/18/99 09:05 COMMENTS: PT ADMITTED AND ORIENTED PER STANDARD

3) 12/18/99 09:11 STRIP REVIEWED BY MD BP121/84 M 97 P 88
4) 12/18/99 09:12 MARK
5) 12/18/99 09:14 COMMENTS: VE BY CNM AT MARK. 4/70...AROM FOR CL FLUID
   AT MARK. PT TOLERATES WELL...IF TRACING REASSURING MAY AMBULATE.
   PT AWARE AND AGREES

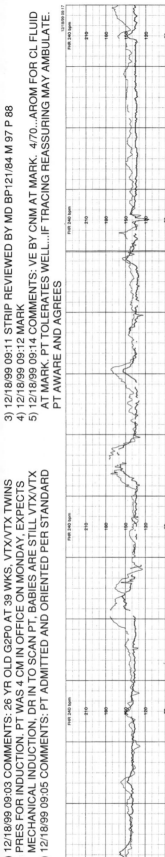

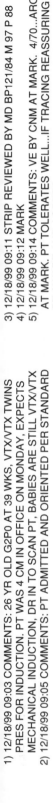

Strip Chart K–1

1) 12/18/99 20:30
   BP 95/61 M 71 P 112
   COMMENTS: PT SLEEPING SOUNDLY.

~ 11 hours later

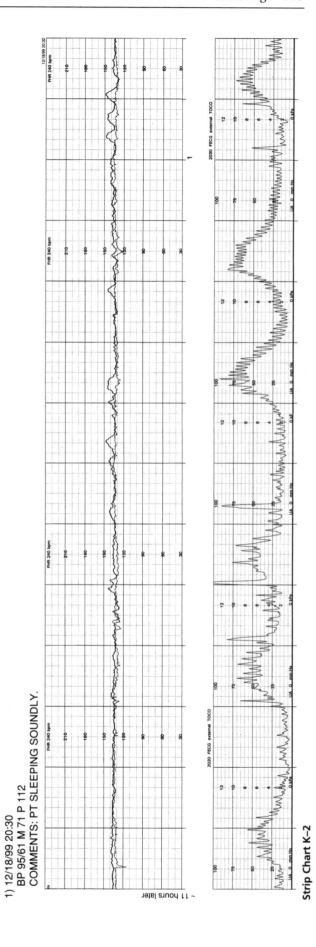

Strip Chart K–2

1) 12/18/99 20:35
MODERATE TO PALPATION; COMMENTS: PT REMAINS COMFORTABLE ON R
SIDE PITOCIN REMAINS @ 4 MU/MIN SM MEC FLUID WITH + B SHOW NOTED;
T 98.5 PO; STRIP REVIEWED BY RN; SIDERAILS UP; CALL BELL IN REACH.

2) 12/18/99 20:45
BP 98/60 M 71 P 106

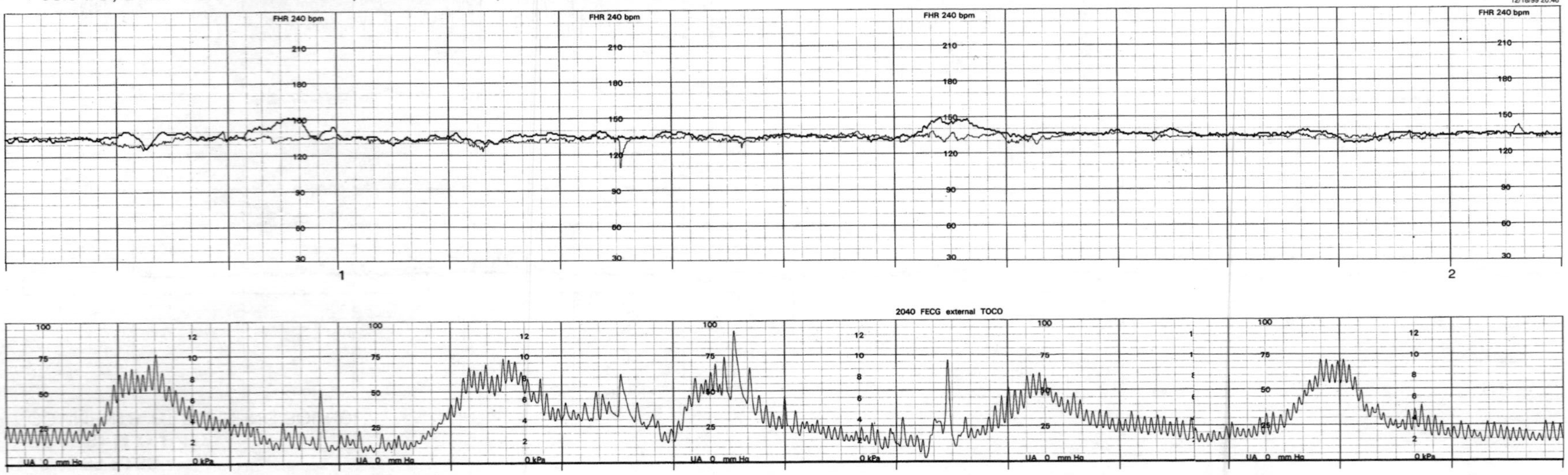

Strip Chart K-3

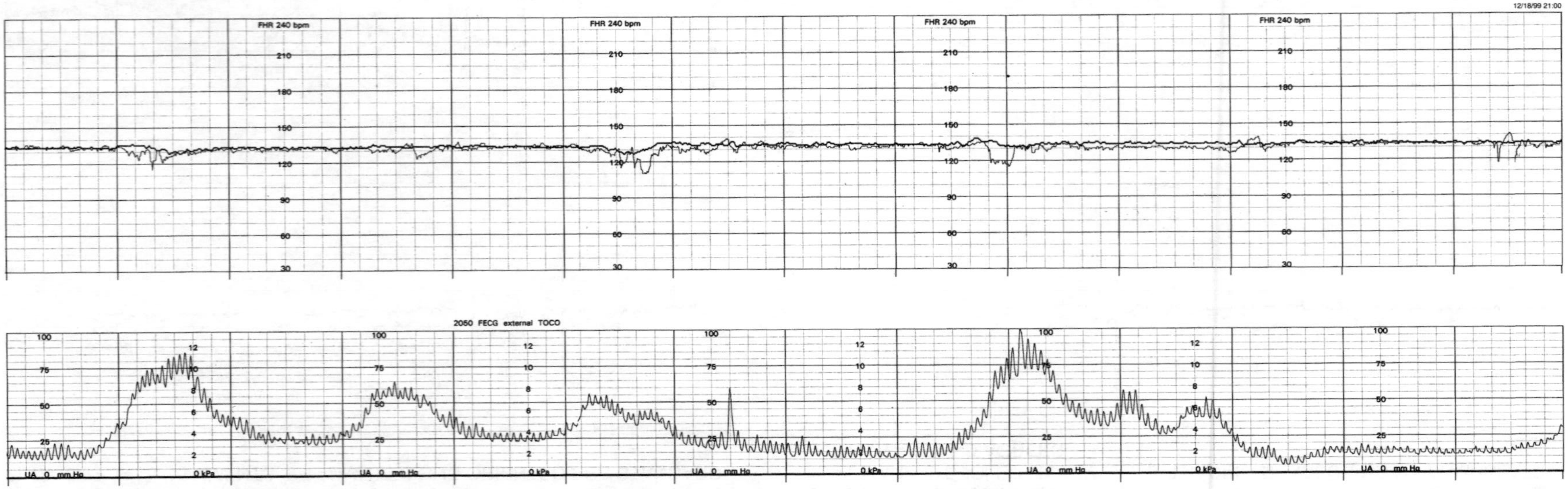

Strip Chart K-4

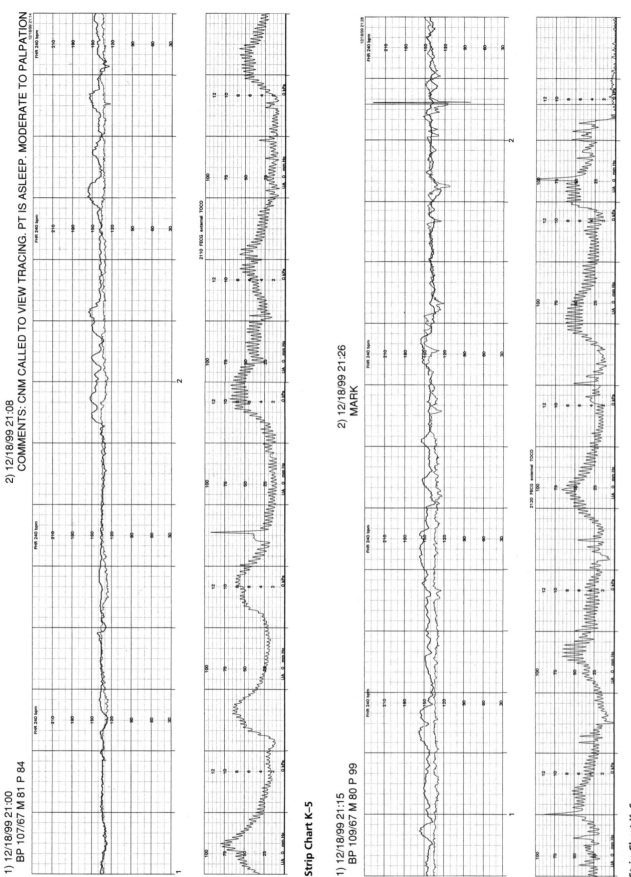

1) 12/18/99 21:00
BP 107/67 M 81 P 84

2) 12/18/99 21:08
COMMENTS: CNM CALLED TO VIEW TRACING. PT IS ASLEEP. MODERATE TO PALPATION

Strip Chart K-5

1) 12/18/99 21:15
BP 109/67 M 80 P 99

2) 12/18/99 21:26
MARK

Strip Chart K-6

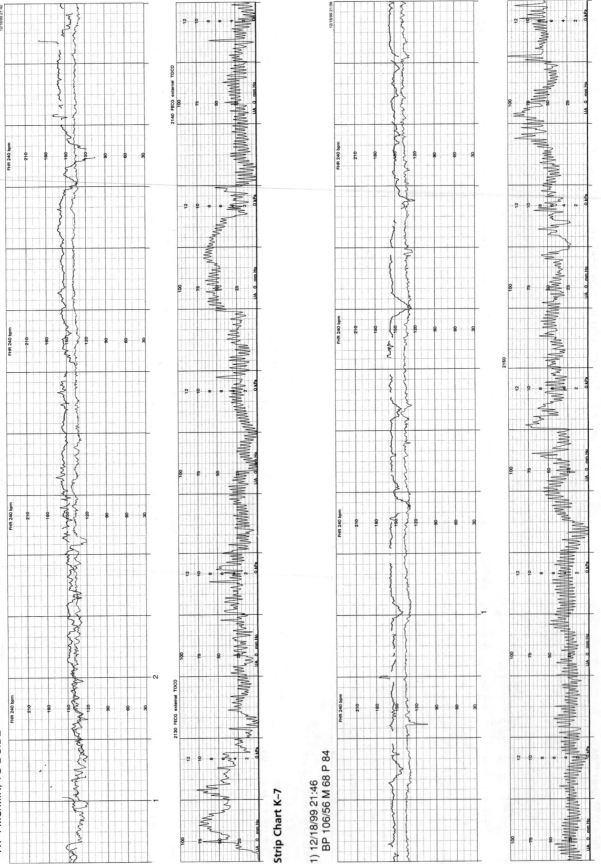

1) 12/18/99 21:29
MODERATE TO PALPATION; COMMENTS: VE AT MARK. FULLY DILATED. PT NOT
FEELING ANY PRESSURE OR CTX. + SHOW, NO FLUID SEEN PITOCIN REMAINS
AT 4 MU/MIN, TO L SIDE

2) 12/18/99 21:31
BP 93/50 M 61 P 94

Strip Chart K–7

1) 12/18/99 21:46
BP 106/56 M 68 P 84

Strip Chart K–8

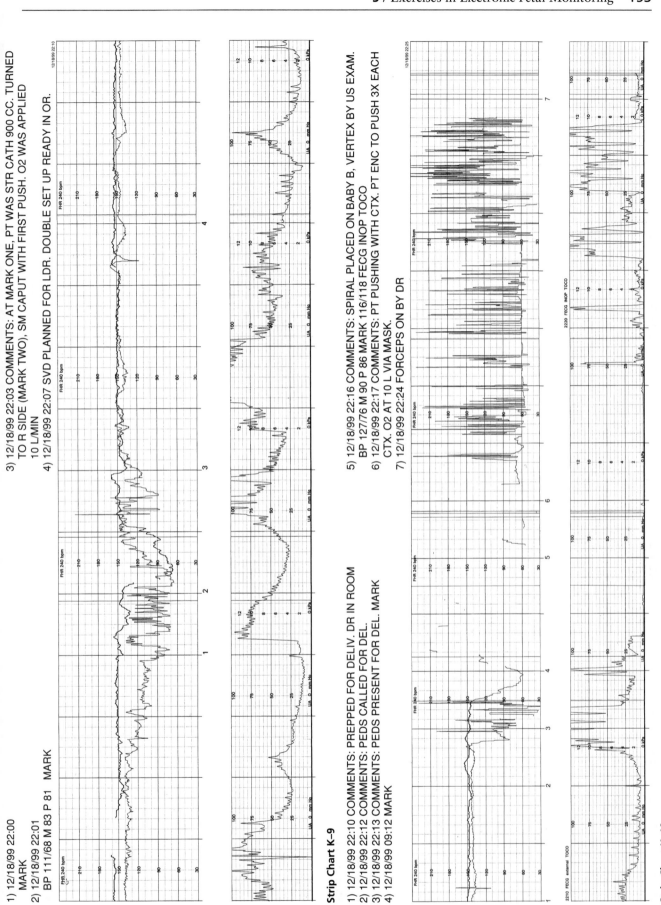

Strip Chart K-9

1) 12/18/99 22:00 MARK
2) 12/18/99 22:01 BP 111/68 M 83 P 81   MARK
3) 12/18/99 22:03 COMMENTS: AT MARK ONE, PT WAS STR CATH 900 CC. TURNED TO R SIDE (MARK TWO), SM CAPUT WITH FIRST PUSH. O2 WAS APPLIED 10 L/MIN
4) 12/18/99 22:07 SVD PLANNED FOR LDR. DOUBLE SET UP READY IN OR.

1) 12/18/99 22:10 COMMENTS: PREPPED FOR DELIV. DR IN ROOM
2) 12/18/99 22:12 COMMENTS: PEDS CALLED FOR DEL.
3) 12/18/99 22:13 COMMENTS: PEDS PRESENT FOR DEL. MARK
4) 12/18/99 09:12 MARK

5) 12/18/99 22:16 COMMENTS: SPIRAL PLACED ON BABY B, VERTEX BY US EXAM. BP 127/76 M 90 P 86 MARK 116/118 FECG INOP TOCO
6) 12/18/99 22:17 COMMENTS: PT PUSHING WITH CTX. PT ENC TO PUSH 3X EACH CTX. O2 AT 10 L VIA MASK.
7) 12/18/99 22:24 FORCEPS ON BY DR

Strip Chart K-10

HX OF PATIENT L: 36 YO, G₁P₀, 40+ WKS, ADMITTED FOR SPONTANEOUS LABOR. SROM AT 1100, CLEAR. 3 CMS ON ADMIT AT 0200.

1) 11/01/00 02:44
   POSITION CHANGE TO L SIDE. HUSBAND MASSAGING PT'S BACK. PT COPING
   W/ CTX EFFECTIVELY.

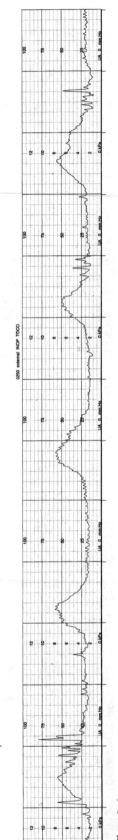

Strip Chart L-1

1) 11/01/00 03:05
   MAT PULSE 94. MONITOR ADJUSTED.

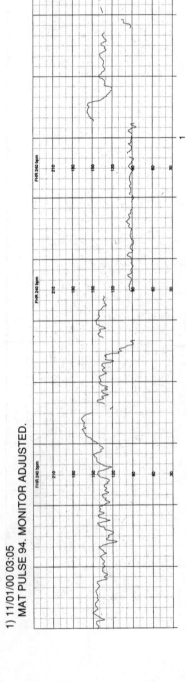

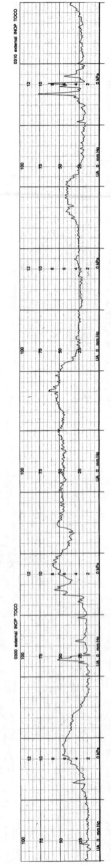

Strip Chart L-2

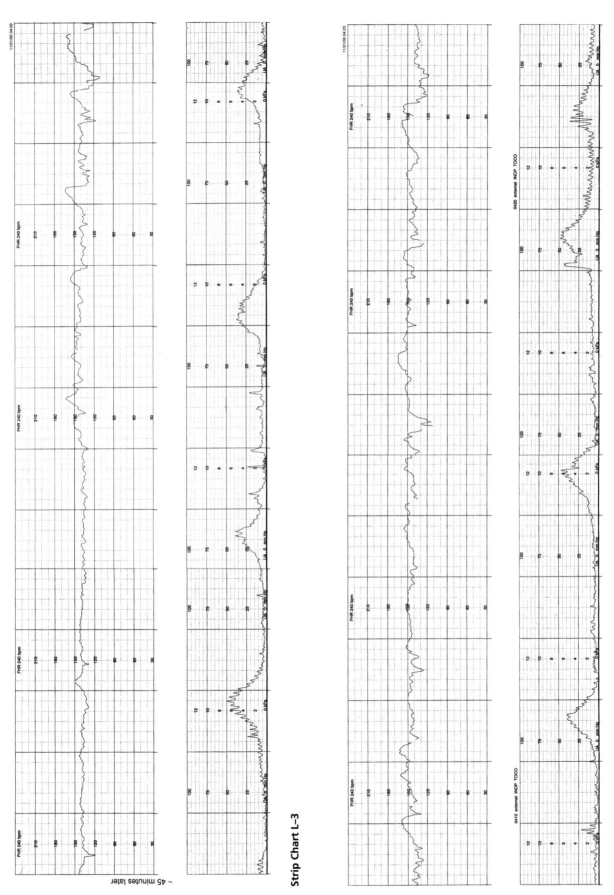

Strip Chart L–3

~ 45 minutes later

Strip Chart L–4

1) 11/01/00 05:27
BP 128/74 P 88 R 20 T 98.9. PT DOZING OFF BETWEEN CTX, USES BREATHING
TECHNIQUES DURING THEM. UCS PALPATE MILD-MODERATE WITH REST IN
BETWEEN.

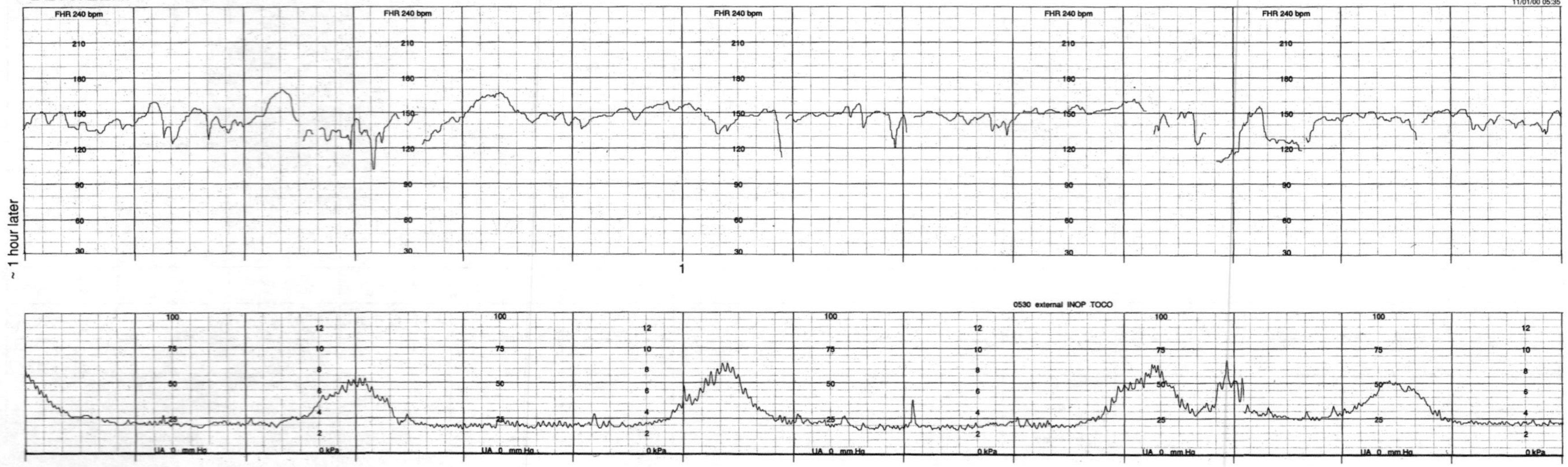

~ 1 hour later

Strip Chart L-5

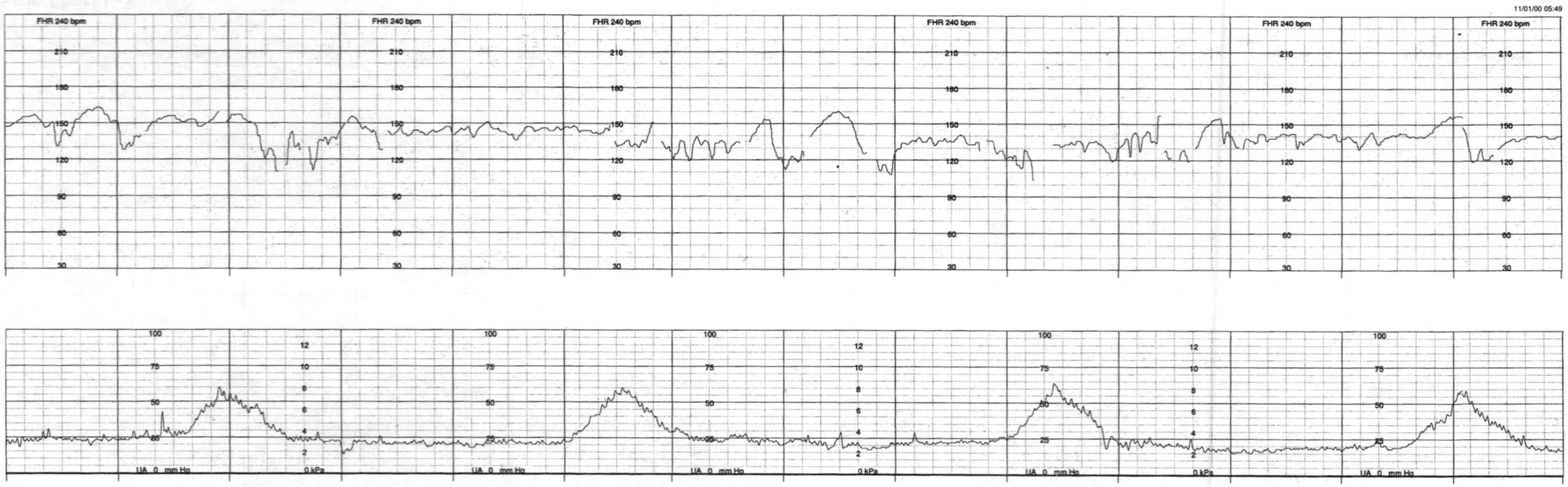

Strip Chart L-6

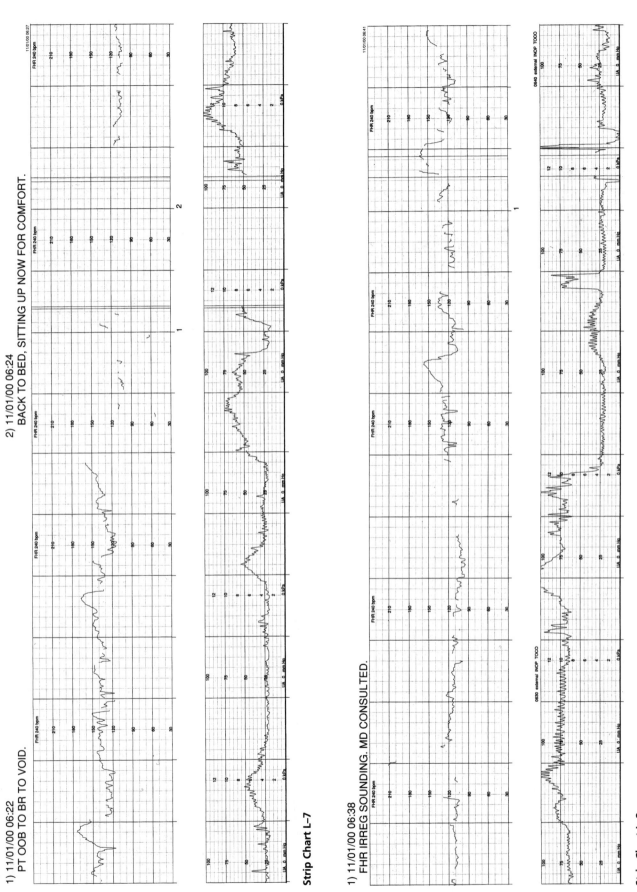

1) 11/01/00 06:22
PT OOB TO BR TO VOID.

2) 11/01/00 06:24
BACK TO BED, SITTING UP NOW FOR COMFORT.

Strip Chart L-7

1) 11/01/00 06:38
FHR IRREG SOUNDING. MD CONSULTED.

Strip Chart L-8

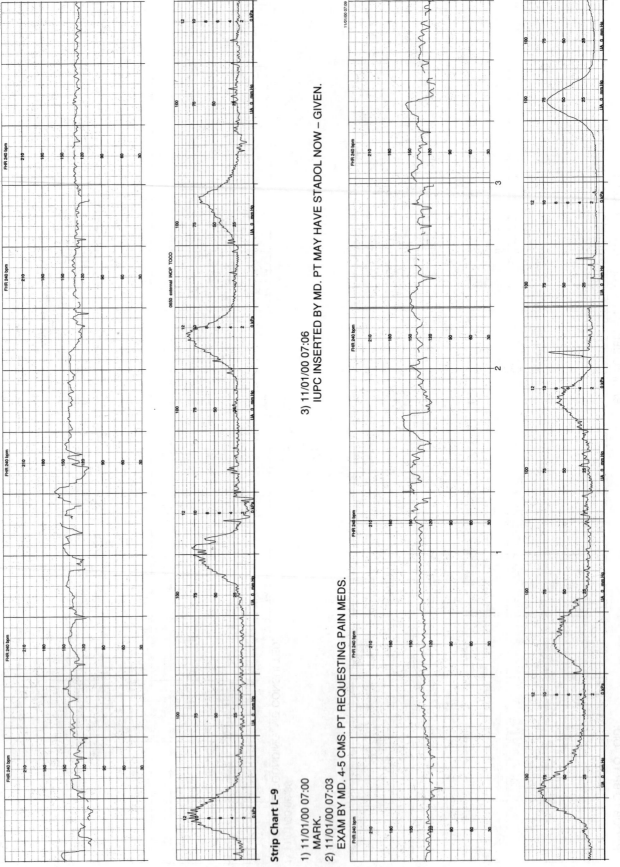

Strip Chart L-9

1) 11/01/00 07:00
   MARK.

2) 11/01/00 07:03
   EXAM BY MD. 4-5 CMS. PT REQUESTING PAIN MEDS.

3) 11/01/00 07:06
   IUPC INSERTED BY MD. PT MAY HAVE STADOL NOW – GIVEN.

Strip Chart L-10

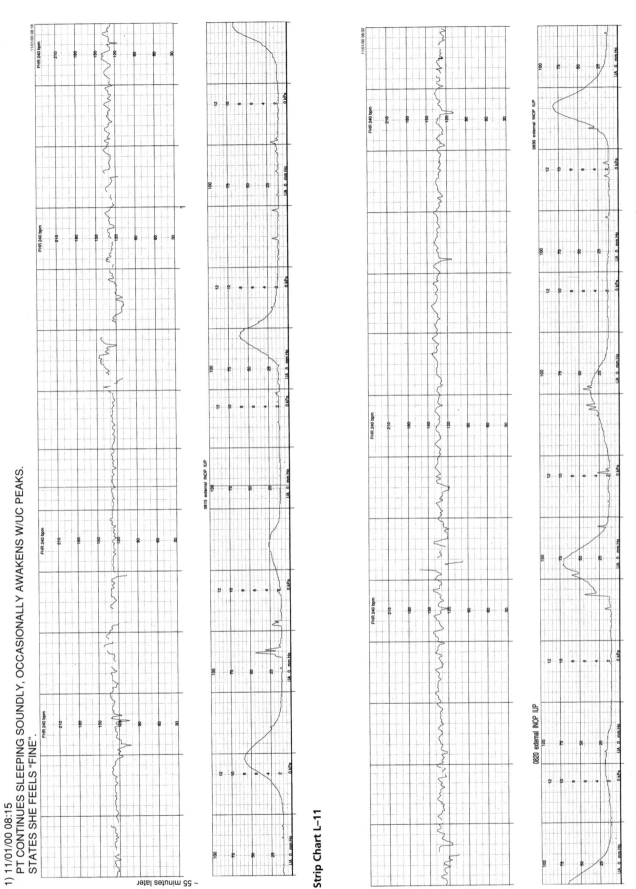

1) 11/01/00 08:15
PT CONTINUES SLEEPING SOUNDLY, OCCASIONALLY AWAKENS W/UC PEAKS.
STATES SHE FEELS "FINE".

~ 55 minutes later

Strip Chart L–11

Strip Chart L–12

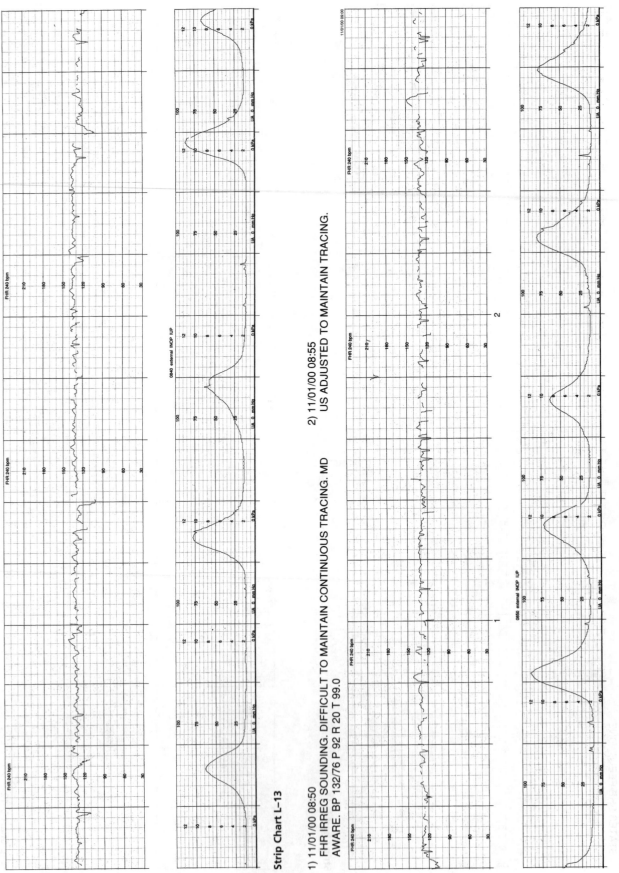

Strip Chart L–13

1) 11/01/00 08:50
FHR IRREG SOUNDING. DIFFICULT TO MAINTAIN CONTINUOUS TRACING. MD
AWARE. BP 132/76 P 92 R 20 T 99.0

2) 11/01/00 08:55
US ADJUSTED TO MAINTAIN TRACING.

Strip Chart L–14

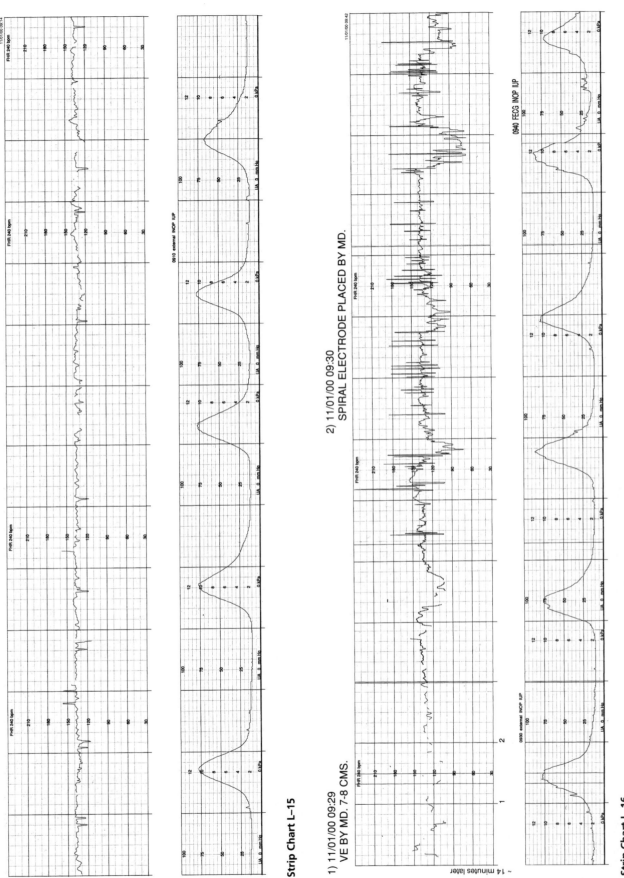

Strip Chart L–15

1) 11/01/00 09:29
VE BY MD. 7-8 CMS.

2) 11/01/00 09:30
SPIRAL ELECTRODE PLACED BY MD.

~14 minutes later

Strip Chart L–16

1) 11/01/00 09:45
PERICARE GIVEN, LINENS CHANGED. COPIOUS CLEAR FLUID W/EXAM. MD
REMAINS AT BEDSIDE OBSERVING FHR. IRREGULARITY DISCUSSED W/PT +
HUSBAND. PT TO LEFT SIDE.

2) 11/01/00 09:46
IUPC REMOVED BY MD.

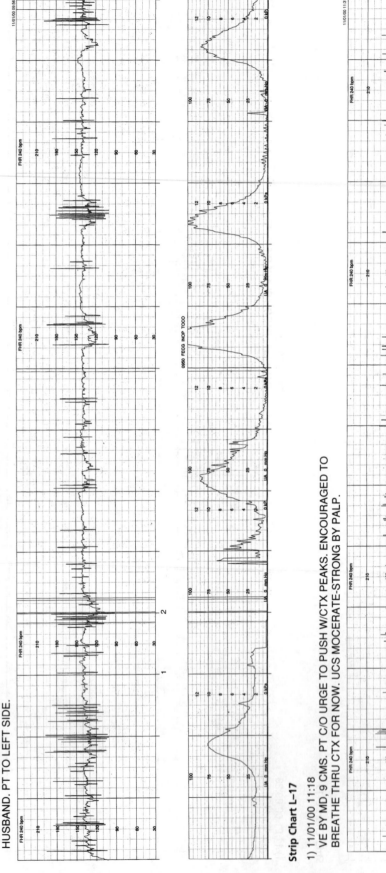

Strip Chart L-17

1) 11/01/00 11:18
VE BY MD, 9 CMS. PT C/O URGE TO PUSH W/CTX PEAKS. ENCOURAGED TO
BREATHE THRU CTX FOR NOW. UCS MOCERATE-STRONG BY PALP.

~ 1 hour 2 minutes later

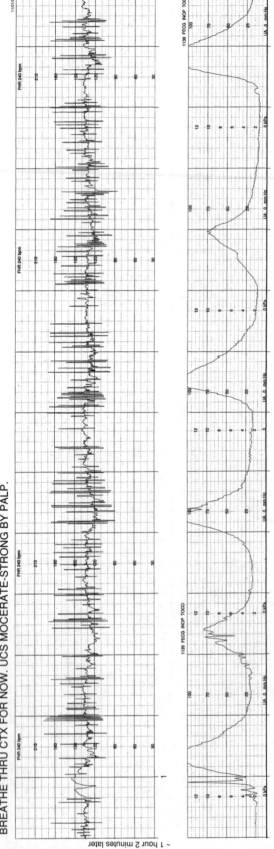

Strip Chart L-18

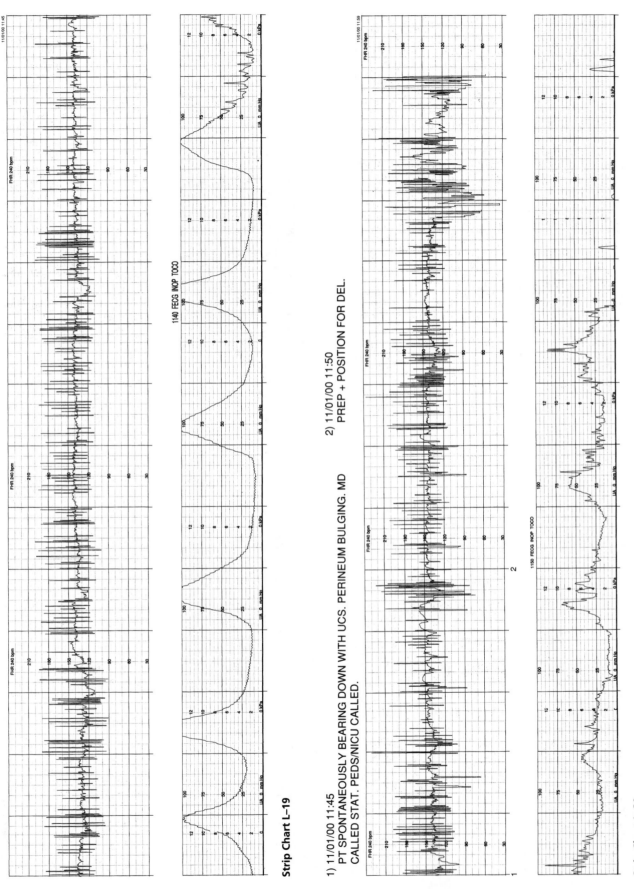

Strip Chart L-19

1) 11/01/00 11:45
PT SPONTANEOUSLY BEARING DOWN WITH UCS. PERINEUM BULGING. MD
CALLED STAT. PEDS/NICU CALLED.

2) 11/01/00 11:50   PREP + POSITION FOR DEL.

Strip Chart L-20

PATIENT M

1) 07/25/00 18:30 COMMENTS: G8 P2 40+ WKS PRESENTS TO TEST ROOM C/O CTX Q 2-3 MINS. DENIES ROM, NO FM TODAY.

2) 07/25/00 18:33 COMMENTS: DR IN TO VIEW STRIP. CONTRACTIONS PALPATE MODERATE. BP 135/77 M 98 P 82

3) 07/25/00 18:39 COMMENTS: EXAM BY DR 4/100/INTACT

4) 07/25/00 18:41 COMMENTS: TO L SIDE.

5) 07/25/00 18:42 COMMENTS: IV LR STARTED WITH 18 G IN R HAND; BLOOD WORK OBTAINED AND SENT.

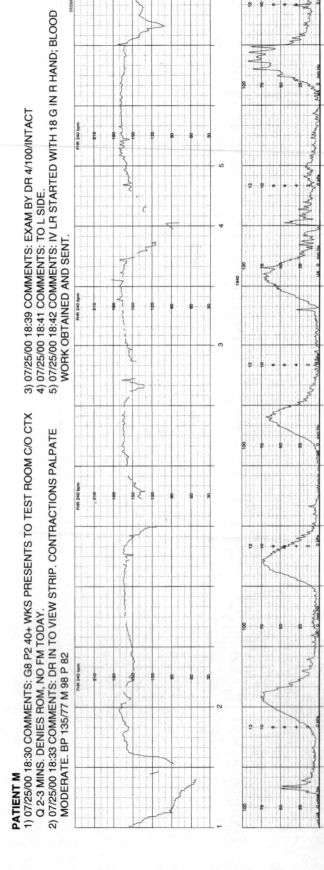

Strip Chart M–1

1) 07/25/00 18:50 COMMENTS: TO L SIDE O2 10 L FACE MASK. REPORT TO LDR. PT TO LDR VIA STRETCHER.

2) 07/25/00 18:52 116/118 EXTERNAL INOP TOCO

3) 07/25/00 18:54 NONE COMMENTS: AT MARK PT. GIVEN O2 10 LITERS VIA MASK

4) 07/25/00 18:55 MARK

5) 07/25/00 18:56 MARK

6) 07/25/00 18:57 COMMENTS: PT POSITIONED ON HANDS AND KNEES.

7) 07/25/00 18:58 COMMENTS: DR IN TO EVAL PT

8) 07/25/00 18:59 COMMENTS: DR IN DISCUSSING PLAN OF CARE

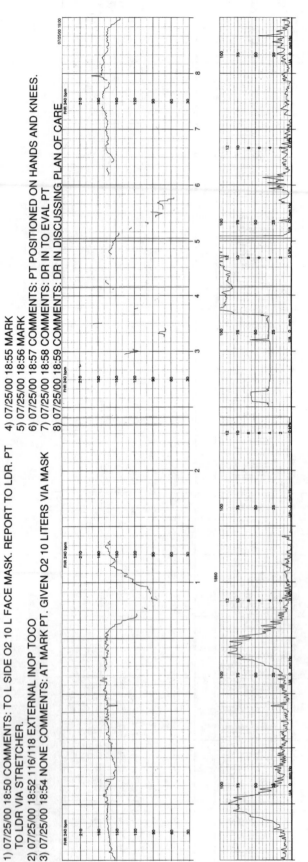

Strip Chart M–2

1) 07/25/00 19:01 COMMENTS: PT SUPINE DR, INSERTING AT MARK, RUPTURED WITH THICK MECONIUM

2) 07/25/00 19:05 COMMENTS: IUPC IN PLACE BY DR.

3) 07/25/00 19:06 COMMENTS: IV BOLUS IN PROGRESS

4) 07/25/00 19:07 COMMENTS: PT ON RT SIDE WITH O2 AT 10 LITERS 07/25/00

5) 07/25/00 19:08 COMMENTS: STARTING AMNIOFUSION 500CC BOLUS

6) 07/25/00 19:14 COMMENTS: PT SUPINE, DR PERFORMS SCALP STIM

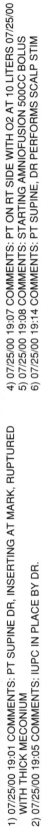
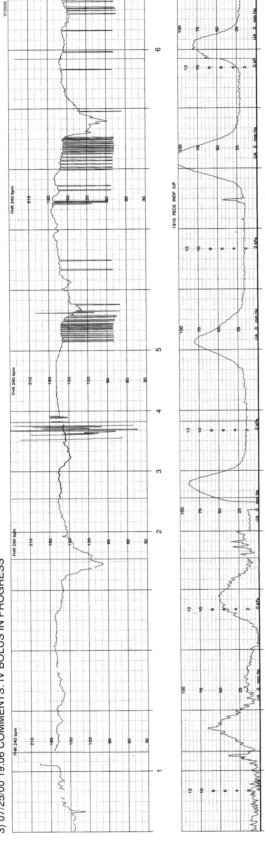
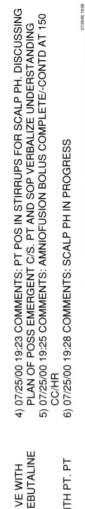

Strip Chart M–3

1) 07/25/00 19:14 COMMENTS: REPORT RECEIVED. PT SUPINE FOR VE WITH SCALP STIM AT MARK. PT TO R SIDE. ORDERS RECEIVED FOR TEBUTALINE MARK

2) 07/25/00 19:17 COMMENTS: TERB .25MG IV PUSH.

3) 07/25/00 19:20 COMMENTS: DR IN RM. DISCUSSING SCALP PH WITH PT. PT CONSENTING.

4) 07/25/00 19:23 COMMENTS: PT POS IN STIRRUPS FOR SCALP PH. DISCUSSING PLAN OF POSS EMERGENT C/S. PT AND SOP VERBALIZE UNDERSTANDING

5) 07/25/00 19:25 COMMENTS: AMNIOFUSION BOLUS COMPLETE/-CONTD AT 150 CC/HR

6) 07/25/00 19:28 COMMENTS: SCALP PH IN PROGRESS

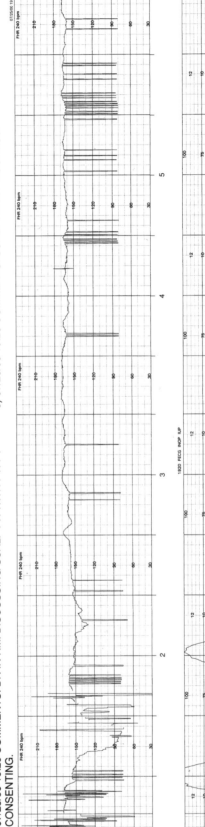
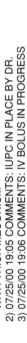

Strip Chart M–4

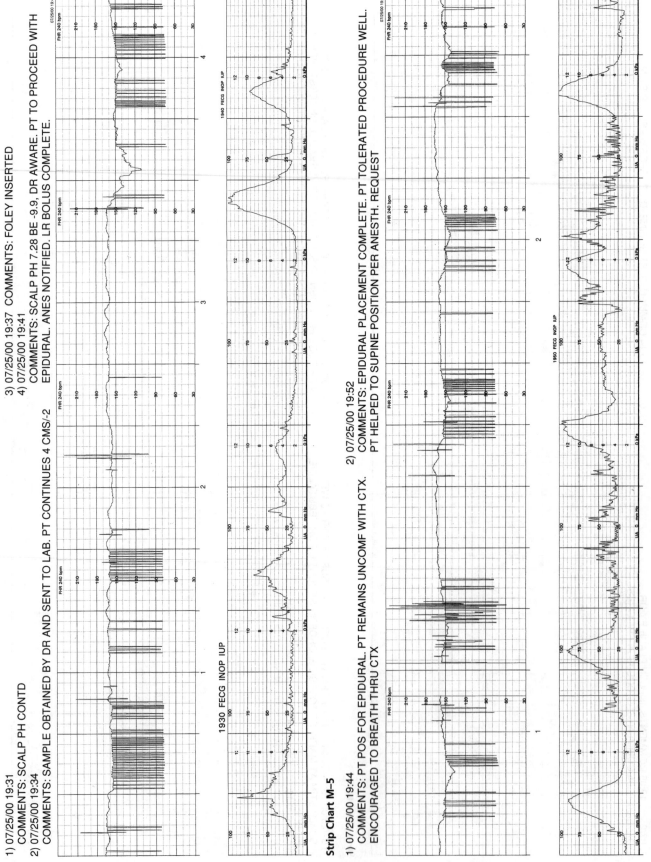

1) 07/25/00 19:31
   COMMENTS: SCALP PH CONTD
2) 07/25/00 19:34
   COMMENTS: SAMPLE OBTAINED BY DR AND SENT TO LAB. PT CONTINUES 4 CMS/-2

3) 07/25/00 19:37   COMMENTS: FOLEY INSERTED
4) 07/25/00 19:41
   COMMENTS: SCALP PH 7.28 BE -9.9, DR AWARE. PT TO PROCEED WITH
   EPIDURAL. ANES NOTIFIED. LR BOLUS COMPLETE.

Strip Chart M–5

1) 07/25/00 19:44
   COMMENTS: PT POS FOR EPIDURAL. PT REMAINS UNCOMF WITH CTX.
   ENCOURAGED TO BREATH THRU CTX

2) 07/25/00 19:52
   COMMENTS: EPIDURAL PLACEMENT COMPLETE. PT TOLERATED PROCEDURE WELL.
   PT HELPED TO SUPINE POSITION PER ANESTH. REQUEST

Strip Chart M–6

1) 07/25/00 19:57
   COMMENTS: VE BY DR. 8CMS/+1. SCALP STIM APPLIED WITH EXAM
2) 07/25/00 19:58   BP 154/104 M 116 P 93
3) 07/25/00 20:01   COMMENTS: PT TURNED TO L SIDE. DR IN RM

4) 07/25/00 20:02
   COMMENTS: PT TO R SIDE. DR DECLARING PT FOR EMERGENT C/S.
5) 07/25/00 20:03   COMMENTS: PT REPOSITION TO BACK FOR PREP
6) 07/25/00 20:04   COMMENTS: PT TO OR

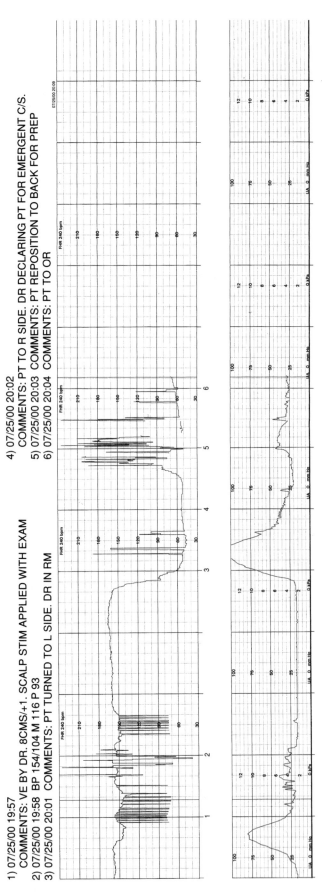

Strip Chart M–7

HX OF PATIENT N: G₃P₂, WITH INCONSISTENT PRENATAL CARE. PRESENTED FOR APPOINTMENT AT ~30 WKS BY DATES. NO COMPLAINTS. PLACED ON EFM FOR ROUTINE TESTING.

1) 09/09/00 14:59 14:11 BP 151/89 M 113 P 87 COMMENTS: PT HELPED TO LOUNGE CHAIR FOR MONITORING. STATES HAVING "BP PROBLEMS" IN PAST.

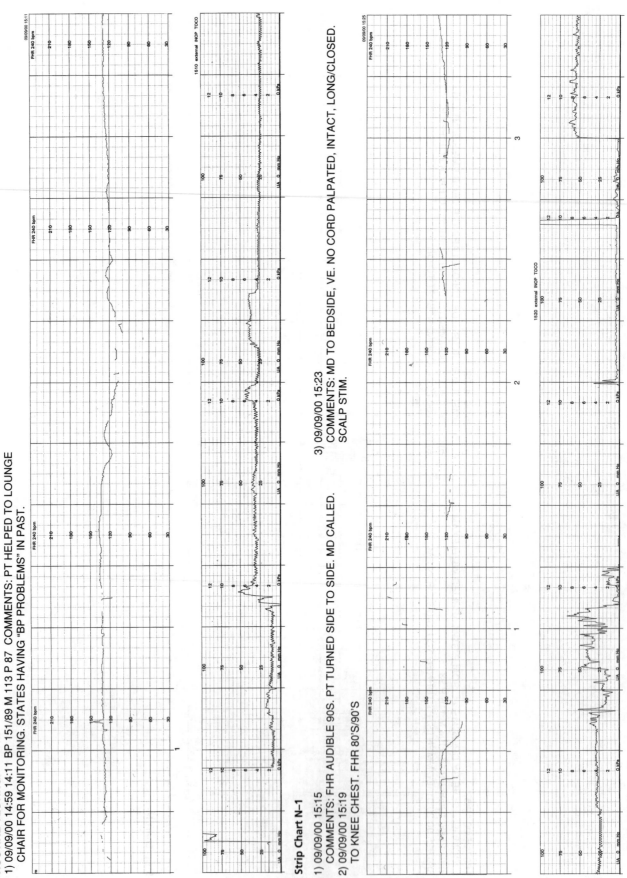

Strip Chart N-1

1) 09/09/00 15:15
COMMENTS: FHR AUDIBLE 90S. PT TURNED SIDE TO SIDE. MD CALLED.

2) 09/09/00 15:19
TO KNEE CHEST. FHR 80'S/90'S

3) 09/09/00 15:23
COMMENTS: MD TO BEDSIDE, VE. NO CORD PALPATED, INTACT, LONG/CLOSED. SCALP STIM.

Strip Chart N-2

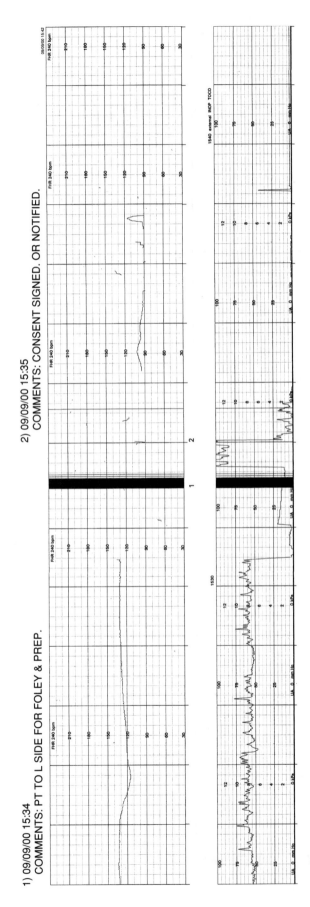

1) 09/09/00 15:34
COMMENTS: PT TO L SIDE FOR FOLEY & PREP.

2) 09/09/00 15:35
COMMENTS: CONSENT SIGNED. OR NOTIFIED.

Strip Chart N-3

HX OF PATIENT O: 37 YO, G2P1, 39+ WKS, MILD PIH. CALLED MD AT 10:00 WITH C/O DECREASED FETAL MOVEMENT. LAST EVALUATION TWO DAYS PRIOR: NST REACTIVE & REASSURING, BPP 8/8.

1) 08/07/03 11:00
   120/170 external INOP INOP TOCO
   Comments: PT ADMITTED TO LDR 6. C/O NO FM TODAY. FOR NST/BPP. GIVEN ORANGE JUICE/CRACKERS.
   BP 143/77 P137 R22

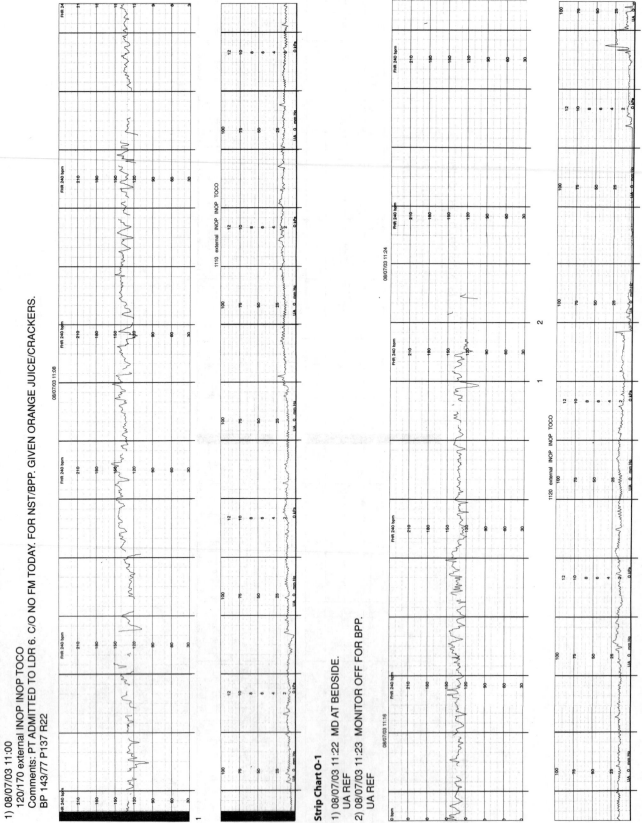

Strip Chart O-1

1) 08/07/03 11:22 MD AT BEDSIDE.
   UA REF
2) 08/07/03 11:23 MONITOR OFF FOR BPP.
   UA REF

Strip Chart O-2

HX OF PATIENT P: 36 YO, G$_3$P$_2$, 37+ WKS. PRESENTS WITH BRIGHT RED VAGINAL BLEEDING X I HOUR; DENIES PAIN, DENIES CONTRACTIONS. ABDOMEN SOFT, NON-TENDER.

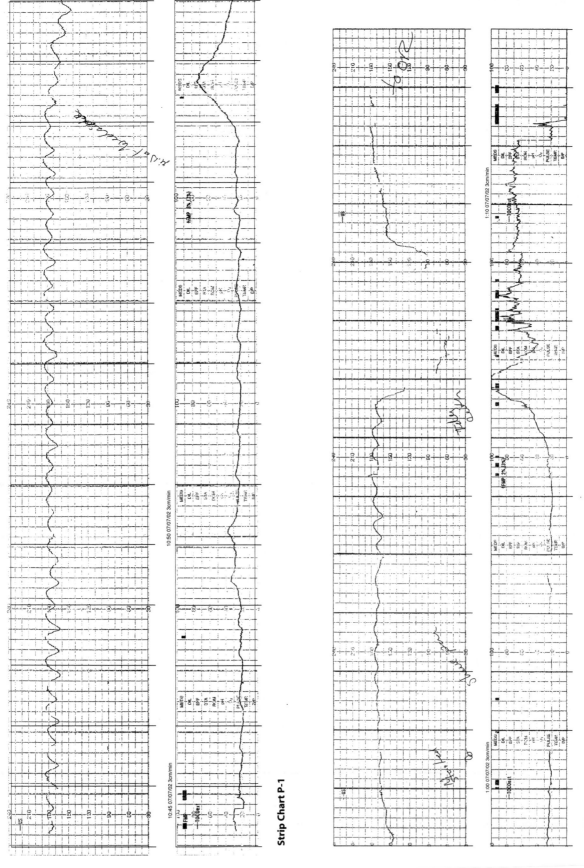

Strip Chart P-1

Strip Chart P-2

Guide to Interpretation

Strip Chart A-1			
Fetal Heart Rate		*Uterine Activity*	
Baseline Rate:	135 bpm	Frequency:	Hyperstimulation
Variability:	Moderate	Duration:	Hyperstimulation
Periodic/Episodic Changes:	Prolonged decelerations	Strength:	Palpate
		Resting Tone:	Palpate

Discussion

- Artifact noted with use of spiral electrode to perform AROM. Spiral electrode should be placed after membranes are either spontaneously or artificially ruptured.
- When no fluid is seen on AROM, it is appropriate to consider the presence of meconium or decreased fluid volume.
- The tocotransducer should be adjusted in order to facilitate interpretation of uterine activity.

Strip Chart A-2			
Fetal Heart Rate		*Uterine Activity*	
Baseline Rate:	135 bpm	Frequency:	Irregular
Variability:	Moderate	Duration:	Indeterminate
Periodic/Episodic Changes:	Variable and prolonged decelerations	Strength:	Indeterminate
		Resting Tone:	Indeterminate

Discussion:

- It appears that uterine hyperstimulation has resulted in a pattern of prolonged deceleration.
- An amnioinfusion was ordered for treatment of variable decelerations. The IUPC (placed during the interval between the two portions of tracing displayed) should be rezeroed.

Strip Chart A-3			
Fetal Heart Rate		*Uterine Activity*	
Baseline Rate:	140 bpm	Frequency:	Irregular
Variability:	Moderate	Duration:	60–90 seconds
Periodic/Episodic Changes:	Variable and prolonged decelerations	Strength:	15–40 mm/Hg
		Resting Tone:	15–20 mm/Hg

Discussion:

- Tocolysis administered to decrease stress of contractions on the fetus.
- Interventions are initiated to improve fetal status while preparation for operative delivery is simultaneously undertaken.

Strip Chart A-4			
Fetal Heart Rate		*Uterine Activity*	
Baseline Rate:	140 bpm	Frequency:	3–4 minutes
Variability:	Minimal	Duration:	90 seconds–3 minutes
Periodic/Episodic Changes:	Variable, late, and prolonged decelerations	Strength:	15–35 mm/Hg
		Resting Tone:	15–20 mm/Hg

Discussion:

• FHR baseline variability has decreased. Interventions do not appear to be effective in improving fetal status.

Strip Chart A-5			
Fetal Heart Rate		*Uterine Activity*	
Baseline Rate:	150 bpm	Frequency:	2½–4 minutes
Variability:	Minimal	Duration:	80 seconds–2 minutes
Periodic/Episodic Changes:	Variable, late, and prolonged decelerations	Strength:	20–60 mm/Hg
		Resting Tone:	15–25 mm/Hg

Discussion:

• The baseline FHR rising and continues to exhibit minimal variability.
• The apparent concern over a lack of fluid return with amnioinfusion is appropriate.

Strip Chart A-6			
Fetal Heart Rate		*Uterine Activity*	
Baseline Rate:	140 bpm	Frequency:	4½–7½ minutes
Variability:	Minimal	Duration:	2½–3½ minutes
Periodic/Episodic Changes:	Variable, late, and prolonged decelerations	Strength:	40–70 mm/Hg
		Resting Tone:	15–25 mm/Hg

Discussion:

• The FHR baseline continues to exhibit nonreassuring signs (minimal variability; variable, late and prolonged decelerations). In such an instance, it may be helpful to use adjunct means to assess fetal acid–base status.

Strip Chart A-7			
Fetal Heart Rate		**Uterine Activity**	
Baseline Rate:	140 bpm	Frequency:	2–4 minutes
Variability:	Minimal	Duration:	2–3 minutes
Periodic/Episodic Changes:	Variable, late, and prolonged decelerations	Strength:	45–65 mm/Hg
		Resting Tone:	25 mm/Hg

Discussion:

- The FHR continues to exhibit nonreassuring signs.
- Cervical progress has been made.
- The fetal acid–base status continues to be unknown.
- These variable decelerations exhibit shoulders.

Strip Chart A-8			
Fetal Heart Rate		**Uterine Activity**	
Baseline Rate:	150 bpm	Frequency:	1½–2 minutes
Variability:	Minimal	Duration:	70 seconds–2 minutes
Periodic/Episodic Changes:	Variable, late, and prolonged decelerations	Strength:	30–100 mm/Hg
		Resting Tone:	35–45 mm/Hg

Discussion

- It is difficult to determine the FHR baseline due to the frequency of contractions and the presence of decelerations.

OUTCOME:

SVD live male at 11:57. Apgars 7/9, nuchal cord × 2. Cord pH 7.21/BE-2. Resuscitation—tactile stimulation, blow-by O_2.

Strip Chart B-1			
Fetal Heart Rate		**Uterine Activity**	
Baseline:	130 bpm	Frequency:	2–3 minutes
Variability:	Minimal	Duration:	60–90 seconds
Periodic/Episodic Changes:	Variable and late decelerations	Strength:	Pushing
		Resting Tone:	Tocotransducer in place—must palpate

Discussion

- *Considerations:*
  - Position changes to assist in rotating fetus to OA and possibly decrease the severity of the variable decelerations.
  - Decrease stress on the fetus by allowing it to passively descend (the patient has an epidural in place).
  - If patient does have a strong urge to push, she can be encouraged not to push with every contraction to allow the fetus recovery time.
  - Amnioinfusion is not an option while the patient is actively pushing.

Strip Chart B-2			
Fetal Heart Rate		*Uterine Activity*	
Baseline:	130 bpm	Frequency:	2–4 minutes
Variability:	Minimal	Duration:	60–90 seconds
Periodic/Episodic Changes:	Variable and late decelerations	Strength:	Pushing
		Resting Tone:	Tocotransducer in place—must palpate

Discussion:

- These variable decelerations exhibit shoulders.

Strip Chart B-3			
Fetal Heart Rate		*Uterine Activity*	
Baseline:	130 bpm	Frequency:	2 minutes
Variability:	Moderate–minimal	Duration:	70–90 seconds
Periodic/Episodic Changes:	Variable and late decelerations	Strength:	Pushing
		Resting Tone:	Tocotransducer in place—must palpate

Discussion:

- Variable decelerations continue to present with shoulders.
- Position changes, not pushing with every contraction, and rest and descend (passive descent) should be considered to minimize the stress of contractions and pushing on the fetus.
- The frequency of the contractions/pushing coupled with the presence of decelerations makes interpretation of the FHR baseline difficult.

Strip Chart B-4			
Fetal Heart Rate		*Uterine Activity*	
Baseline:	140 bpm	Frequency:	2–4 minutes
Variability:	Minimal	Duration:	70–110 seconds
Periodic/Episodic Changes:	Variable and late decelerations	Strength:	Tocotransducer in place—must palpate
		Resting Tone:	Tocotransducer in place—must palpate

Discussion

- It is difficult to determine the characteristics of the FHR without a clear recording of uterine activity—the tocotransducer should be adjusted.
- The FHR is improving with the discontinuation of pushing efforts.

Strip Chart B-5			
Fetal Heart Rate		*Uterine Activity*	
Baseline:	125 bpm	Frequency:	2½–3 minutes
Variability:	Minimal	Duration:	90 seconds–2 minutes
Periodic/Episodic Changes:	Acceleration; early, late, and variable decelerations	Strength:	Tocotransducer in place—must palpate
		Resting Tone:	Tocotransducer in place—must palpate

Strip Chart B-6			
Fetal Heart Rate		*Uterine Activity*	
Baseline:	150 bpm	Frequency:	2–4 minutes
Variability:	Minimal	Duration:	90 seconds–2½ minutes
Periodic/Episodic Changes:	Variable and late decelerations	Strength:	Pushing
		Resting Tone:	Tocotransducer in place—must palpate

Discussion:

• FHR decelerations reappear when pushing is resumed.

OUTCOME:

Live female at 17:38. Cord pH 7.35/BE–5.0, Apgars 8/9. 3487 grams (7 lbs 11 oz). Spontaneous cry, no resuscitation necessary.

Strip Chart C		
Fetal Heart Rate		*Uterine Activity*
Baseline FHR:	Persistent supraventricular tachycardia (SVT) is present. The FHR as recorded on the strip chart is half the rate noted by auscultation and sonographic examination (half-counting).	No contraction activity is noted during observation of this 28-week gestation.
Periodic/Episodic Changes:	It is difficult to tell whether occasional irregularities of the FHR are due to dysrhythmia or if decelerations of the FHR are present.	

Discussion:

• Continous electronic fetal monitoring accomplished through use of an ultrasound transducer may not be the most effective means for monitoring the fetus with a dysrhythmia. As this example demonstrates, the rapid heart rate of this fetus with SVT exceeds the processing capabilities of this mode of monitoring. This results in half-counting of the FHR as it is recorded on the strip chart. Both rapidity and irregularity of the FHR pose a challenge to maintaining a continuous and useful FHR tracing.

Strip Chart D-1			
Fetal Heart Rate		*Uterine Activity*	
Baseline:	135 bpm	Frequency:	Indeterminate
Variability:	Moderate	Duration:	Indeterminate
Periodic/Episodic Changes:	Indeterminate	Strength:	Tocotransducer in place—must palpate
		Resting Tone:	Tocotransducer in place—must palpate

Discussion:

- The tocotransducer needs to be adjusted so that uterine activity can be recorded and assessed.
- Without uterine activity data, it is not possible to accurately assess the FHR baseline, variability, or the presence of periodic/episodic changes. In this case, gaps in the data should be considered suspicious and may be suggestive of decelerations.

Strip Chart D-2			
Fetal Heart Rate		*Uterine Activity*	
Baseline:	140 bpm	Frequency:	1–1½ minutes
Variability:	Moderate	Duration:	40 seconds–2 minutes
Periodic/Episodic Changes:	None	Strength:	Tocotransducer in place—must palpate
		Resting Tone:	Tocotransducer in place—must palpate

Strip Chart D-3			
Fetal Heart Rate		*Uterine Activity*	
Baseline:	140 bpm	Frequency:	2–3 minutes
Variability:	Minimal	Duration:	70–110 seconds
Periodic/Episodic Changes:	Accelerations; variable decelerations	Strength:	Moderate by palpation
		Resting Tone:	Tocotransducer in place—must palpate

Strip Chart D-4			
Fetal Heart Rate		*Uterine Activity*	
Baseline:	Indeterminate	Frequency:	Unknown
Variability:	Indeterminate	Duration:	Unknown
Periodic/Episodic Changes:	Indeterminate	Strength:	Tocotransducer in place—must palpate
		Resting Tone:	Tocotransducer in place—must palpate

Discussion:

- The tocotransducer has not been readjusted since the patient's last position change. Lack of uterine activity data makes assessment of FHR baseline and periodic/episodic changes difficult.
- The gaps in the data continue to be suspicious and may be suggestive of decelerations.

Strip Chart D-5			
Fetal Heart Rate		*Uterine Activity*	
Baseline:	135 bpm	Frequency:	1–2 minutes?
Variability:	Moderate?	Duration:	50–100 seconds?
Periodic/Episodic Changes:	Accelerations? Decelerations?	Strength:	Tocotransducer in place—must palpate
		Resting Tone:	Tocotransducer in place—must palpate

Discussion:

- Because uterine activity remains unclear, it is impossible to definitively determine the FHR baseline, variability, and the presence of periodic/episodic changes.
- Uterine contractions appear to be recorded as an inverted waveform.

Strip Chart D-6			
Fetal Heart Rate		*Uterine Activity*	
Baseline:	145 bpm	Frequency:	Unknown
Variability:	Moderate?	Duration:	Unknown
Periodic/Episodic Changes:	Decelerations?	Strength:	Tocotransducer in place—must palpate
		Resting Tone:	Tocotransducer in place—must palpate

Strip Chart D-7			
Fetal Heart Rate		*Uterine Activity*	
Baseline:	140–150 bpm?	Frequency:	Unknown
Variability:	Moderate?	Duration:	Unknown
Periodic/Episodic Changes:	Decelerations?	Strength:	Moderate by palpation
		Resting Tone:	Tocotransducer in place—must palpate

Discussion:

- The FHR tracing is strongly suspicious of decelerations, but their type is indeterminate as there is no definitive uterine activity data available.

Strip Chart D-8			
Fetal Heart Rate		*Uterine Activity*	
Baseline:	Indeterminate	Frequency:	Unknown—hyperstimulation?
Variability:	Indeterminate	Duration:	Unknown—hyperstimulation?
Periodic/Episodic Changes:	Prolonged deceleration?	Strength:	Tocotransducer in place—must palpate
		Resting Tone:	Tocotransducer in place—must palpate

Discussion:

- While the data presented is unclear, this tracing is strongly suspicious of uterine hyperstimulation resulting in a prolonged deceleration. This patient needs closer observation, particularly since Cervidil is in place. The external transducers need to be attended to more closely, and if a clinically significant signal cannot be obtained, internal monitoring should be considered. Additionally, the care provider should be made aware of the suspicious findings.

Strip Chart D-9			
Fetal Heart Rate		*Uterine Activity*	
Baseline:	140 bpm?	Frequency:	Unknown
Variability:	Minimal?	Duration:	Unknown
Periodic/Episodic Changes:	Decelerations?	Strength:	Tocotransducer in place—must palpate
		Resting Tone:	Tocotransducer in place—must palpate

Strip Chart D-10			
Fetal Heart Rate		*Uterine Activity*	
Baseline:	150 bpm?	Frequency:	Unknown—hyperstimulation?
Variability:	Minimal?	Duration:	Unknown—hyperstimulation?
Periodic/Episodic Changes:	Decelerations?	Strength:	Tocotransducer in place—must palpate
		Resting Tone:	Tocotransducer in place—must palpate

Discussion:

- The tracing continues to be of poor quality. Without uterine activity data, it is impossible to accurately determine the fetal or maternal response to the induction.

Strip Chart D-11			
Fetal Heart Rate		*Uterine Activity*	
Baseline:	150 bpm?	Frequency:	Unknown—hyperstimulation?
Variability:	Minimal?	Duration:	Unknown—hyperstimulation?
Periodic/Episodic Changes:	Decelerations?	Strength:	Tocotransducer in place—must palpate
		Resting Tone:	Tocotransducer in place—must palpate

Discussion

- The uterine activity pattern continues to appear suspicious for hyperstimulation. Closer monitoring is indicated.

Strip Chart D-12			
Fetal Heart Rate		*Uterine Activity*	
Baseline:	145 bpm?	Frequency:	Unknown—hyperstimulation?
Variability:	Minimal?	Duration:	Unknown—hyperstimulation?
Periodic/Episodic Changes:	Prolonged decelerations?	Strength:	Tocotransducer in place—must palpate
		Resting Tone:	Tocotransducer in place—must palpate

Discussion:

- The tracing remains strongly suspicious for uterine hyperstimulation resulting in prolonged decelerations.

Strip Chart D-13

Fetal Heart Rate		Uterine Activity	
Baseline:	140 bpm?	Frequency:	Unknown—hyperstimulation?
Variability:	Minimal?	Duration:	Unknown—hyperstimulation?
Periodic/Episodic Changes:	Decelerations?	Strength:	Tocotransducer in place—must palpate
		Resting Tone:	Tocotransducer in place—must palpate

Discussion:
- Accurate assessment of the tracing continues to be impeded by lack of data.

Strip Chart D-14

Fetal Heart Rate		Uterine Activity	
Baseline:	Indeterminate	Frequency:	Unknown—hyperstimulation?
Variability:	Indeterminate	Duration:	Unknown—hyperstimulation?
Periodic/Episodic Changes:	Indeterminate	Strength:	Tocotransducer in place—must palpate
		Resting Tone:	Tocotransducer in place—must palpate

Discussion:
- The gaps in the FHR data are particularly worrisome, as Cervidil remains in place and there is suspicion of hyperstimulation.

Strip Chart D-15

Fetal Heart Rate		Uterine Activity	
Baseline:	135 bpm?	Frequency:	Unknown—hyperstimulation?
Variability:	Minimal?	Duration:	Unknown—hyperstimulation?
Periodic/Episodic Changes:	Indeterminate	Strength:	Tocotransducer in place—must palpate
		Resting Tone:	Tocotransducer in place—must palpate

Discussion:
- The FHR baseline is not recording for a significant period of time. Data that can possibly be regarded as representing the FHR baseline is decreased from the previously determined baseline rate.

Strip Chart D-16			
Fetal Heart Rate		*Uterine Activity*	
Baseline:	135 bpm?	Frequency:	Unknown
Variability:	Minimal?	Duration:	Unknown
Periodic/Episodic Changes:	Prolonged deceleration	Strength:	Tocotransducer in place—must palpate
		Resting Tone:	Tocotransducer in place—must palpate

Discussion:

• Prolonged deceleration noted with VE and AROM. Internal monitoring initiated.

Strip Chart D-17			
Fetal Heart Rate		*Uterine Activity*	
Baseline:	160 bpm	Frequency:	1–2½ minutes
Variability:	Minimal	Duration:	40–60 seconds
Periodic/Episodic Changes:	Early and late decelerations	Strength:	20–85 mm/Hg
		Resting Tone:	15–25 mm/Hg

Discussion:

• The FHR baseline is rising.
• Uterine hyperstimulation is apparent. Tocolytics should be considered.

Strip Chart D-18			
Fetal Heart Rate		*Uterine Activity*	
Baseline:	160 bpm	Frequency:	1–1½ minutes
Variability:	Minimal	Duration:	70–90 seconds
Periodic/Episodic Changes:	Early, late, and variable decelerations	Strength:	30–55 mm/Hg
		Resting Tone:	20–30 mm/Hg

Discussion

• The FHR baseline continues to rise and is presently tachycardic.

Strip Chart D-19			
Fetal Heart Rate		*Uterine Activity*	
Baseline:	140 bpm	Frequency:	1–1½ minutes
Variability:	Minimal	Duration:	50–70 seconds
Periodic/Episodic Changes:	Early, variable, and late decelerations	Strength:	20–75 mm/Hg
		Resting Tone:	15–30 mm/Hg

Discussion:

• Uterine hyperstimulation continues to negatively impact the FHR.

Strip Chart D-20			
Fetal Heart Rate		*Uterine Activity*	
Baseline:	145 bpm	Frequency:	1–2 minutes
Variability:	Minimal	Duration:	60–80 seconds
Periodic/Episodic Changes:	Early, variable, late, and prolonged decelerations	Strength:	30–75 mm/Hg
		Resting Tone:	15–30 mm/Hg

Discussion:

• There appears to be no improvement in the FHR with the interventions attempted (position change, IV, and O_2).

Strip Chart D-21			
Fetal Heart Rate		*Uterine Activity*	
Baseline:	150 bpm?	Frequency:	1–2 minutes
Variability:	Minimal?	Duration:	60–80 seconds
Periodic/Episodic Changes:	Early, variable, late, and prolonged decelerations	Strength:	35–75 mm/Hg
		Resting Tone:	15–25 mm/Hg

Discussion:

• It is difficult to accurately determine the FHR baseline due to the frequency of contractions and decelerations.

• The patient is a primigravida and has progressed from 4 cm to full dilation in ~1 hour and 20 minutes.

Strip Chart D-22			
Fetal Heart Rate		*Uterine Activity*	
Baseline:	140 bpm?	Frequency:	1–1½ minutes
Variability:	Minimal?	Duration:	50–90 seconds
Periodic/Episodic Changes:	Early, variable, late, and prolonged decelerations	Strength:	45–70 mm/Hg
		Resting Tone:	15–25 mm/Hg

Strip Chart D-23			
Fetal Heart Rate		*Uterine Activity*	
Baseline:	155 bpm?	Frequency:	1–2½ minutes
Variability:	Minimal?	Duration:	60–70 seconds
Periodic/Episodic Changes:	Early and late decelerations	Strength:	40–75 mm/Hg
		Resting Tone:	20–30 mm/Hg

Discussion:

• Uterine hyperstimulation continues to negatively impact the FHR and makes interpretation of the tracing difficult.

Strip Chart D-24			
Fetal Heart Rate		**Uterine Activity**	
Baseline:	Indeterminate	Frequency:	1–1½ minutes
Variability:	Indeterminate	Duration:	70–90 seconds
Periodic/Episodic Changes:	Early, variable, late, and prolonged decelerations	Strength:	Pushing
		Resting Tone:	20–30 mm/Hg

Discussion

• The frequency of uterine contractions and decelerations impedes accurate determination of the baseline FHR.

OUTCOME:

Live female at 14:45. Apgars 5/7. Resuscitation: positive pressure ventilation with 100% O_2, tactile stimulation, and blow-by O_2. One hour postnally, the baby was tachypneic, had ↓ O_2 saturation, ↓ sugars, and was sent to the NICU. A full recovery eventually occurred.

Strip Chart E-1			
Fetal Heart Rate		**Uterine Activity**	
Baseline:	140 bpm	Frequency:	1½–3 minutes
Variability:	Minimal	Duration:	60–100 seconds
Periodic/Episodic Changes:	Early decelerations	Strength:	60–80 mm/Hg
		Resting Tone:	20–35 mm/Hg

Discussion:

• There is no acceleration noted coincident with the VE. It would be beneficial to perform assessment of fetal acid–base status, particularly as oxytocin is infusing.

Strip Chart E-2			
Fetal Heart Rate		**Uterine Activity**	
Baseline:	150 bpm	Frequency:	1½–2½ minutes
Variability:	Minimal	Duration:	80–90 seconds
Periodic/Episodic Changes:	Early, late, and prolonged decelerations	Strength:	55–80 mm/Hg
		Resting Tone:	25–35 mm/Hg

Discussion:

• As the FHR continues to demonstrate nonreassuring signs (minimal variability, late and prolonged decelerations), it would be helpful to have more information about the fetal status.

Strip Chart E-3			
Fetal Heart Rate		*Uterine Activity*	
Baseline:	150 bpm	Frequency:	1–3 minutes
Variability:	Minimal	Duration:	90 seconds–2 minutes
Periodic/Episodic Changes:	Early, late, and prolonged decelerations	Strength:	40–80 mm/Hg
		Resting Tone:	20–35 mm/Hg

Discussion:

- The oxytocin infusion had been continued despite the nonreassuring FHR tracing, but is now appropriately discontinued and the MD notified.
- The position changes, IV bolus, and O_2 are appropriate interventions. Tocolytics may also assist with intrauterine resuscitation.

Strip Chart E-4			
Fetal Heart Rate		*Uterine Activity*	
Baseline:	155 bpm	Frequency:	2–4½ minutes
Variability:	Minimal	Duration:	70–110 seconds
Periodic/Episodic Changes:	Early and late decelerations	Strength:	55–80 mm/Hg
		Resting Tone:	20–25 mm/Hg

Strip Chart E-5			
Fetal Heart Rate		*Uterine Activity*	
Baseline:	150 bpm	Frequency:	1½–3 minutes
Variability:	Minimal	Duration:	70–90 seconds
Periodic/Episodic Changes:	Early decelerations: induced acceleration	Strength:	50–80 mm/Hg
		Resting Tone:	20–25 mm/Hg

Discussion:

- The acceleration that occurred as a result of scalp stimulation is reassuring, as it is suggestive that the fetus is not presently experiencing acidosis.
- The patient has dilated 1 cm this hour.

Strip Chart E-6			
Fetal Heart Rate		*Uterine Activity*	
Baseline:	150 bpm	Frequency:	1½–3 minutes
Variability:	Minimal	Duration:	60–80 seconds
Periodic/Episodic Changes:	Early and late decelerations	Strength:	20–70 mm/Hg
		Resting Tone:	15–35 mm/Hg

Discussion:

- The oxytocin infusion is restarted despite the nonreassuring FHR tracing, as the response to scalp stimulation seems to have reassured the clinicians about fetal status.

Strip Chart E-7			
Fetal Heart Rate		**Uterine Activity**	
Baseline:	150 bpm	Frequency:	1–3 minutes
Variability:	Minimal	Duration:	70–110 seconds
Periodic/Episodic Changes:	Late? and early decelerations	Strength:	15–70 mm/Hg
		Resting Tone:	15–20 mm/Hg

Discussion:

- Due to the frequency of the contractions, it is difficult to distinguish whether or not late decelerations are occurring.
- Coupling of contractions/hyperstimulation is present.
- The oxytocin is increased, despite FHR and uterine activity patterns.

Strip Chart E-8			
Fetal Heart Rate		**Uterine Activity**	
Baseline:	145 bpm	Frequency:	1–4 minutes
Variability:	Minimal	Duration:	60 seconds—3 minutes
Periodic/Episodic Changes:	Induced acceleration × 1; prolonged deceleration × 1	Strength:	20–70 mm/Hg
		Resting Tone:	15–20 mm/Hg

Discussion:

- It is difficult to determine the FHR baseline due to the frequency of the contractions.
- The patient has progressed 3 cm this hour.
- An acceleration of the FHR is noted with scalp stimulation, a reassuring finding.

Strip Chart E-9			
Fetal Heart Rate		**Uterine Activity**	
Baseline:	150 bpm	Frequency:	1–4 minutes
Variability:	Minimal	Duration:	60–110 seconds
Periodic/Episodic Changes:	Late and prolonged decelerations	Strength:	20–70 mm/Hg
		Resting Tone:	15–30 mm/Hg

Discussion:

- The oxytocin infusion is discontinued in response to the deceleration pattern.
- Uterine hyperstimulation continues.
- The FHR appears to respond to patient positioning to right lateral.

Strip Chart E-10			
Fetal Heart Rate		**Uterine Activity**	
Baseline:	150 bpm	Frequency:	1–3½ minutes
Variability:	Minimal	Duration:	70 seconds–2 minutes
Periodic/Episodic Changes:	Early and late? decelerations	Strength:	55–85 mm/Hg
		Resting Tone:	15–30 mm/Hg

Discussion:
- Due to the frequency of the contractions, it is difficult to distinguish the deceleration pattern.

Strip Chart E-11			
Fetal Heart Rate		**Uterine Activity**	
Baseline:	140 bpm	Frequency:	2–3½ minutes
Variability:	Minimal	Duration:	70 seconds–3 minutes
Periodic/Episodic Changes:	Early and late decelerations	Strength:	35–70 mm/Hg
		Resting Tone:	15–30 mm/Hg

Discussion:
- The oxytocin infusion is restarted.
- The FHR continues to have nonreassuring elements present and to lack reassuring components.

Strip Chart E-12			
Fetal Heart Rate		**Uterine Activity**	
Baseline:	140 bpm	Frequency:	1½–2½ minutes
Variability:	Minimal	Duration:	90 seconds–3 minutes
Periodic/Episodic Changes:	Late and prolonged decelerations	Strength:	30–80 mm/Hg
		Resting Tone:	15–45 mm/Hg

Discussion:
- It is difficult to determine the FHR baseline due to the frequency of contractions.
- The oxytocin infusion is discontinued as a result of the prolonged deceleration.
- The FHR is not responding well to maternal bearing down efforts.

Strip Chart E-13			
Fetal Heart Rate		**Uterine Activity**	
Baseline:	160 bpm	Frequency:	2–2½ minutes
Variability:	Minimal	Duration	90 seconds–4 minutes
Periodic/Episodic Changes:	Early, late, and prolonged decelerations	Strength:	25–80 mm/Hg
		Resting Tone:	15–25 mm/Hg

Discussion:
- The FHR baseline appears to be rising.

Strip Chart E-14

Fetal Heart Rate		Uterine Activity	
Baseline:	155 bpm	Frequency:	1½–3½ minutes
Variability:	Minimal	Duration:	70 seconds–2 minutes
Periodic/Episodic Changes:	Early and late decelerations	Strength:	20–80 mm/Hg
		Resting Tone:	15–20 mm/Hg

Strip Chart E-15

Fetal Heart Rate		Uterine Activity	
Baseline:	155 bpm	Frequency:	1–3 minutes
Variability:	Minimal	Duration:	60 seconds–4 minutes
Periodic/Episodic Changes:	Early, late, variable, and prolonged decelerations	Strength:	10–70 mm/Hg
		Resting Tone:	20–25 mm/Hg

Discussion:

- Uterine hyperstimulation is present, and the FHR continues to be nonreassuring.
- As there is no apparent acceleration with scalp stimulation, a fetal scalp blood sample is currently in progress.

Strip Chart E-16

Fetal Heart Rate		Uterine Activity	
Baseline:	160 bpm	Frequency:	1½–4½ minutes
Variability:	Minimal	Duration:	70 seconds–2 minutes
Periodic/Episodic Changes:	Early, late, and prolonged decelerations	Strength:	15–85 mm/Hg
		Resting Tone:	15–30 mm/Hg

Discussion:

- The result of fetal scalp blood sample demonstrates that the fetus is not acidotic.

Strip Chart E-17

Fetal Heart Rate		Uterine Activity	
Baseline:	160 bpm	Frequency:	1½–4½ minutes
Variability:	Minimal	Duration:	60 seconds–3 minutes
Periodic/Episodic Changes:	Late and prolonged decelerations	Strength:	30–85 mm/Hg
		Resting Tone:	15–35 mm/Hg

Discussion:

- The FHR baseline continues to rise.
- The oxytocin infusion continues to be increased.

Strip Chart E-18			
Fetal Heart Rate		**Uterine Activity**	
Baseline:	165 bpm	Frequency:	2–3 minutes
Variability:	Minimal	Duration:	80 seconds–3 minutes
Periodic/Episodic Changes:	Variable, late, and prolonged decelerations	Strength:	55–70 mm/Hg
		Resting Tone:	15–40 mm/Hg

Discussion:

- The FHR is consistently better when the patient is on her right side.
- The oxytocin infusion is discontinued with prolonged decelerations secondary to uterine hyperstimulation.

Strip Chart E-19			
Fetal Heart Rate		**Uterine Activity**	
Baseline:	170 bpm	Frequency:	1½–3½ minutes
Variability:	Minimal	Duration:	80 seconds–3 minutes
Periodic/Episodic Changes:	Early and late decelerations	Strength:	30–85 mm/Hg
		Resting Tone:	15–35 mm/Hg

Discussion:

- The FHR baseline has been progressively rising and is now tachycardic.

Strip Chart E-20			
Fetal Heart Rate		**Uterine Activity**	
Baseline:	170 bpm	Frequency:	1½–3 minutes
Variability:	Minimal	Duration:	80 seconds–3 minutes
Periodic/Episodic Changes:	Early and late decelerations	Strength:	30–70 mm/Hg
		Resting Tone:	25–35 mm/Hg

Discussion:

- The result of the fetal scalp blood sample demonstrates acidosis. A vacuum extraction is initiated and accomplished.
- Preparations for delivery included arranging for back-up with the OR for a possible failed vacuum attempt and pediatric back-up for neonatal care.

OUTCOME:

Live male at 3:45. Cord pH 7.16 / BE-12. Apgars 5/7/9. Resuscitation: positive pressure ventilation with 100% O_2, blow-by O_2, and tactile stimulation.

Strip Chart F-1			
Fetal Heart Rate		**Uterine Activity**	
Baseline:	165 bpm	Frequency:	2–3 minutes
Variability:	Minimal	Duration:	90–110 seconds
Periodic/Episodic Changes:	Variable and late decelerations	Strength:	40–75 mm/Hg
		Resting Tone:	25–30 mm/Hg

Discussion:

- The oxytocin infusion rate is increased, despite:
  - Tachycardic FHR baseline
  - Increased uterine resting tone

Strip Chart F-2			
Fetal Heart Rate		**Uterine Activity**	
Baseline:	165 bpm	Frequency:	2–3 minutes
Variability:	Minimal	Duration:	90 seconds–2½ minutes
Periodic/Episodic Changes:	Variable and late decelerations	Strength:	35–65 mm/Hg
		Resting Tone:	30–35 mm/Hg

Discussion:

- The frequency of contractions and late deceleration pattern pose a challenge to interpretation of the FHR baseline.
- The uterine resting tone continues to be increased.
- The FHR is beginning to rise at the end of this segment of tracing.

Strip Chart F-3			
Fetal Heart Rate		**Uterine Activity**	
Baseline:	170 bpm	Frequency:	2–3 minutes
Variability:	Minimal	Duration:	80 seconds–2 minutes
Periodic/Episodic Changes:	Variable and late decelerations	Strength:	40–65 mm/Hg
		Resting Tone:	25–35 mm/Hg

Discussion:

- The FHR baseline is tachycardic and continuing to rise. Fetal acid–base status should be evaluated.
- The oxytocin infusion continues, despite a nonreassuring tracing. Discontinuation of infusion and initiation of intrauterine resuscitation measures should be considered, as should notification of the care provider and any other necessary personnel.

Strip Chart F-4			
Fetal Heart Rate		**Uterine Activity**	
Baseline:	165 bpm?	Frequency:	1½–2 minutes
Variability:	Minimal	Duration:	90 seconds–2 minutes
Periodic/Episodic Changes:	Late, variable, and prolonged decelerations	Strength:	25–65 mm/Hg
		Resting Tone:	25–35 mm/Hg

Strip Chart F-5			
Fetal Heart Rate		**Uterine Activity**	
Baseline:	60 bpm?	Frequency:	2–3 minutes
Variability:	Minimal	Duration:	60–100 seconds
Periodic/Episodic Changes:	Variable and late decelerations	Strength:	60–80 mm/Hg
		Resting Tone:	20–35 mm/Hg

Discussion:
- It is helpful to have documented information regarding the audible FHR during this time as a continuous recording is not available.
- The heart rate recorded at the end of the tracing that occurs within the 120–150 range is maternal.

OUTCOME:

Male delivered at 14:03. Apgars 0/0. A full neonatal code ensued and was successful. The neonate went to NICU for observation—no negative sequelae noted, discharged home with patient.

Strip Chart G-1			
Fetal Heart Rate		**Uterine Activity**	
Baseline Rate:	145 bpm	Frequency:	2½–3½ minutes
Variability:	Moderate–minimal	Duration:	100–130 seconds
Periodic/Episodic Changes:	Variable, late, and prolonged decelerations	Strength:	60–80 mm/Hg
		Resting Tone:	20–30 mm/Hg

Discussion:
- The FHR baseline can only be determined toward the end of this segment of the tracing, due to the frequency of contractions and presence of late decelerations.
- Fetal arterial oxygen saturation monitoring ($FSpO_2$) is being utilized, as noted by the dotted line appearing in the uterine activity portion of the strip chart. $FSpO_2$ was approved for use by the FDA in 2000 as an adjunct method of fetal assessment. It did not achieve widespread clinical use as it did not meet the objectives of reducing cesarean delivery rates and improving newborn status. It does provide interesting information from research and educational perspectives, hence the presentation of this example. Values below 30% may be representative of significant metabolic acidosis.
- The position change implemented appears to have had a positive impact on fetal status.
- The presence of uterine hyperstimulation should be considered.

Strip Chart G-2			
Fetal Heart Rate		*Uterine Activity*	
Baseline Rate:	140 bpm	Frequency	2–3 minutes
Variability:	Moderate	Duration:	90–100 seconds
Periodic/Episodic Changes:	Variable decelerations	Strength:	70–80 mm/Hg
		Resting Tone:	20–25 mm/Hg

Discussion:

- $FSpO_2$ remains ≥45.
- Variable decelerations are less prominent in appearance since the patient's position was changed.
- The strip chart paper needs to be changed (as indicated by black squares appearing at the bottom of the strip chart).

Strip Chart G-3			
Fetal Heart Rate		*Uterine Activity*	
Baseline Rate:	140 bpm	Frequency:	2–3 minutes
Variability:	Moderate	Duration:	100 seconds–2 minutes
Periodic/Episodic Changes:	Variable and late decelerations	Strength:	75 mm/Hg
		Resting Tone:	25 mm/Hg

Discussion:

- $FSpO_2$ remains ≥40.

Strip Chart G-4			
Fetal Heart Rate		*Uterine Activity*	
Baseline Rate:	145 bpm	Frequency:	1½–3 minutes
Variability:	Minimal	Duration:	90 seconds–3½ minutes (hyperstimulation)
Periodic/Episodic Changes:	Variable and late decelerations	Strength:	35–80 mm/Hg
		Resting Tone:	20–40 mm/Hg

Discussion:

- $FSpO_2$ remains ≥35.
- It is of interest to note the decrease in $FSpO_2$ concurrent with the uterine hyperstimulation.

Strip Chart G-5			
Fetal Heart Rate		*Uterine Activity*	
Baseline Rate:	150 bpm	Frequency:	1½–3 minutes
Variability:	Minimal	Duration:	90 seconds–3½ minutes
Periodic/Episodic Changes:	Variable and late decelerations	Strength:	45–75 mm/Hg
		Resting Tone:	20–30 mm/Hg

Discussion:

- Repositioning the patient for examination appears to negatively impact the FHR.
- $FSpO_2$ >30.

Strip Chart G-6			
Fetal Heart Rate		*Uterine Activity*	
Baseline Rate:	150 bpm	Frequency:	1½–3½ minutes
Variability:	Minimal	Duration:	90–100 seconds
Periodic/Episodic Changes:	?Early, variable, and late decelerations	Strength:	50–70 mm/Hg
		Resting Tone:	20–30 mm/Hg

Discussion:

- $FSpO_2$ ≥45.
- Uterine hyperstimulation is present.

OUTCOME:

C-birth at 23:50 for lack of progress, nonreassuring FHR tracing, and $FSpO_2$ < 30 with episodes of hyperstimulation. Live male, Apgars 5/7/9. Resuscitation: tactile stimulation, positive pressure ventilation with 100% O_2, blow-by O_2.

Strip Chart H-1			
Fetal Heart Rate		*Uterine Activity*	
Baseline:	160 bpm	Frequency:	4–5 minutes
Variability:	Moderate	Duration:	80–110 seconds
Periodic/Episodic Changes:	Late and (mild) variable decelerations	Strength:	Mild per palpation
		Resting Tone:	Tocotransducer in place—must palpate

Strip Chart H-2			
Fetal Heart Rate		**Uterine Activity**	
Baseline:	160 bpm	Frequency:	2–5 minutes
Variability:	Moderate	Duration:	80–110 seconds
Periodic/Episodic Changes:	Late and (mild) variable decelerations	Strength:	Tocotransducer in place—must palpate
		Resting Tone:	Tocotransducer in place—must palpate

Discussion:

• This tracing could be confusing if the FHR baseline is not the first parameter determined and/or if it is not accurately assessed. Cursory assessment might lead to the incorrect assumption that the FHR baseline is in the 135–145 range with accelerations present.

Strip Chart H-3			
Fetal Heart Rate		**Uterine Activity**	
Baseline:	160 bpm	Frequency:	Irregular
Variability:	Moderate	Duration:	80 seconds–2½ minutes
Periodic/Episodic Changes:	Late and (mild) variable decelerations	Strength:	Tocotransducer in place—must palpate
		Resting Tone:	Tocotransducer in place—must palpate

Strip Chart H-4			
Fetal Heart Rate		**Uterine Activity**	
Baseline:	160 bpm	Frequency:	4½–5 minutes
Variability:	Moderate	Duration:	80 seconds–2 minutes
Periodic/Episodic Changes:	Late and (mild) variable decelerations	Strength:	Tocotransducer in place—must palpate
		Resting Tone:	Tocotransducer in place—must palpate

Strip Chart H-5			
Fetal Heart Rate		**Uterine Activity**	
Baseline:	160 bpm	Frequency:	1½–3 minutes
Variability:	Moderate	Duration:	80–100 seconds
Periodic/Episodic Changes:	Late and (mild) variable decelerations	Strength:	Tocotransducer in place—must palpate
		Resting Tone:	Tocotransducer in place—must palpate

Strip Chart H-6			
Fetal Heart Rate		*Uterine Activity*	
Baseline:	160 bpm	Frequency:	1½–2½ minutes
Variability:	Minimal	Duration:	30–100 seconds
Periodic/Episodic Changes:	Late and (mild) variable decelerations	Strength:	Tocotransducer in place—must palpate
		Resting Tone:	Tocotransducer in place—must palpate

Discussion:

• This tracing is not only a nonreactive NST, it is also a positive CST. Therefore, the status of this fetus requires further testing/investigation in a timely manner.

Strip Chart I-1			
Fetal Heart Rate		*Uterine Activity*	
Baseline:	130 bpm	Frequency:	1½–2 minutes
Variability:	Moderate	Duration:	70–90 seconds
Periodic/Episodic Changes:	Accelerations variable decelerations	Strength:	Tocotransducer in place—must palpate
		Resting Tone:	Tocotransducer in place—must palpate

Discussion:

• The tracing needs to be monitored closely as contractions are occurring too frequently. It may be necessary to use intervention (eg, stop oxytocin, administer terbutaline) to slow contraction pattern.

Strip Chart I-2			
Fetal Heart Rate		*Uterine Activity*	
Baseline:	125 bpm	Frequency	1–1½ minutes
Variability:	Moderate	Duration:	70–90 seconds
Periodic/Episodic Changes:	Acceleration, variable decelerations	Strength:	Moderate to palpation
		Resting Tone:	Tocotransducer in place—must palpate

Strip Chart I-3			
Fetal Heart Rate		*Uterine Activity*	
Baseline:	125 bpm	Frequency:	1½–2 minutes
Variability:	Moderate	Duration:	50–100 seconds
Periodic/Episodic Changes:	Prolonged deceleration	Strength:	Tocotransducer in place—must palpate
		Resting Tone:	Tocotransducer in place—must palpate

Discussion:
- Prolonged deceleration appears to have recovered with position change.

Strip Chart I-4			
Fetal Heart Rate		*Uterine Activity*	
Baseline:	130 bpm	Frequency:	1½–2 minutes
Variability:	Moderate	Duration:	70–110 seconds
Periodic/Episodic Changes:	Early decelerations	Strength:	Moderate to palpation
		Resting Tone:	Uterus palpates "soft" between UCs

Discussion:
- Uterine hyperstimulation pattern continues.

Strip Chart I-5			
Fetal Heart Rate		*Uterine Activity*	
Baseline:	125 bpm	Frequency:	1½–4 minutes
Variability:	Moderate	Duration:	60–90 seconds
Periodic/Episodic Changes:	Variable decelerations	Strength:	Tocotransducer in place—must palpate
		Resting Tone:	Tocotransducer in place—must palpate

Discussion:
- The decelerations noted in this segment of tracing were immediately preceded by accelerations. This type of acceleration pattern, known as "shoulders," only occurs with variable decelerations.

Strip Chart I-6			
Fetal Heart Rate		**Uterine Activity**	
Baseline:	125 bpm	Frequency:	1–5 minutes
Variability:	Moderate	Duration:	50–90 seconds
Periodic/Episodic Changes:	Variable deceleration?	Strength:	Moderate to palpation
		Resting Tone:	Uterus palpates "soft" between UCs

Strip Chart I-7			
Fetal Heart Rate		**Uterine Activity**	
Baseline:	145 bpm	Frequency:	1–3 minutes
Variability:	Moderate–minimal	Duration:	60 seconds–2 minutes
Periodic/Episodic Changes:	Early, variable, and late decelerations	Strength:	Tocotransducer in place—must palpate
		Resting Tone:	Tocotransducer in place—must palpate

Discussion:

- The oxytocin, which has been started sometime in the early morning, should be discontinued as the FHR baseline has risen from its earlier rate, the variability has decreased, and late decelerations are present. It is appropriate to notify the care provider of these changes so that the patient can be further evaluated. Other measures to promote intrauterine resuscitation (eg, position changes, O_2, fluid bolus) should also be considered.

Strip Chart I-8			
Fetal Heart Rate		**Uterine Activity**	
Baseline:	140 bpm	Frequency:	1½–3 minutes
Variability:	Minimal	Duration:	80–110 seconds
Periodic/Episodic Changes:	Early and variable decelerations	Strength:	Tocotransducer in place—must palpate
		Resting Tone:	Tocotransducer in place—must palpate

Strip Chart I-9			
Fetal Heart Rate		**Uterine Activity**	
Baseline:	140 bpm	Frequency:	1½–3 minutes
Variability:	Minimal	Duration:	70 seconds–2 minutes
Periodic/Episodic Changes:	Early, variable, and late decelerations	Strength:	Tocotransducer in place—must palpate
		Resting Tone:	Tocotransducer in place—must palpate

Strip Chart I-10			
Fetal Heart Rate		**Uterine Activity**	
Baseline:	145 bpm	Frequency:	1–3½ minutes
Variability:	Minimal	Duration:	70 seconds–2 minutes
Periodic/Episodic Changes:	Early, variable, and late decelerations	Strength:	Moderate to palpation
		Resting Tone:	Uterus palpates with "rest" between UCs

Discussion:

- The oxytocin continues to be increased, despite the increase in FHR baseline, decreased variability, and presence of late decelerations. Fetal acid–base status should be further evaluated and measures to promote intrauterine resuscitation (eg, decrease contraction pattern, position changes, O$_2$) should also be considered.

Strip Chart I-11			
Fetal Heart Rate		**Uterine Activity**	
Baseline:	145 bpm	Frequency:	1½–3 minutes
Variability:	Moderate	Duration:	90–100 seconds
Periodic/Episodic Changes:	Variable decelerations	Strength:	Tocotransducer in place—must palpate
		Resting Tone:	Tocotransducer in place—must palpate

Discussion:

- The patient's positioning seems to have affected the ultrasound transducer signal. Without the information that the audible signal from the electronic fetal monitor provides, it is not possible to know for certain what the gaps and fluctuations in the data represent. The data displayed may either be halving or doubling of the FHR, or wide variations in the FHR that are actually occurring.

Strip Chart I-12			
Fetal Heart Rate		*Uterine Activity*	
Baseline:	140 bpm	Frequency:	1½–3½ minutes
Variability:	Moderate to minimal	Duration:	80–110 seconds
Periodic/Episodic Changes:	Accelerations?; early, variable, late, decelerations; prolonged deceleration	Strength:	Tocotransducer in place—must palpate
		Resting Tone:	Tocotransducer in place—must palpate

Discussion:

- Appropriately, a spiral electrode was placed in order to more accurately monitor the FHR. No cervical progress has been made in the past hour. Attempt to avoid supine hypotension has been made by wedging the patient to her left side (maternal/fetal condition should prevail over anesthetic distribution). The FHR baseline is not stable during this period. It appears to be continuously rising as the fetus attempts recovery. Discontinuing the oxytocin to assist with intrauterine resuscitation would be advisable.

Strip Chart I-13			
Fetal Heart Rate		*Uterine Activity*	
Baseline:	145 bpm	Frequency:	1½–2 minutes
Variability:	Minimal–moderate	Duration:	80 seconds–2 minutes
Periodic/Episodic Changes:	Early, variable, and late decelerations	Strength:	Tocotransducer in place—must palpate
		Resting Tone:	Tocotransducer in place—must palpate

Discussion:

- The variability of the FHR baseline appears minimal during the first segment of tracing. During the second half of this tracing, frequent variable decelerations almost give the FHR baseline variability a marked appearance. Position changes and amnioinfusion may be helpful in alleviating the severity and occurrence of the variable deceleration pattern.
- The presence of uterine hyperstimulation should be addressed (ie, discontinuation of oxytocin).

Strip Chart I-14			
Fetal Heart Rate		*Uterine Activity*	
Baseline:	145 bpm	Frequency:	1–1½ minutes
Variability:	Moderate	Duration:	50–90 seconds
Periodic/Episodic Changes:	Early, variable, and late decelerations	Strength:	Tocotransducer in place—must palpate
		Resting Tone:	Tocotransducer in place—must palpate

Discussion:

- The tocotransducer needs to be adjusted in order to accurately evaluate the tracing. It appears that uterine hyperstimulation continues.

Strip Chart I-15			
Fetal Heart Rate		**Uterine Activity**	
Baseline:	150 bpm	Frequency:	1–2½ minutes
Variability:	Minimal	Duration:	70–110 seconds
Periodic/Episodic Changes:	Variable and late decelerations	Strength:	Moderate–strong to palpation
		Resting Tone:	Tocotransducer in place—must palpate

Strip Chart I–16			
Fetal Heart Rate		**Uterine Activity**	
Baseline:	125 bpm	Frequency:	1–3 minutes
Variability:	Marked	Duration:	40 seconds–2 minutes
Periodic/Episodic Changes:	Prolonged deceleration	Strength:	Tocotransducer in place—must palpate
		Resting Tone:	Tocotransducer in place—must palpate

Discussion:

- It appears that the position change had a negative effect on the FHR, as did the contractions (which occur too frequently). Intrauterine resuscitation was initiated.

Strip Chart I–17			
Fetal Heart Rate		**Uterine Activity**	
Baseline:	145 bpm	Frequency:	2–4 minutes
Variability:	Minimal	Duration:	80–90 seconds
Periodic/Episodic Changes:	Early, late, and variable decelerations	Strength:	Tocotransducer in place—must palpate
		Resting Tone:	Tocotransducer in place—must palpate

Strip Chart I–18			
Fetal Heart Rate		*Uterine Activity*	
Baseline:	150 bpm	Frequency:	1–2½ minutes
Variability:	Minimal–moderate	Duration:	70 seconds–2 minutes
Periodic/Episodic Changes:	Variable and late decelerations	Strength:	Tocotransducer in place—must palpate
		Resting Tone:	Tocotransducer in place—must palpate

Discussion:

- The patient has made little cervical change in past 2½ hours. Insertion of an IUPC may be helpful in assisting with assessment of labor and would also provide means for administrating an amnioinfusion.
- Assurance of fetal-acid–base status should be attained before re-starting the oxytocin infusion.

Strip Chart I–19			
Fetal Heart Rate		*Uterine Activity*	
Baseline:	150 bpm	Frequency:	1–3 minutes
Variability:	Minimal–moderate	Duration:	1½–4 minutes
Periodic/Episodic Changes:	Variable and late decelerations; prolonged deceleration	Strength:	Tocotransducer in place—must palpate
		Resting tone:	Tocotransducer in place—must palpate

Discussion:

- A period of hyperstimulation is present, negatively affecting the FHR. Interventions aimed at intrauterine resuscitation are performed.

Strip Chart I–20			
Fetal Heart Rate		*Uterine Activity*	
Baseline:	155 bpm	Frequency:	1½–3 minutes
Variability:	Moderate	Duration:	1½–2 minutes
Periodic/Episodic Changes:	Early, late, and variable decelerations	Strength:	Tocotransducer in place—must palpate
		Resting tone:	Tocotransducer in place—must palpate

Discussion:

- The FHR baseline has increased.

Strip Chart I–21

Fetal Heart Rate		Uterine Activity	
Baseline:	150 bpm	Frequency:	2–3 minutes
Variability:	Moderate–minimal	Duration:	70–90 seconds
Periodic/Episodic Changes:	Early, late, and variable decelerations	Strength:	Tocotransducer in place—must palpate
		Resting tone:	Tocotransducer in place—must palpate

Discussion:

- The oxytocin infusion has been stopped to promote perfusion to the fetus and then restarted in an effort to continue labor progress. Reassurance of fetal acid–base status is needed prior to restarting the oxytocin, as is closer evaluation of labor.

Strip Chart I–22

Fetal Heart Rate		Uterine Activity	
Baseline:	150 bpm	Frequency:	2–3 minutes
Variability:	Moderate–marked	Frequency:	1½–2 minutes
Periodic/Episodic Changes:	Variable and late decelerations	Strength:	Strong to palpation
		Resting tone:	Tocotransducer in place—must palpate

Discussion:

- The patient is a VBAC who has not made any cervical change in a number of hours, despite the occurrence of contractions that are strong to palpation. Additionally, the fetus does not appear to be tolerating the stress of uterine contractions. In order to continue with this trial of labor, the fetal acid–base status and the contraction pattern should be further investigated.

Strip Chart I–23

Fetal Heart Rate		Uterine Activity	
Baseline:	145 bpm	Frequency:	1½ –3 minutes
Variability:	Moderate	Duration:	1½–2 minutes
Periodic/Episodic Changes:	Variable and late decelerations; prolonged deceleration	Strength:	Tocotransducer in place—must palpate
		Resting Tone:	Tocotransducer in place—must palpate

Strip Chart I–24

Fetal Heart Rate		Uterine Activity	
Baseline:	135 bpm	Frequency:	2½–3 minutes
Variability:	Moderate	Duration:	1½–2 minutes
Periodic/Episodic Changes:	Early, variable, and late decelerations; accelerations?	Strength:	Tocotransducer in place—must palpate
		Resting Tone:	Tocotransducer in place—must palpate

Strip Chart I-25

Fetal Heart Rate		Uterine Activity	
Baseline:	135 bpm	Frequency	2–4 minutes
Variability:	Moderate–marked	Duration:	1–2 minutes
Periodic/Episodic Changes:	Early, variable, and late decelerations; accelerations	Strength:	Tocotransducer in place—must palpate
		Resting Tone:	Tocotransducer in place—must palpate

Discussion:

• The acceleration noted with scalp stimulation suggests that the fetus is not presently hypoxic/acidotic.

Strip Chart I-26

Fetal Heart Rate		Uterine Activity	
Baseline:	135 bpm	Frequency:	2–3 minutes
Variability:	Moderate–marked	Duration:	60–100 seconds
Periodic/Episodic Changes:	Early, variable, and late decelerations; accelerations?	Strength:	Tocotransducer in place—must palpate
		Resting Tone:	Tocotransducer in place—must palpate

OUTCOME:

Live female by repeat cesarean birth at 11:05, tight nuchal cord × 1, Apgars 8/9, 8 lbs, 8 oz. Resuscitation: suction on the perineum and at warmer, blow-by O_2, and tactile stimulation.

Strip Chart J-1			
Fetal Heart Rate		*Uterine Activity*	
Baseline:	160 bpm	Frequency:	1–3½ minutes
Variability:	Minimal–absent	Duration:	1–2 minutes
Periodic/Episodic Changes:	Late decelerations	Strength:	Tocotransducer in place—must palpate
		Resting Tone:	Tocotransducer in place—must palpate

Discussion:

- The tocotransducer needs to be adjusted to facilitate interpretation of the tracing.
- The oxytocin is increased, despite the presence of a nonreassuring FHR (borderline tachycardia, minimal–absent variability, late decelerations). Steps should be taken at this time to improve the fetal condition, including decreasing the stress of contractions on the fetus by discontinuing the oxytocin infusion.

Strip Chart J-2			
Fetal Heart Rate		*Uterine Activity*	
Baseline:	160 bpm	Frequency:	1½–3½ minutes
Variability:	Minimal–absent	Duration:	80 seconds
Periodic/Episodic Changes:	Late decelerations	Strength:	Moderate to palpation
		Resting Tone:	Tocotransducer in place—must palpate

Discussion:

- Maternal BP is low. Patient may be hypotensive due to recent epidural placement.

Strip Chart J-3			
Fetal Heart Rate		*Uterine Activity*	
Baseline:	160 bpm	Frequency:	1½–2 minutes
Variability:	Minimal–absent	Duration:	1–3 minutes
Periodic/Episodic Changes:	Late and variable decelerations	Strength:	Moderate to palpation
		Resting Tone:	Tocotransducer in place—must palpate

Discussion:

- An attempt to assess fetal acid–base status is made with scalp stimulation. While the FHR does increase, it does not accelerate per criteria. A spiral electrode is placed to monitor the fetus more closely.
- The tocotransducer is now adjusted to show a more clear view of uterine activity, which may be excessive and bears close observation.

Strip Chart J-4			
Fetal Heart Rate		*Uterine Activity*	
Baseline:	165 bpm	Frequency:	2–3½ minutes
Variability:	Minimal	Duration:	80 seconds–2½ minutes
Periodic/Episodic Changes:	Late and variable decelerations	Strength:	Moderate–strong to palpation
		Resting Tone:	Tocotransducer in place—must palpate

Discussion:

- It is clear that the practitioners are concerned about the patient's condition and attempts at intrauterine resuscitation are being made (oxytocin infusion discontinues, position changes, O_2 in place).

Strip Chart J-5			
Fetal Heart Rate		*Uterine Activity*	
Baseline:	160 bpm	Frequency	2–5 minutes
Variability:	Minimal	Duration:	100 seconds
Periodic/Episodic Changes:	Late decelerations	Strength:	Tocotransducer in place—must palpate
		Resting Tone:	Tocotransducer in place—must palpate

Discussion:

- Interventions appear to be having a positive effect on the FHR.

Strip Chart J-6			
Fetal Heart Rate		*Uterine Activity*	
Baseline:	155 bpm	Frequency:	5 minutes
Variability:	Minimal	Duration:	1½–3 minutes
Periodic/Episodic Changes:	Late decelerations; acceleration with scalp stimulation	Strength:	Mild–moderate to palpation
		Resting Tone:	Tocotransducer in place—must palpate

Discussion:

- The fetus seems to be responding to the interventions. The acceleration noted with scalp stimulation is a sign that the fetus is likely not acidotic. It is clear from the annotations on the tracing that the maternal/fetal condition is being closely monitored during this tenuous period.
- The patient's BP appears to be recovering.

Strip Chart J-7

Fetal Heart Rate		Uterine Activity	
Baseline:	150 bpm	Frequency:	4½–6 minutes
Variability:	Absent–minimal	Duration:	1½–3 minutes
Periodic/Episodic Changes:	Late decelerations	Strength:	Tocotransducer in place—must palpate
		Resting Tone:	Tocotransducer in place—must palpate

Discussion:

- It is important to note that although the FHR drops below the baseline by only a few bpm, these decreases represent late decelerations continuing to occur.
- It appears that the nurse is sufficiently concerned about the tracing and its management to have activated the chain of command.

Strip Chart J-8

Fetal Heart Rate		Uterine Activity	
Baseline:	155 bpm	Frequency:	1½–4 minutes
Variability:	Minimal–moderate	Duration:	80 seconds–3 minutes
Periodic/Episodic Changes:	Late and variable decelerations; accelerations with scalp stimulation	Strength:	Mild–moderate to palpation
		Resting Tone:	"Soft" between contractions

Discussion:

- The patient's temperature is beginning to rise. This can occur as a side effect of an epidural. The fetus does respond well to scalp stimulation with an acceleration and transient improvement of its FHR baseline variability. The change in position to accommodate the examination may explain the change in depth and appearance of the subsequent decelerations.

Strip Chart J-9

Fetal Heart Rate		Uterine Activity	
Baseline:	160 bpm	Frequency:	2½–3½ minutes
Variability:	Minimal	Duration:	2–3 minutes
Periodic/Episodic Changes:	Late and variable decelerations	Strength:	Tocotransducer in place—must palpate
		Resting Tone:	Tocotransducer in place—must palpate

Discussion:

- Fetal acid–base status is re-evaluated by scalp stimulation. The fetus continues to appear not to be acidotic.
- No cervical change has been made and it has been decided to place an IUPC to monitor the labor more closely.

Strip Chart J-10			
Fetal Heart Rate		**Uterine Activity**	
Baseline:	165 bpm	Frequency:	1½–3 minutes
Variability:	Minimal	Duration:	70 seconds–2 minutes
Periodic/Episodic Changes:	Late and variable decelerations	Strength:	Tocotransducer in place—must palpate
		Resting Tone:	Tocotransducer in place—must palpate

Discussion:

- FHR baseline is now tachycardic.
- While the oxytocin infusion had been restarted per orders, it has not been increased.

Strip Chart J-11			
Fetal Heart Rate		**Uterine Activity**	
Baseline:	165 bpm	Frequency:	2–3½ minutes
Variability:	Minimal	Duration:	1½–2 minutes
Periodic/Episodic Changes:	Late decelerations	Strength:	20–70 mm/Hg
		Resting Tone:	30 mm/Hg

Discussion:

- Uterine resting tone bears consideration as it should be maintained <25 mm/Hg.

Strip Chart J-12			
Fetal Heart Rate		**Uterine Activity**	
Baseline:	160 bpm	Frequency:	1½–4 minutes
Variability:	Minimal	Duration:	60–80 seconds
Periodic/Episodic Changes:	Late and variable decelerations; acceleration with scalp stimulation	Strength:	20–65 mm/Hg
		Resting Tone:	25–30 mm/Hg

Discussion:

- The oxytocin infusion was discontinued once again, likely out of concern for fetal status. Fetal status is reassessed with scalp stimulation and the fetus does not appear to be acidotic at this time.

Strip Chart J-13

Fetal Heart Rate		Uterine Activity	
Baseline:	160 bpm	Frequency:	4–4½ minutes
Variability:	Minimal	Duration:	1½–2 minutes
Periodic/Episodic Changes:	Late decelerations	Strength:	15–50 mm/Hg
		Resting Tone:	25–30 mm/Hg

Strip Chart J-14

Fetal Heart Rate		Uterine Activity	
Baseline:	155 bpm	Frequency:	5 minutes
Variability:	Absent–minimal	Duration:	1½–3 minutes
Periodic/Episodic Changes:	Late deceleration	Strength:	15–65 mm/Hg
		Resting Tone:	25 mm/Hg

Discussion:

- A fetal scalp blood sample is being attempted for the purpose of determining fetal acid–base status. The presence of caput can be problematic for this procedure, as it may falsely lower the pH result.

Strip Chart J-15

Fetal Heart Rate		Uterine Activity	
Baseline:	165 bpm	Frequency:	2½–4 minutes
Variability:	Minimal–moderate	Duration:	70 seconds–2½ minutes
Periodic/Episodic Changes:	Late decelerations	Strength:	15–25 mm/Hg
		Resting Tone:	25 mm/Hg

Strip Chart J-16

Fetal Heart Rate		Uterine Activity	
Baseline:	155 bpm	Frequency:	3½–5 minutes
Variability:	Minimal	Duration:	80–90 seconds
Periodic/Episodic Changes:	Late decelerations	Strength:	45–70 mm/Hg
		Resting Tone:	15–20 mm/Hg

Discussion:

- The result of the fetal scalp blood sample confirms that, despite the nonreassuring FHR tracing, the fetus is not acidotic. The oxytocin infusion was restarted at a lower rate than it had previously been infusing.
- The fluid bolus given earlier seems to have assisted in stabilizing the patient's blood pressure and temperature.

Strip Chart J-17			
Fetal Heart Rate		*Uterine Activity*	
Baseline:	155 bpm	Frequency:	2–5 minutes
Variability:	Minimal	Duration:	80 seconds–3 minutes
Periodic/Episodic Changes:	Late decelerations	Strength:	25–60 mm/Hg
		Resting Tone:	15–20 mm/Hg

Strip Chart J-18			
Fetal Heart Rate		*Uterine Activity*	
Baseline:	160 bpm	Frequency:	2–4 minutes
Variability:	Minimal	Duration:	1–2 minutes
Periodic/Episodic Changes:	Late decelerations	Strength:	10–50 mm/Hg
		Resting Tone:	15–20 mm/Hg

Strip Chart J-19			
Fetal Heart Rate		*Uterine Activity*	
Baseline:	160 bpm	Frequency:	3–4½ minutes
Variability:	Minimal	Duration:	1–2 minutes
Periodic/Episodic Changes:	Late decelerations	Strength:	25–75 mm/Hg
		Resting Tone:	20–25 mm/Hg

Discussion:

- While the FHR does increase somewhat with scalp stimulation (at marks "1" and "2"), accelerations do not result. Artifact is produced during the second attempt at scalp stimulation due to the examiner's contact with the spiral electrode causing interference in the signal.
- The oxytocin infusion has been increased and the patient has made cervical change. Fetal status must continue to be assessed as reassurance could not be gained from scalp stimulation.

Strip Chart J-20			
Fetal Heart Rate		*Uterine Activity*	
Baseline:	155 bpm	Frequency:	2½–4 minutes
Variability:	Minimal	Duration:	1–1½ minutes
Periodic/Episodic Changes:	Late decelerations	Strength:	35–85 mm/Hg
		Resting Tone:	15–35 mm/Hg

Strip Chart J-21

Fetal Heart Rate		Uterine Activity	
Baseline:	155 bpm	Frequency:	2–4 minutes
Variability:	Minimal	Duration:	70–80 seconds
Periodic/Episodic Changes:	Late decelerations	Strength:	20–70 mm/Hg
		Resting Tone:	15–25 mm/Hg

Discussion:

- Scalp stimulation produces an acceleration that doesn't quite meet criteria and therefore does not provide reassurance. The oxytocin infusion is discontinued and fetal scalp blood sampling is planned.
- It is notable that the fetal scalp blood sample seems to be taken with the patient turned to her back. While it can be technically challenging, this procedure should be attempted with the patient in a side-lying position to prevent a further decrease in uterine perfusion that may result from supine hypotension.

Strip Chart J-22

Fetal Heart Rate		Uterine Activity	
Baseline:	160 bpm	Frequency:	4–5 minutes
Variability:	Minimal	Duration:	60–100 seconds
Periodic/Episodic Changes:	Late decelerations	Strength:	20–60 mm/Hg
		Resting Tone:	25–30 mm/Hg

Strip Chart J-23

Fetal Heart Rate		Uterine Activity	
Baseline:	155 bpm	Frequency:	1½–5 minutes
Variability:	Minimal	Duration:	90 seconds
Periodic/Episodic Changes:	Late decelerations	Strength:	40–55 mm/Hg
		Resting Tone:	15–20 mm/Hg

Discussion:

- The result of the fetal scalp blood sampling shows that the fetus is not acidotic. The oxytocin infusion is therefore restarted.

Strip Chart J-24

Fetal Heart Rate		Uterine Activity	
Baseline:	150 bpm	Frequency:	2½–4 minutes
Variability:	Minimal	Duration:	80 seconds–2 minutes
Periodic/Episodic Changes:	Late decelerations	Strength:	50–65 mm/Hg
		Resting Tone:	20–25 mm/Hg

Discussion:

- Oncoming RN appropriately palpates maternal abdomen to ensure that the IUPC reading is accurate.

Strip Chart J-25			
Fetal Heart Rate		*Uterine Activity*	
Baseline:	160 bpm	Frequency:	2–4 minutes
Variability:	Minimal	Duration:	1½–2 minutes
Periodic/Episodic Changes:	Late decelerations	Strength:	30–70 mm/Hg
		Resting Tone:	25–30 mm/Hg

Discussion:

- The patient is now fully dilated.
- While the FHR does increase with scalp stimulation, it still does not manage an acceleration. Another fetal scalp blood sample is therefore taken.
- Oxytocin remains infusing at the same rate (7 mU/min.) at which it had last been restarted. As cervical progress occurred for this patient, it was not necessary to increase the rate and risk further stress on the fetus.

Strip Chart J-26			
Fetal Heart Rate		*Uterine Activity*	
Baseline:	160 bpm	Frequency:	1–4 minutes
Variability:	Minimal	Duration:	80 seconds–2½ minutes
Periodic/Episodic Changes:	Late decelerations	Strength:	40–70 mm/Hg
		Resting Tone:	25–30 mm/Hg

Discussion:

- The results of the fetal scalp blood sampling were reassuring; therefore the patient's course of labor will be allowed to continue.

Strip Chart J-27			
Fetal Heart Rate		*Uterine Activity*	
Baseline:	165 bpm	Frequency:	3–4 minutes
Variability:	Minimal	Duration:	80 seconds–2½ minutes
Periodic/Episodic Changes:	Late decelerations	Strength:	15–70 mm/Hg
		Resting Tone:	25–30 mm/Hg

Discussion:

- Consideration should be given to allowing the fetus to descend without active pushing by the patient in order to minimize the amount of stress on the fetus during second stage.

Strip Chart J-28			
Fetal Heart Rate		**Uterine Activity**	
Baseline:	160 bpm	Frequency:	2–4 minutes
Variability:	Minimal	Duration:	1½–2 minutes
Periodic/Episodic Changes:	Late decelerations	Strength:	Pushing
		Resting Tone:	25–30 mm/Hg

Discussion:

- Although an epidural is in place, consideration should be given to patient positioning during pushing. It may still be possible to assist her to a modified squat position by utilizing available equipment (eg, bed controls, birth ball, squatting bar) and personnel (including support persons). Squatting may hasten second stage and assist in avoiding the effects of supine hypotension on the fetus.

Strip Chart J-29			
Fetal Heart Rate		**Uterine Activity**	
Baseline:	165 bpm	Frequency:	3–5 minutes?
Variability:	Minimal	Duration:	? seconds (pushing)
Periodic/Episodic Changes:	Late and prolonged decelerations	Strength:	Pushing
		Resting Tone:	20–30 mm/Hg

Discussion:

- Pushing has increased the depth and length of the decelerations. The nurse appears to recognize this and turns the patient to her right side to push. This intervention does appear to lessen the depth and length of the decelerations.
- With each effort, the patient is pushing for an extended amount of time. Her pushing does not appear to be co-ordinated with uterine activity, a problem particular to directed pushing. It may be helpful to allow the fetus to descend until the patient has the urge to push spontaneously and can better coordinate her bearing down efforts with the occurrence of contractions. Reassurance of fetal status can continue to be obtained in the same manner that it had been during first stage labor.

Strip Chart J-30			
Fetal Heart Rate		**Uterine Activity**	
Baseline:	165 bpm	Frequency:	Minutes?
Variability:	Minimal	Duration:	Seconds?
Periodic/Episodic Changes:	Late and prolonged decelerations	Strength:	Pushing
		Resting Tone:	20–30 mm/Hg

Discussion:

- The combination of frequent, uncoordinated pushing efforts and contractions poses a challenge to interpretation of the tracing in regard to FHR baseline rate, variability, and uterine activity patterns.

Strip Chart J-31			
Fetal Heart Rate		**Uterine Activity**	
Baseline:	170 bpm?	Frequency:	Unknown (not monitored)
Variability:	Minimal?	Duration:	Unknown (not monitored)
Periodic/Episodic Changes:	Late decelerations?	Strength:	Unknown (not monitored)
		Resting Tone:	Unknown (not monitored)

Discussion:

- It was decided that delivery of the fetus could be hastened by use of forceps at this time. Internal monitors were removed and the fetus was delivered.
- Without uterine activity data, it is difficult to determine with certainty the FHR baseline, variability, and periodic/episodic changes.

OUTCOME:

22:55 live female by forceps. Cord pH 7.28, BE −3. Apgars 9/9. Resuscitation: suction, O_2, tactile stimulation.

Strip Chart K-1				
Fetal Heart Rate			**Uterine Activity**	
	A	*B*	Frequency:	3–4 minutes
Baseline:	140 bpm	135 bpm	Duration:	2–2½ minutes
Variability:	Moderate	Moderate–minimal	Strength:	Tocotransducer in place—must palpate
Periodic/Episodic Changes:	Accelerations; mild variable decelerations	Accelerations	Resting Tone:	Tocotransducer in place—must palpate

Discussion:

- Fetus "A" is represented by the lighter density recording.

Strip Chart K-2				
Fetal Heart Rate			**Uterine Activity**	
	A	*B*	Frequency:	1½–3 minutes
Baseline:	130 bpm	135 bpm	Duration:	1–2 minutes
Variability:	Minimal	Moderate–minimal	Strength:	Tocotransducer in place—must palpate
Periodic/Episodic Changes:	Early decelerations, mild variable decelerations	None	Resting Tone:	Tocotransducer in place—must palpate

Discussion:

- "A" is now being monitored internally with a spiral electrode. Small increases of "B's" FHR above the baseline do not meet criteria for accelerations.

Strip Chart K-3				
Fetal Heart Rate			**Uterine Activity**	
	A	B	Frequency:	2–2½ minutes
Baseline:	135 bpm	135 bpm	Duration:	2–2½ minutes
Variability:	Minimal	Minimal	Strength:	Moderate to palpation
Periodic/Episodic Changes:	Early decelerations, mild variable decelerations	Accelerations	Resting Tone:	Tocotransducer in place—must palpate

Strip Chart K-4				
Fetal Heart Rate			**Uterine Activity**	
	A	B	Frequency:	2–5 minutes
Baseline:	130 bpm	135 bpm	Duration:	2–3 minutes
Variability:	Minimal	Minimal	Strength:	Tocotransducer in place—must palpate
Periodic/Episodic Changes:	Early, late, and variable decelerations	Early decelerations	Resting Tone:	Tocotransducer in place—must palpate

Strip Chart K-5				
Fetal Heart Rate			**Uterine Activity**	
	A	B	Frequency:	1½–3½ minutes
Baseline:	130 bpm	140 bpm	Duration:	1½–2 minutes
Variability:	Minimal	Moderate–minimal	Strength:	Moderate to palpation
Periodic/Episodic Changes:	Early decelerations	Accelerations	Resting Tone:	Tocotransducer in place—must palpate

Strip Chart K-6				
Fetal Heart Rate			**Uterine Activity**	
	A	B	Frequency:	2–3 minutes
Baseline:	135 bpm	145 bpm	Duration:	2–2½ minutes
Variability:	Minimal	Moderate	Strength:	Tocotransducer in place—must palpate
Periodic/Episodic Changes:	Early, late, and variable decelerations	None	Resting Tone:	Tocotransducer in place—must palpate

Discussion:

- In regard to "A": readjustment of the tocotransducer to eliminate artifact (or utilization of an IUPC) would assist with interpretation of the tracing by better demonstrating the timing of decelerations in relation to contractions.
- In regard to "B": the increases of the FHR above the baseline do not meet criteria for accelerations.

Strip Chart K-7				
Fetal Heart Rate			**Uterine Activity**	
	A	B	Frequency:	Tocotransducer needs to be adjusted
Baseline:	135 bpm?	155 bpm?	Duration:	Tocotransducer needs to be adjusted
Variability:	Minimal	Moderate	Strength:	Moderate to palpation
Periodic/Episodic Changes:	Decelerations present, type is indeterminate	Variable decelerations	Resting Tone:	Must palpate

Discussion:

- Without uterine activity data, it is not possible to accurately interpret the FHR baseline rate (and therefore the variability) or the type of periodic/episodic changes present. It does, however, appear that the baseline FHR of "B" has risen significantly.

Strip Chart K-8				
Fetal Heart Rate			**Uterine Activity**	
	A	B	Frequency:	Tocotransducer needs to be adjusted
Baseline:	140 bpm	160 bpm	Duration:	Tocotransducer needs to be adjusted
Variability:	Minimal	Minimal	Strength:	Tocotransducer in place—must palpate
Periodic/Episodic Changes:	Decelerations present, type is indeterminate	Variable decelerations	Resting Tone:	Tocotransducer in place—must palpate

Discussion:

- It remains difficult to determine with certainty the FHR baseline rate and variability, or the type of periodic/episodic changes present due to lack of useful uterine activity data.

Strip Chart K-9				
Fetal Heart Rate			**Uterine Activity**	
	A	B	Frequency:	2 minutes
Baseline:	145 bpm	150 bpm	Duration:	1–2 minutes
Variability:	Minimal	Minimal	Strength:	Tocotransducer in place—must palpate
Periodic/Episodic Changes:	Prolonged deceleration; early, variable, and late decelerations	Variable deceleration	Resting Tone:	Tocotransducer in place—must palpate

Strip Chart K-10

	Fetal Heart Rate		Uterine Activity	
	A	B	Frequency:	Tocotransducer needs to be adjusted
Baseline:	140 bpm	150 bpm, then terminal bradycardia	Duration:	Tocotransducer needs to be adjusted
Variability:	Minimal	Minimal	Strength:	Must palpate
Periodic/Episodic Changes:		Resting Tone:	Must palpate	

OUTCOME:

- "A" female delivered spontaneously at 22:14. Apgars 7/9. 2665 grams (5 lbs, 14 oz). Resuscitation: ET suctioning, blow-by O_2, tactile stimulation.
- "B" delivered at 22:26 by forceps. pH 6.975, pCO_2 132.8, pO_2 25, BE −5.5. Apgars 5/9. 2466 grams (5 lbs, 7 oz). Resuscitation: positive pressure ventilation with 100% O_2, blow-by O_2, tactile stimulation.

Strip Chart L-1

	Fetal Heart Rate		Uterine Activity
Baseline:	135 bpm	Frequency:	2–3 minutes
Variability:	Moderate	Duration:	80 seconds–2 minutes
Periodic/Episodic Changes:	Accelerations; variable decelerations	Strength:	Tocotransducer in place—must palpate
		Resting Tone:	Tocotransducer in place—must palpate

Discussion:

- Despite the presence of mild variable decelerations, the tracing is reassuring.

Strip Chart L-2

	Fetal Heart Rate		Uterine Activity
Baseline:	135 bpm	Frequency:	3 minutes
Variability:	Moderate	Duration:	1–2 minutes
Periodic/Episodic Changes:	Accelerations; variable decelerations	Strength:	Tocotransducer in place—must palpate
		Resting Tone:	Tocotransducer in place—must palpate

Discussion:

- It appears that the maternal pulse was erroneously recorded for a period of time.

Strip Chart L-3			
Fetal Heart Rate		*Uterine Activity*	
Baseline:	140 bpm	Frequency:	3–4 minutes
Variability:	Moderate	Duration:	1–1½ minutes
Periodic/Episodic Changes:	Accelerations; variable decelerations	Strength:	Tocotransducer in place—must palpate
		Resting Tone:	Tocotransducer in place—must palpate

Strip Chart L-4			
Fetal Heart Rate		*Uterine Activity*	
Baseline:	150 bpm	Frequency:	2–4 minutes
Variability:	Moderate	Duration:	1–1½ minutes
Periodic/Episodic Changes:	Variable decelerations	Strength:	Tocotransducer in place—must palpate
		Resting Tone:	Tocotransducer in place—must palpate

Strip Chart L-5			
Fetal Heart Rate		*Uterine Activity*	
Baseline:	145 bpm	Frequency:	2–4 minutes
Variability:	Moderate	Duration:	1 minute
Periodic/Episodic Changes:	Accelerations; variable decelerations	Strength:	Mild–moderate by palpation
		Resting Tone:	"Rest" present

Discussion:

• While the FHR tracing continues to be reassuring, it warrants observation as the FHR has risen slightly and the variable decelerations seem to be starting to increase in severity. At this point, position changes may be helpful in alleviating some of the variable decelerations.

Strip Chart L-6			
Fetal Heart Rate		*Uterine Activity*	
Baseline:	145 bpm	Frequency:	3½–4 minutes
Variability:	Moderate	Duration:	60–70 seconds
Periodic/Episodic Changes:	Variable decelerations	Strength:	Tocotransducer in place—must palpate
		Resting Tone:	Tocotransducer in place—must palpate

Strip Chart L-7			
Fetal Heart Rate		*Uterine Activity*	
Baseline:	135 bpm	Frequency:	2–4 minutes
Variability:	Moderate	Duration:	1–2 minutes
Periodic/Episodic Changes:	Accelerations; variable decelerations	Strength:	Tocotransducer in place—must palpate
		Resting Tone:	Tocotransducer in place—must palpate

Discussion:

• Prior to and immediately following patient's trip to the bathroom, the FHR appears to be 105–115 bpm. There are no annotations to clarify if this is accurate or another occurrence of the maternal signal recording on the FHR tracing.

Strip Chart L-8			
Fetal Heart Rate		*Uterine Activity*	
Baseline:	120 bpm	Frequency:	3–3½ minutes
Variability:	Moderate	Duration:	1–1½ minutes
Periodic/Episodic Changes:	Accelerations; variable decelerations, late decelerations?	Strength:	Tocotransducer in place—must palpate
		Resting Tone:	Tocotransducer in place—must palpate

Discussion:

• It is difficult to assess the timing of FHR decelerations (to determine whether late decelerations are occurring) due to a lack of clear uterine activity data. The tocotransducer is readjusted at the end of this segment of tracing.

Strip Chart L-9			
Fetal Heart Rate		*Uterine Activity*	
Baseline:	135 bpm	Frequency:	3–4 minutes
Variability:	Moderate	Duration:	1–1½ minutes
Periodic/Episodic Changes:	Accelerations; variable decelerations	Strength:	Tocotransducer in place—must palpate
		Resting Tone:	Tocotransducer in place—must palpate

Strip Chart L-10			
Fetal Heart Rate		*Uterine Activity*	
Baseline:	135 bpm	Frequency:	2–5 minutes
Variability:	Moderate	Duration:	1–1½ minutes
Periodic/Episodic Changes:	Accelerations; variable decelerations	Strength:	Tocotransducer in place—must palpate
		Resting Tone:	Tocotransducer in place—must palpate

Discussion:

• There continues to be a possibility that late decelerations are present, but they do not occur in any consistent manner. The FHR tracing warrants observation.

Strip Chart L-11			
Fetal Heart Rate		*Uterine Activity*	
Baseline:	130 bpm	Frequency:	3½–4½ minutes
Variability:	Moderate	Duration:	1–1½ minutes
Periodic/Episodic Changes:	Variable and late? decelerations	Strength:	15–55 mm/Hg
		Resting Tone:	10 mm/Hg

Strip Chart L-12			
Fetal Heart Rate		*Uterine Activity*	
Baseline:	135 bpm	Frequency:	2–5 minutes
Variability:	Moderate	Duration:	1–1½ minutes
Periodic/Episodic Changes:	Variable and late decelerations	Strength:	25–60 mm/Hg
		Resting Tone:	10–15 mm/Hg

Strip Chart L-13			
Fetal Heart Rate		*Uterine Activity*	
Baseline:	135 bpm	Frequency:	2–4½ minutes
Variability:	Moderate	Duration:	1–1½ minutes
Periodic/Episodic Changes:	Variable and late decelerations	Strength:	50–75 mm/Hg
		Resting Tone:	10 mm/Hg

Strip Chart L-14			
Fetal Heart Rate		*Uterine Activity*	
Baseline:	130 bpm	Frequency:	2–3 minutes
Variability:	Moderate–minimal	Duration:	90 seconds
Periodic/Episodic Changes:	Late decelerations and variable decelerations	Strength:	50–80 mm/Hg
		Resting Tone:	10–15 mm/Hg

Strip Chart L-15			
Fetal Heart Rate		*Uterine Activity*	
Baseline:	135 bpm	Frequency:	2½–3 minutes
Variability:	Minimal	Duration:	1–1½ minutes
Periodic/Episodic Changes:	Early decelerations; variable decelerations?	Strength:	55–70 mm/Hg
		Resting Tone:	10–15 mm/Hg

Discussion:

- The FHR has taken on a markedly different appearance from when the patient was admitted. The variability is diminished (butorphanol was, however, administered 2 hours prior), there are no longer accelerations, and there are now brief, odd fluctuations both above and below the baseline FHR. Also, the nurse has noted that the FHR is "irregular-sounding" and that it is difficult to maintain a continuous recording. Application of a spiral electrode to rule out dysrhythmia may be helpful. Auscultation of the FHR with a fetoscope or visualization with M-mode sonography may also assist with evaluation of this fetus.

Strip Chart L-16			
Fetal Heart Rate		*Uterine Activity*	
Baseline:	135 bpm	Frequency:	2½–3 minutes
Variability:	Moderate	Duration:	1–1½ minutes
Periodic/Episodic Changes:	Variable decelerations	Strength:	50–65 mm/Hg
		Resting Tone:	10 mm/Hg

Discussion:

- The variable decelerations, which began occurring with greater depth and frequency during contractions following the cervical exam. This may be due to positioning and/or fluid loss during the exam.

Strip Chart L-17			
Fetal Heart Rate		*Uterine Activity*	
Baseline:	140 bpm	Frequency:	2–3 minutes
Variability:	Minimal	Duration:	1½–2 minutes
Periodic/Episodic Changes:	Variable decelerations	Strength:	Tocotransducer in place—must palpate
		Resting Tone:	Tocotransducer in place—must palpate

Discussion:

• Although the FHR tracing does not have the "typical" presentation of a dysrhythmia (usually more organized-appearing deflections), the audible irregularities assist in determining its presence. At this point, sonographic examination may be helpful in determining the etiology of the dysrhythmia and allow for any special preparations needed for delivery to be made.

• The FHR baseline is still visible relatively clearly through the dysrhythmia.

Strip Chart L-18			
Fetal Heart Rate		*Uterine Activity*	
Baseline:	135 bpm	Frequency:	2–3 minutes
Variability:	Moderate	Duration:	1½–2 minutes
Periodic/Episodic Changes:	Variable and late decelerations	Strength:	Moderate—strong by palpatation
		Resting Tone:	Tocotransducer in place—must palpate

Discussion:

• An acceleration is noted as a response to the cervical examination, a reassuring indication that the fetus is not likely to be experiencing acidosis.

Strip Chart L-19			
Fetal Heart Rate		*Uterine Activity*	
Baseline:	140 bpm	Frequency:	2–3 minutes
Variability:	Moderate–minimal	Duration:	1½–2 minutes
Periodic/Episodic Changes:	Variable and late decelerations	Strength:	Tocotransducer in place—must palpate
		Resting Tone:	Tocotransducer in place—must palpate

Strip Chart L-20			
Fetal Heart Rate		*Uterine Activity*	
Baseline:	145 bpm	Frequency:	2 minutes
Variability:	Moderate–minimal	Duration:	1½–2 minutes
Periodic/Episodic Changes:	Variable decelerations	Strength:	Tocotransducer in place—must palpate
		Resting Tone:	Tocotransducer in place—must palpate

OUTCOME:

11:58 SVD of live female over intact perineum. Apgars 7/8; taken to NICU for observation. No structural anomalies detected. Periods of PVCs persisted for less than 1 week and then ceased. Neonate was discharged home with monitoring on day 8.

Strip Chart M-1			
Fetal Heart Rate		*Uterine Activity*	
Baseline:	165 bpm	Frequency:	2–3 minutes
Variability:	Minimal	Duration:	1–1½ minutes
Periodic/Episodic Changes:	Variable and late decelerations	Strength:	Moderate to palpation
		Resting Tone:	Tocotransducer in place—must palpate

Discussion:

- It is quickly recognized that this patient needs to be admitted for more intensive care (states no fetal movement, has nonreassuring FHR tracing, laboring). An IV is started, blood work is sent, and the patient is transferred to L&D.

Strip Chart M-2			
Fetal Heart Rate		*Uterine Activity*	
Baseline:	170 bpm	Frequency:	No data available
Variability:	Moderate	Duration:	No data available
Periodic/Episodic Changes:	Variable and late decelerations	Strength:	Must palpate
		Resting Tone:	Must palpate

Strip Chart M-3			
Fetal Heart Rate		*Uterine Activity*	
Baseline:	170 bpm	Frequency:	2–3 minutes
Variability:	Minimal	Duration:	1–1½ minutes
Periodic/Episodic Changes:	Late and variable decelerations	Strength:	70–85 mm/Hg
		Resting Tone:	15–20 mm/Hg

Discussion:

- The FHR is tachycardic. When membranes are ruptured, thick meconium is present. Internal monitors (spiral electrode and IUPC) are placed to more closely monitor the fetus. Scalp stimulation is used to evaluate the fetus—no acceleration is achieved.
- Position changes, IV fluid bolus, O$_2$, and amnioinfusion are employed to improve fetal status. The amnioinfusion should decrease the frequency and severity of the variable decelerations and also serve to thin the meconium.

Strip Chart M-4			
Fetal Heart Rate		*Uterine Activity*	
Baseline:	170 bpm	Frequency:	Irregular?—signal seems to be interrupted; fetal scalp blood sampling procedure
Variability:	Minimal	Duration:	60–70 seconds?—signal seems to be interrupted; fetal scalp blood sampling procedure
Periodic/Episodic Changes:	Variable and late decelerations	Strength:	15–80 mm/Hg?—signal seems to be interrupted; fetal scalp blood sampling procedure
		Resting Tone:	15–20 mm/Hg

Discussion:

- The disruption in the FHR recording is likely to be artifact, as it is occurring mainly during procedures and events that may cause interference with the contact of the spiral electrode.
- Further attempts at intrauterine resuscitation are being made by administering terbutaline to decrease the stress of uterine activity on the fetus.
- Although technically challenging, it is optimal to perform fetal scalp blood sampling with the patient in a side-lying position to promote uterine perfusion.

Strip Chart M-5			
Fetal Heart Rate		*Uterine Activity*	
Baseline:	165 bpm	Frequency:	1½–4½ minutes
Variability:	Minimal	Duration:	1½–2 minutes
Periodic/Episodic Changes:	Variable and late decelerations	Strength:	25–80 mm/Hg
		Resting Tone:	10–20 mm/Hg

Discussion:

- While the pH result of the fetal scalp blood sampling is within normal range, the base excess is borderline for acidosis. The results are reassuring enough to allow labor to continue under close observation and with timely reevaluation.

Strip Chart M-6			
Fetal Heart Rate		*Uterine Activity*	
Baseline:	160 bpm	Frequency:	2–4 minutes
Variability:	Minimal	Duration:	1–2 minutes
Periodic/Episodic Changes:	Early and late decelerations	Strength:	70–75 mm/Hg
		Resting Tone:	15–30 mm/Hg

Discussion:

- Post epidural placement, consideration to patient positioning should include the effect of supine positioning on both the patient and the fetus. Modified positioning, with the patient wedged to one side or the other, is preferable to supine. If lateral positioning is best for the fetus, the patient can be turned frequently to assist with equalizing epidural coverage.

Strip Chart M-7			
Fetal Heart Rate		*Uterine Activity*	
Baseline:	160 bpm	Frequency:	× 2
Variability:	Minimal	Duration:	80–90 seconds
Periodic/Episodic Changes:	Early and late decelerations; prolonged deceleration	Strength:	60–85 mm/Hg
		Resting Tone:	15–20 mm/Hg

Discussion:

- There are a variety of reasons to consider regarding why the FHR would decelerate under such conditions, such as:
  - Rapid cervical progress and fetal descent (patient went from 4 to 8 cms and −2 to +1 in ~23 minutes), which may have caused a vagal response in the fetus as the head descended.
  - Hypotension due to 1) supine positioning, or 2) epidural. While a BP had been recently obtained (and was increased rather than decreased), it may have been helpful to have obtained a BP during this time.
  - Stress of uterine contractions—the effects of the terbutaline given earlier may be diminishing.
  - Cord prolapse, abruption, uterine rupture.

OUTCOME:

20:25. Live male by cesarean birth. Cord pH 6.99/BE −14 (values indicative of metabolic acidosis). Apgars 7/8. Resuscitation: ET suctioning (no meconium below the cords), blow-by O_2, tactile stimulation.

Strip Chart N-1			
Fetal Heart Rate		*Uterine Activity*	
Baseline:	130 bpm	Frequency:	× 1?
Variability:	Minimal–absent	Duration:	No data available
Periodic/Episodic Changes:	Prolonged deceleration	Strength:	No data available
		Resting Tone:	No data available

Strip Chart N-2			
Fetal Heart Rate		*Uterine Activity*	
Baseline:	130 bpm	Frequency:	No data available
Variability:	Minimal–absent	Duration:	No data available
Periodic/Episodic Changes:	Prolonged decelerations?	Strength:	No data available
		Resting Tone:	No data available

Discussion:

- There appears to be some double-counting of the FHR during decelerations. The actual FHR as noted by the clinician is likely obtained per the electronic fetal monitor's audible signal.
- There is no acceleration with scalp stimulation to reassure the clinicians of normal fetal acid–base status. It is important to understand the scalp stimulation is a test that is done to see if the fetus can accelerate its heart rate above its baseline rate. This test is correctly initiated when the FHR is at baseline and not in the midst of deceleration.

Strip Chart N-3			
Fetal Heart Rate		*Uterine Activity*	
Baseline:	130 bpm	Frequency:	No data available
Variability:	Absent	Duration:	No data available
Periodic/Episodic Changes:	Prolonged decelerations	Strength:	No data available
		Resting Tone:	No data available

Discussion:

- It may have been prudent in this case to perform a sonographic examination shortly after this patient was admitted and the FHR tracing appeared nonreassuring. This may have helped to rule out the presence of anomalies.

OUTCOME:

15:49. Live female with multiple anomalies incompatible with life, including hypoplastic lungs. Neonatal death ensued at 2 hours.

Strip Chart O-1			
Fetal Heart Rate		*Uterine Activity*	
Baseline:	135 bpm	Frequency:	None
Variability:	Moderate	Duration:	
Periodic/Episodic Changes:	Variable decelerations	Strength:	
		Resting Tone:	

Discussion:

• Use of orange juice or other similar interventions to hasten the time to achieving a reactive tracing is not an evidence-based practice.

• Patient's c/o no fetal movement and similarity between the recorded data on the strip chart and the MHR should prompt further investigation (see Chapters 2 and 3).

Strip Chart O-2			
Fetal Heart Rate		*Uterine Activity*	
Baseline:	135 bpm	Frequency:	None
Variability:	Moderate	Duration:	
Periodic/Episodic Changes:	Variable decelerations	Strength:	
		Resting Tone:	

OUTCOME:

No fetal cardiac activity observed during sonographic evaluation. A primary cesarean birth was performed immediately. 11:46 3615-gram male, Apgars 0/0, clear fluid, tight nuchal cord × 2. Cord pH 6.70, BE –24. Resuscitation: full code unsuccessful. Recorded heart rate was maternal.

Strip Chart P-1			
Fetal Heart Rate		*Uterine Activity*	
Baseline:	Indeterminate (sinusoidal pattern)	Frequency:	Irregular
Variability:	Absent (sinusoidal pattern)	Duration:	2½ minutes
Periodic/Episodic Changes:	Late deceleration	Strength:	Tocotransducer in place—must palpate
		Resting Tone:	

Strip Chart P-2			
Fetal Heart Rate		*Uterine Activity*	
Baseline:	170 bpm	Frequency:	Irregular
Variability:	Absent (sinusoidal pattern)	Duration:	2+ minutes
Periodic/Episodic Changes:	Prolonged deceleration	Strength:	Tocotransducer in place—must palpate
		Resting Tone:	

OUTCOME:

An emergent cesarean birth was performed. When the uterus was opened, vasa previa was observed. 11:30 3500-gram female, clear fluid, nuchal cord × 2, Apgars 0/1/5. Cord pH 7.03. A full neonatal code was successful. Infant to NICU; required sodium bicarb to correct metabolic acidosis. Low hematocrit (due to fetal bleeding from vasa previa) required transfusion of PRBCs. Velamentous insertion of the cord later noted by pathology.

6 | Legal Issues in Electronic Fetal Monitoring

Rebecca Cady, JD

Litigation of Obstetric Cases

Litigation involving claims of substandard care during labor and delivery (L&D) has become commonplace in our society. Griffin, Heland, Esser, and Jones (1998) reported that obstetric care was involved in 61.2% of claims. The 2006 American College of Obstetricians and Gynecologists (ACOG) Survey on Professional Liability showed similar results. Respondents to this survey reported a claim rate of 62.1% during the period of January 2003 through December 2005. Of those claims, the most frequent primary allegation was neurologically impaired infant (30.8%). The second most frequent allegation was stillbirth/neonatal death (15.8%).

Beckman (1996) examined malpractice claims, including allegations of nursing negligence, filed from 1988 through 1993. Of 747 cases alleging nursing negligence, 17.4% pertain to an adverse outcome in the L&D area. The primary cause of fetal injury was linked with inadequate communication of nursing assessment data to the physician. Failure to detect fetal distress in a timely manner due to infrequent assessment of the electronic fetal monitor tracing caused greater than half of the injuries in cases that alleged nursing negligence. Failure to promptly inform the physician of fetal distress caused serious injury to 35 newborns and resulted in 16 deaths. Other causes of injury included failure to implement the chain of command in a timely manner when the physician did not respond appropriately to fetal distress, inadequate fetal assessment, and medication errors. Fetal monitoring interpretation and management are still common issues in litigation over adverse outcomes in pregnancy (Miller, 2005). Additionally, electronic fetal monitoring (EFM) plays a well-documented role in perinatal morbidity and mortality. As of July 2004, 77% of sentinel events involving perinatal death or permanent disability reported to the Joint Commission on Accreditation of Hospital Organizations (JCAHO) involved nonreassuring fetal status, and 34% involved a root cause of inadequate EFM (JCAHO, 2004). Even if L&D nurses are not personally named as defendants in an obstetric lawsuit, they still become involved in the litigation process as percipient witnesses to the care rendered to the patient and fetus by the defendant health care providers. In the claims reported by the ACOG Survey, the categorization of the codefendants included hospitals (42.3%), nurses (12%), and nurse-midwives (3.8%) (ACOG, 2006).

Importance of the Strip Chart to Obstetric Case Litigation

Often the most critical piece of evidence in a birth injury case is the strip chart. Eighty-four percent of monitored labors in the United States are monitored via EFM (Chez, Harvey, and Harvey, et al., 2000). Seventy percent of all claims concerning intrapartum care in relation to brain damage are based on the cardiotocogram and electronic fetal monitor (Symonds, 1994). One of the most common allegations in suits against obstetrics and gynecology (OB/GYN) physicians is improper treatment of fetal distress (Bentley-Lewis, 1996). Greenwald (1998, p. 19) noted, "No tool is more universally used to demonstrate alleged negligence in obstetric claims than the electronic fetal monitor." Miller (2005) noted that common system errors related to the use of intrapartum EFM include knowledge deficits, communication failures, and fear of conflict. Therefore, all nurses working in this area must be aware of the legal implications of the tasks they perform related to EFM. These include monitor placement and removal, interpretation of the strip chart data, response to abnormal patterns, documentation, communication of findings to the care provider, and troubleshooting the equipment. Simpson (2000) identified key components of a risk management plan regarding EFM:

- Common EFM language in all professional communication and medical record documentation
- Joint nurse–physician education about EFM
- Competent care providers
- Collaboration and mutual respect among care providers
- Clear definition for fetal well-being and assessment of fetal well-being on admission
- Ongoing assessment and determination of fetal well-being during labor
- Appropriate use of intrauterine resuscitation techniques
- Accurate monitoring of fetal heart rate and uterine activity via EFM
- Accurate interpretation of EFM data
- Organizational resources and systems to support clinically timely interventions when the fetal heart rate is nonreassuring
- Continuation of EFM until birth
- Neonatal resuscitation team in attendance at birth if any question of fetal compromise
- Interdisciplinary case reviews for near misses and adverse outcomes

Costs and Outcome of Obstetric Lawsuits

An obstetric claims study by Farmers Insurance Group Companies' Professional Liability Division found that between the years 1991 and 1995, L&D claims represented slightly over 6% of the hospital and physician claims occurring in the top seven areas of frequency. These same claims, however, accounted for more than 11% ($37,665,836) of the total dollars spent for indemnity, expenses, and reserves (Rommal, 1996). More than 50% of damages awarded in all health care malpractice cases consisted of settlements and compensation for obstetric malpractice (Fiesta, 1994a).

According to the ACOG Survey, the respondents reported that 67.4% of claims were dropped or settled without payment (on behalf of the physician); 37.3% were dropped by the defendant; 13% were dismissed by the court; and 17.1% were settled without payment by the obstetrician/gynecologist. Of the outcomes involving payment, 20% of the claims settled prior to the start of trial or before a verdict; 3.4% of the claims closed through arbitration; and 10.2% of the claims closed through jury or court verdict (ACOG, 2006).

The general public's familiarity with medical malpractice settlements or judgments occurs primarily through media reports or dramatic re-enactments of the more sensational multimillion-dollar verdicts. However, the reality is that the average for all paid claims reported in this survey was $504,925. For the neurologically impaired infant requiring long-term care, the average payment was $1,150,687/case (ACOG, 2006).

Why Do So Many Patients Sue?

Stolte and associates (Stolte, Myers, & Owen, 1994) believe that the use of technologies such as EFM results in higher patient expectations and, therefore, increases the chances for litigation. McRae (1999) notes that the expectation of EFM technology has grown to include its ability to prevent fetal neurologic damage and unnecessary surgical delivery. Such beliefs abound, despite evidence that EFM has failed to reduce the rate of cerebral palsy (Gimovsky, 1994; Nelson et al., 1996; Sandmire, 1990; Schifrin, 1994; Symonds, 1994). One author believes that much of the blame placed on EFM should be assigned to those who make clinical decisions (Paul, 1994), whereas others contend that the problem rests with a lack of consistent reliable terminology (Flamm, 1994).

Clinical Competency and Interpretation of Fetal Strip Charts

Failing to understand and/or interpret information presented by the electronic fetal monitor clearly falls below the standard of care (Schifrin, 1993). In determining whether a nurse has been negligent in the care of a particular patient, one of the questions to be asked is whether the nurse's actions complied with nationally recognized standards for L&D nursing. Fiesta (1994b) noted that nursing standards tend to be more uniform than those for physicians, which may make it easier to establish negligence against a nurse. McRae (1999) noted that, although some courts allow for reasonable judgment by the physician as the standard in malpractice negligence, obstetric nurses have no such privilege for practice decisions. This creates a double standard and may serve to strengthen the physician's defense while weakening that of the nurse. Nurses, therefore, need to ensure that they are intimately familiar with the professional standards and guidelines for EFM. Failure to follow such practice guidelines is likely to lead to a finding of liability if a patient incurs harm.

Despite many advances in obstetric care over the past 20 years, EFM skills are still not being obtained or maintained by all nurses working in the L&D area. As early as 1986, the Nurses Association of the American College of Obstetricians and Gynecologists (NAACOG) mandated that maintaining the quality of individual practice was an inherent responsibility of the professional nurse. The Association of Women's Health, Obstetric and Neonatal Nurses (AWHONN, 2000) continues to maintain the position that only registered nurses (RNs) with expertise in EFM should initi-

ate and evaluate the technology. Nurses should also complete a course of study that includes the core competencies.

Hospitals can be held liable for having nurses who are not proficient in EFM skills perform such duties. JCAHO (1996) requires that an orientation be provided and an assessment conducted on each staff member's ability to fulfill specific job responsibilities, the purpose being to familiarize staff with their jobs and work environment before undertaking patient care duties. As this relates to EFM, staff nurses in L&D (or other areas that perform EFM) should not be allowed to care for monitored patients independently until certain skill criteria are met (AWHONN, 2006).

CASE EXAMPLES: FAILURE TO ADEQUATELY MONITOR EFM

McRae (1993) reported a case in which a 27-year-old G_1P_0 was admitted to the hospital at 38 weeks' gestation, with a blood pressure of 160/100. On admission assessment, the cervix was 2 cm dilated, 65% effaced, and the fetus presented in vertex position at -3 station. The patient was contracting every 3 to 4 minutes. The patient reported a history of elevated blood pressure that preceded hospital admission by 2 weeks. She was noted to have $+1$ edema and $+3$ deep tendon reflexes.

Two hours after her admission, magnesium sulfate was administered to the patient intravenously. Five hours post admission, the nursing staff initiated external EFM. At that time, the patient's blood pressure was 144/86, and the fetal heart rate (FHR) baseline was determined to be 144. Over the next 4 hours, the patient continued to contract every 3 to 5 minutes. The nurses documented the FHR as being within the range of 120 and 144, but failed to document any further EFM assessment. There was no report of baseline variability or the presence or absence of periodic changes. The membranes were artificially ruptured, and a spiral electrode was applied. It was documented that the fluid was clear.

Four hours later (13 hours post admission), the nurse changed the maternal position to the left side. At this time, the medical record reflects the patient's blood pressure to be 150/90 and the FHR at 152. No further information about the FHR was documented at that time. Four more hours passed, and an oxytocin infusion was initiated. The patient's blood pressure was 170/110, and the FHR was noted to be 130. It was recorded in the nurses' notes that maternal position was changed several times, but that the oxytocin infusion continued despite documentation of tetanic contractions. The physician ordered preoperative blood work for a possible cesarean birth.

Four hours from the time the oxytocin infusion began, the patient achieved complete dilation. At that time, EFM was discontinued and no further fetal assessment was made until delivery, which occurred 35 minutes later. Upon delivery, seizure activity of the neonate was noted. No Apgar scores were recorded.

At no time during the > 21 hours of labor did the nursing staff document an adequate assessment and evaluation of fetal status. Interestingly, the fetal strip charts were "lost," as were the hospital's policy and procedure manuals. The nurse expert for the patient opined that the care provided by the nurses was below the standard of care in the following respects: Failing to adequately assess, interpret, and document fetal status with the use of EFM; failure to assess and document the color of amniotic fluid for the duration of the labor; failure to intervene and discontinue oxytocin in the presence of tetanic contractions; and failure to document the FHR during the final 35 minutes of labor. The jury agreed and found for the plaintiff.

McRae (1993) reported another case in which staff failed to adequately perform EFM assessment. In this case, a 22-year-old G_1P_0 was admitted at 39 weeks' gestation reporting SROM 18 hours before admission. Because she was not contracting and was only fingertip dilated, an elective induction was begun 2 hours after admission. At this time, an external EFM was placed. Two hours later, frequent contractions and an obvious decrease in long-term variability were apparent. Although tetanic contractions ensued, the nurses continued to increase the oxytocin every 15 minutes. Five hours after oxytocin was begun, the nursing staff doubled and continued to increase the oxytocin. Two hours after that, a spiral electrode was placed and the tocodynamometer was removed and never reapplied. Twice during the next 20 minutes, the nurses changed maternal position and documented contractions of 90 to 100 seconds' duration, with only 15 seconds between contractions. Over the next hour, several more position changes were performed. The oxytocin was decreased, discontinued, and then restarted within a 20-minute period. Short-term variability became diminished. After 16.5 hours of oxytocin infusion, a female infant was delivered with Apgars of 2 and 5. The plaintiff's expert nurse opined that the nurses' care was below the standard of care for the following reasons: Failure to adequately monitor fetal status, failure to adequately document the color of the amniotic fluid, failure to question the use of oxytocin, failure to challenge inappropriate medical management, failure to administer proper amounts of oxytocin, failure to discontinue oxytocin in light of tetanic contractions, and failure to follow protocols set forth by The Association of Women's Health, Obstetric, and Neonatal Nurses (AWHONN) regarding oxytocin administration and the nurse's role in EFM. This case was settled out of court for a substantial amount of money to care for the severely handicapped child.

McRae (1993) reported a case regarding inadequate EFM assessment of twin pregnancy. In that case, a 30-year-old G_1P_0 with twin gestation was admitted in labor at term after an uneventful pregnancy. On admission, she was having moderately intense contractions every 2 to 3 minutes, the cervix was 5 to 6 cm dilated, and the FHR was 160 bpm in the left upper quadrant and 130 bpm in the right lower quadrant. A spiral electrode was applied to twin A shortly after admission. There was no nursing assessment of FHR variability, but both FHR baseline rates were documented as being within normal range. For some reason during the labor, the fetuses were not monitored for the same length of time; twin A was recorded for 100 minutes, and twin B for only 84 minutes. Despite a rapidly progressing labor, the nursing staff not only failed to record observations of FHR but also left the patient alone for an hour at the change of shift, immediately after documentation of a deep, prolonged deceleration. The physician also left the patient alone after having observed the deceleration and ordering an IV to be started. The physician was not notified until 45 minutes later that the FHR tracing indicated a worsening problem. Twin B developed persistent and repetitive decelerations that occurred for more than 60 minutes without intervention. Finally, a cesarean birth was performed. Twin A was delivered in good condition and is healthy. Twin B was born with Apgars of 0 and 1 and required vigorous resuscitation. The initial arterial blood gas was 6.76. The infant suffered the neurologic sequelae of asphyxia. Clearly, the "care" rendered to this patient was far below what the standard requires. This case was settled out of court.

Inter- and Intraobserver Variation in Interpretation of the Fetal Strip Chart

Even nurses and care providers who have been well trained and are proficient in EFM can be inconsistent in how they interpret FHR tracings. For example, a 1998 study (Borgatta, Shrout, & Divon, 1988) revealed that when five perinatologists reviewed 50 strip charts from nonstress tests (NSTs) and then re-reviewed the same FHR tracings, only 11 were classified as the same at both readings by the same perinatologist. Nurses also have the same difficulty. Chez, et al. (1990) found that 16% of nurses interpreted the NST as reactive when it was not. Devane and Lalor (2005) noted that midwives demonstrated the same inter- and intraobserver variability, and suggested that this was an intrinsic characteristic of the interpretation of intrapartum EFM. Murray (1996) discovered that physicians do not necessarily have greater accuracy in interpreting strip charts than do nurses, and that both nurses and physicians have been known to have difficulty in agreeing on interpretation when reviewing the same FHR tracing. Even health care providers who

believe they are experts in EFM interpretation can reach different conclusions from the same strip chart. Cohen et al. (1982) presented 14 different FHR patterns to 12 "experts" in the United States. There was nearly perfect agreement on five FHR tracings, fair agreement on five others, and marked disagreement over the remaining four. Nielson and colleagues (1986) had four experienced obstetricians assess 50 thirty-minute-long FHR tracings. Only 11 of the strip charts were assessed by all four obstetricians in the same way, and 20% were assessed differently when reviewed by the same obstetricians 2 months later. Simpson (2000) noted that this variation continues to be a problem, and that this phenomenon especially affects interpretations suggesting fetal compromise.

These studies illustrate how and why both parties in a given lawsuit can find experts willing to testify under oath, some saying the FHR tracings were normal, with others testifying that the same FHR tracings were abnormal. Unfortunately, in many lawsuits involving neurologic damage, the jury must weigh the testimony of two experts who may be equally qualified but testify to two diametrically opposed findings. The expert for the plaintiff will testify that the strip chart showed fetal distress and will attempt to prove that the resulting neonatal condition was caused by the providers' negligence. The expert for the defendants will testify that the strip chart did not show fetal distress and, even if it did, that the resulting condition was not caused by any action or inaction on the part of the defendants. When presented with a child who has profound damage and will require a lifetime of care, the jury is likely to be seduced by the argument that the injuries could not have resulted from natural processes and is likely to find the health care providers negligent.

CASE EXAMPLES: FAILURE TO PROPERLY MONITOR

Rommal (1996) reports an unpublished case regarding failing to properly monitor. The patient was a primigravida at term gestation who arrived in L&D on an extremely busy night. All the rooms were occupied, so she had to wait to be put into a labor room. The patient was alert and oriented, and complaining of constant uterine pain. The admission note indicated that the fetus was tachycardic at 170 bpm, and that no regular uterine contractions were palpated. The patient reported leaking watery, bloody fluid and feeling decreased fetal movement for 8 to 10 hours. Forty-five minutes after her arrival, she was placed in a labor room. After 15 minutes, the EFM was applied by a scrub technician. The RN entered the labor room 15 minutes later and noticed that the FHR was down to 60 to 70 bpm and had been so for the previous 10 minutes. An emergency cesarean birth was performed, and an abruptio placentae was found. The neonate had Apgars of 0 and 3 and suffered profound neurologic damage. A lawsuit was filed against the hospital. The nurse testified at her deposition that she suspected the patient was abrupting, but she was busy with a second patient in active labor and was trying to get a third patient discharged so she could get the patient in question into bed. The nurse was found negligent for her failure to notify her nurse manager and ask for immediate help in assessing the patient with a possible abruptio placentae, as well as failing to notify the physician of the patient's condition in a timely manner.

In another case, an L&D nurse was called by a physician and informed that a patient was coming to the L&D suite. The physician also told the nurse that the fetus was in a breech position and a cesarean birth was likely to be performed. The physician was present when the patient arrived at the hospital and the nurse placed her in a labor room. The physician examined the patient, confirmed that the fetus was in a breech position, and told the nurse that a cesarean birth was needed due to the breech presentation. Because the physician was in the room with the patient and speaking in a nonurgent manner, the nurse left the room and began preparing for the cesarean birth. When the nurse returned to the room and listened to the FHR for the first time, she discovered that FHR decelerations were present. An emergency cesarean birth was performed, but the child was born with severe physical and cognitive defects. In this case, the jury found that the nurse was not excused from completing an initial assessment of the patient (not performed until an hour after her arrival in L&D) based on the physician's appraisal of patient condition. The jury awarded the patient $3 million. The patient's expert witnesses convinced the jury that the duty to assess was an independent nursing function that could not be delegated even to the physician (*McMillan et al. v. Frye Regional Medical Center et al.,* 1992).

National Standards

AWHONN first published nursing standards for clinical responsibilities in performing EFM in 1980. Nursing actions outlined by this standard included observing, assessing, evaluating, and intervening in accordance with the data received from the monitor. This standard indicated that nurses would be expected to identify the baseline rate, bradycardia, and tachycardia; to assess variability; to identify accelerations and early, late, and variable decelerations; and to report ominous patterns to the physician. AWHONN subsequently published guidelines related to EFM in the form of a position statement entitled "Nursing Responsibilities in Implementing Intrapartum Fetal Heart Rate Monitoring" in 1980, which was reaffirmed in 1994. This publication clearly delineated the nurse's role in EFM and was followed by the position statement "Fetal Assessment" in 2000. AWHONN's instructional book, *Fetal Heart Monitoring Principles and Practices* (revised 2003) expounds on the nurse's role in EFM in greater detail. The position statement was updated in 2000 to include the use of intermittent auscultation. To assist hospitals in providing the necessary components for EFM education, AWHONN has published guidelines for education program content (2006). These guidelines include competence practice, didactic course outlines, learner assessment/ongoing competence validation, terminology, and documentation.

Assessment and documentation of nurses' competence in antepartum and intrapartum FHR and uterine contraction monitoring should be performed as recommended by AWHONN to reduce liability. The nurse must demonstrate knowledge of maternal–fetal physiology; competency in interpretation of the baseline FHR, including variability; periodic/episodic changes of the FHR; uterine activity; and an understanding of the technology used (AWHONN, 2006). The nurse's ability to function independently and accomplish the skills necessary for fetal surveillance should be validated. AWHONN (2000)

> strongly advises that all nurses who perform fetal assessment during the antepartum or intrapartum period complete a course of study that includes the physiologic interpretation of EFM data and its implications for labor support. This course should include instruction in both cognitive and psychomotor skill validations of standardized core competencies used in auscultation, electronic monitoring of the FHR and evaluation of uterine activity.

CASE EXAMPLE: INADEQUATELY TRAINED/INCOMPETENT STAFF

In a case reported by Feutz-Harter (1994), a California hospital settled out of court for $2.15 million in an obstetric case involving an L&D nurse who had graduated from nursing school only 4 months earlier. The plaintiff's allegations focused on the extreme inexperience of the nurse and the failure of the hospital to properly supervise the novice employee. The nurse testified that she realized that something was wrong when she began to have difficulty obtaining a technically adequate FHR pattern. Unfortunately, the nurse failed to adequately articulate this problem to other health care team members. As a result, a delay occurred in delivery, and the infant was born with severe neurologic damage.

Antepartum Observation and Testing

It is important that patients undergoing antepartum evaluation receive adequate observation and monitoring. This may include obtaining a tracing of FHR and uterine activity of at least 20 to 30 minutes' duration, depending on hospital policy. Whether antepartum testing is performed in the hospital or in an outpatient setting, it becomes part of the medical record (Rommal, 1996). There should be evidence that a provider has personally reviewed the strip

chart and that the interpretation is documented within a reasonable period of time. A reasonable period of time has been defined by case law (Rommal, 1996) as being within 24 hours of the test.

CASE EXAMPLE: ANTEPARTUM TESTING

A patient with a postterm pregnancy was having twice-weekly NSTs. During one NST, the patient had a spontaneous contraction with a single late-appearing deceleration, which the nurse noted in the outpatient record. The rest of the FHR tracing appeared reactive, and the nurse called the physician and reported the NST as normal. At this hospital, nurses routinely performed all antepartum test interpretation. The nurse noted on the outpatient record that she advised the physician of the patient's condition. The physician later stated that the nurse never told him of the single deceleration, and that had she told him, he would have induced the patient's labor that same day. Instead, the patient was sent home and returned in labor several days later. At that time, the FHR tracing demonstrated a flat FHR baseline and persistent late decelerations. The neonate presented at birth with severe neurologic damage, including quadriplegia and mental retardation. The jury found that the physician was not negligent; however, it found the hospital liable because the nurse had not provided the physician with full information about the patient (Rubsamen, 1993).

Standardized Terminology

One of the problems with determining the significance of potentially normal and abnormal variations on FHR tracings has been a lack of standardized terminology describing components of FHR patterns. A great deal of work has been done in the past several years toward creating a uniform set of terms for describing FHR patterns. The National Institutes of Health held a research-planning workshop in 1995–1996 to develop standardized and unambiguous definitions for FHR tracings (National Institute of Child Health and Human Development Research Planning Workshop [NICHD], 1997). Participants in this workshop agreed with current definitions of a normal fetal heart rate tracing, ie, "normal baseline rate, normal (moderate FHR variability, presence of accelerations, and absence of decelerations)" (NICHD, 1997). They also concurred that such a tracing is a good predictor of a normally oxygenated fetus. Participants assented that several patterns are "predictive of current or impending fetal asphyxia so severe that the fetus is at risk for neurologic and other fetal damage, or death" (NICHD, 1997). Such patterns include "recurrent late or variable decelerations or substantial bradycardia, with absent FHR variability" (NICHD, 1997). Notably, however, participants made "no a priori assumptions . . . of the putative etiology of the patterns or their relationship to hypoxemia or metabolic acidemia" (NICHD, 1997). Participants did not propose guidelines for clinical management, pending additional research. ACOG (2005) endorsed the clinical application of this nomenclature in 2005. AWHONN (2006) has integrated this nomenclature into their educational courses. Steps facilities can take to ensure consistent communication regarding EFM data include the following:

- Choose one language to be used in all communication about EFM.
- Educate all members of the perinatal team about the EFM language that has been selected, with physicians and nurses learning together. Support periodic continuing education as science and evidence develop.
- Consider certification in EFM for all members of the perinatal team.
- Revise all medical record forms and electronic system pick-lists to correlate with the selected language (Simpson, 2004).

Hospital Policies

JCAHO requires that hospitals have in place policies and procedures for EFM (JCAHO, 1996). Care must be taken when creating and updating policies on a regular basis to ensure that they comply with the standards of the profession. These policies should be updated at least yearly, to ensure that they keep pace with current re-

search findings and recommendations. Institutional policies must, at a minimum, require conduct that meets the nationally recognized standard of care.

Some institutions create policies that reflect conduct higher than the standard of care. This can pose legal problems for several reasons. First, if the policy creates unreasonable expectations of staff, then it is likely to be disregarded or followed only in part. This can present a danger to patients, due to lack of uniformity of care and the possibility that inexperienced personnel will make poor choices in caregiving when acting outside the scope of the policy. Second, many experienced plaintiff attorneys will routinely request copies of the hospital policies and procedures applicable to the care the patient received. If the nursing staff has not followed the institution's policies and procedures, then the plaintiff's attorney is likely to make the argument that "they didn't even follow their own procedures." They will also argue that, by adopting the policy or procedure in question, the hospital acknowledged that this would be the standard of care for its employees. This is an argument that juries find seductive and which often leads to large verdicts in cases of neurologic compromise. It also points out the need to carefully store copies of outdated policies as they are revised and updated. If a case were to go to trial, it would only be just for clinicians to be held accountable to the standards of care as they existed at the time the incident occurred. The nurse must keep in mind both the professional guidelines and standards as well as the facility's procedures when performing tasks related to EFM (Mahlmeister, 2000).

State Law

Most states' nurse practice acts are very broadly worded and do not deal specifically with the skill of EFM. Each nurse does need to be aware of the nurse practice act in the state or states in which he or she practices. EFM, however, is clearly a patient care function that cannot be delegated by the RN to an unlicensed individual, because its use and interpretation require skills that are only acknowledged to be possessed by registered nurses.

Responses to Nonreassuring Fetal Heart Rate Patterns

Once a nonreassuring FHR pattern is present on the strip chart and recognized by the nurse, the issue becomes the nurse's response. Koniak-Griffin (1999) stated that nurses who fail to recognize or ignore a progressively deteriorating or ominous FHR tracing do not possess the competency to perform in the L&D area. Competent nursing practice includes classification of EFM findings, implementation of appropriate interventions, and identification of clinical situations that indicate the need for timely notification of the provider (AWHONN, 2006).

The "30-Minute Rule"

What has become known as the "30-minute rule" indicates that, once a decision is made to perform a cesarean birth, the incision should occur within 30 minutes of the decision (American Academy of Pediatrics [AAP] & ACOG, 2002). All facilities are expected to meet current guidelines for beginning the surgery within 30 minutes of the decision to perform a surgical delivery. Health care providers need to be aware that this "30-minute rule" is not a safety net. There are some situations that warrant immediate intervention, such as uterine rupture. If significant risk factors are present, or obvious deterioration in the patient or fetal condition precedes the call for a cesarean birth, juries have found health care providers negligent for failing to deliver an infant in less time than 30 minutes (AAP & ACOG, 2002).

Even if delivery is accomplished in less than 30 minutes, the child may still suffer injuries. In a study by Chauhan et al. (1997), outcomes were measured for patients who had cesarean births performed for a primary indication of fetal distress. In 52% of the patients, the decision-to-incision time was 30 minutes; the time exceeded 30 minutes in the remaining patients. This study revealed that three adverse outcomes were observed more frequently in association with decision-to-incision times greater than 30 minutes: lower mean umbilical arterial pH; pH under 7.00; and admission to the neonatal intensive care unit (NICU). The study also revealed that, when the incision was made longer than 30 minutes after the decision, there was no apparent adverse neonatal or infant outcome. The researchers concluded that, although a decision-to-incision time less than 30 minutes is a desirable goal for the fetus possibly in distress, failure to achieve this goal was not associated with a measurable negative impact on newborn outcome. Other researchers have also reached the same conclusions. Roemer and Rommermann-Heger (1992) observed no association between the time interval from decision to incision and neonatal acidosis in 168 neonates delivered by emergency cesarean delivery. Schauberger et al. (1994) reported that the incidence of Apgar scores under 6 at 5 minutes was significantly higher if the decision-to-incision time was under 30 minutes. The researchers found no increase in neonatal morbidity and mortality when the time exceeded 30 minutes. Regardless of these findings, it is imperative to practice in accordance with the "30-minute rule" as it is the standard to which clinicians will likely be held accountable.

Predictive Value of Nonreassuring FHR Tracings

Chez et al. (2000) noted that EFM technology came to be widely accepted before proof existed of its efficacy and safety. ACOG (2005) noted that the various methods of intrapartum EFM currently used are not effective in predicting or preventing adverse long-term neurologic outcomes. They also stated that management of nonreassuring FHR patterns does not appear to affect the risk of subsequent cerebral palsy, due to the fact that neurologic abnormalities infrequently result from subtle events occurring during L&D. Conversely, most hypoxic and asphyxic episodes do not result in irreversible neurologic damage. One author questioned whether, given the fact that EFM has not been demonstrated to improve perinatal mortality for low-risk women compared to intermittent auscultation, informed consent should be obtained prior to initiating continuous EFM (Wood, 2003). However, strip charts continue to be used as key pieces of evidence in obstetric malpractice suits despite recognition of the limitations of electronic monitoring in the professional literature.

Communication to Physician/Chain of Command

Every institution should have a written chain of command policy that designates whom the nurse should notify if there is a disagreement with the provider as to the plan of care. Examples of such dissent can occur in relation to FHR pattern interpretation, the use of oxytocin or other medications, or any management plan. Mahlmeister (1996, p. 36) notes that nurses must: (1) be familiar with the established lines of authority in the institution, (2) know when to activate the chain of command, and (3) recognize when it is appropriate to move up a chain of command should there be a delay in or inappropriate response to requests for help. She also indicates that, in carrying out affirmative duty acts, the nurse must demonstrate timeliness, persistence, use of the chain of command process, and continuity of care.

If the FHR tracing is observed to be nonreassuring, the nurse must first implement nursing interventions and then notify the care provider. Mahlmeister (1996) notes that a growing number of licensing boards for registered nursing have created administrative rules and regulations, position statements, or advisories to guide nurses in implementing care provider orders. Mahlmeister (1996) gives as an example section 217.11(5) of the Texas rules and regulations relating to professional nurse education, licensure, and practice, which states,

> The registered nurse shall clarify any order or treatment regimen that the nurse has reason to believe is inaccurate, nonefficacious or contraindicated by consulting with the appropriate licensed practitioner and notifying the ordering practitioner when the registered nurse makes the decision not to administer the medication or treatment.

Additionally, the American Medical Association (AMA) recognizes that nurses have a duty to exercise professional nursing judgment in carrying out care provider orders. In its 1994 code of ethics, the AMA declares,

> Where orders appear to the nurse to be in error or contrary to customary medical and nursing practice, the physician has an ethical obligation to hear the nurse's concern and explain those

orders. In emergencies, when prompt action is necessary and the physician is not immediately available, in the performance of reasonable care a nurse may be justified in acting contrary to the physician's orders for the safety of the patient. (AMA, 1994)

Nurses are legally obligated to act in a positive manner when the patient's well-being is in jeopardy (Murphy, 1987). "If the primary care provider is unavailable to respond in a timely manner, the institutional process should be utilized to ensure appropriate patient evaluation" (AWHONN, 2000).

CASE EXAMPLES: COMMUNICATION WITH CARE PROVIDER

The case of *Fairfax Hospital System, Inc. v. McCarty*, 419 SE 2d 621 (VA 1992) illustrates a nurse's failure to provide timely notice to the physician. In this case, the nurse's failure to recognize and react to fetal distress, including her failure to timely notify the attending physician, was found to be a substantial breach of the standard of care. This nurse either failed to observe or failed to recognize signs of fetal distress that, according to expert testimony, first appeared on the strip chart at approximately 8:29 PM. Experts further testified that by 8:37 PM, the fetus was in distress and that the applicable standard of care required the nurse to institute nursing interventions and notify the physician to expedite delivery. The nurse did not notify the physician until 8:50 PM, at the earliest. According to the physician, the nurse reported decelerations in the FHR but did not indicate that there was any emergency. Experts testified that the nurse's failure to act delayed delivery and caused the infant's poor outcome.

The case of *Campbell v. Centinella Hospital Medical Center* (1994) exemplifies that nurses are held accountable for communicating with physicians about fetal distress and notifying the neonatologist in a timely manner. The plaintiff, an 18-year-old woman, was admitted to the hospital at 6 AM in labor. Oxytocin augmentation was started at noon. Although the FHR was initially normal, at 6 PM a prolonged deceleration to 60 bpm occurred and lasted for 8 minutes. The physician was in attendance at this time. Subsequently, repeated severe variable and late decelerations were observed over the next 2 hours. The patient was taken to the delivery room at 8 PM. FHR monitoring was not conducted for the 22 minutes preceding the vaginal birth because a monitor was not available in the delivery room. The infant had an initial Apgar score of zero and required CPR by the respiratory therapist and nurses in the delivery room. A neonatologist did not examine the infant until 9 PM. The plaintiff's attorney asserted that the defendant hospital's obstetric nurses failed to recognize fetal distress; failed to take actions that would have led to a cesarean birth; failed to assess the FHR in the delivery room, which would have shown terminal bradycardia; and failed to promptly call the neonatologist, which resulted in delayed treatment of the infant's acidosis. The hospital argued that the obstetric nurses deferred to the judgment of the physician and to his interpretation of the strip chart; that the physician was in charge, and, therefore, the nurses could not intervene and order a cesarean birth; and that delayed treatment of the acidosis was not the cause of the infant's injury. The physician settled before trial for nearly $1 million. The hospital went to trial, which resulted in a verdict for the plaintiff in excess of $10 million. The jury did not believe that the nurses could defer all judgment to the physician. The jury felt the nurses were required to act independently to protect the well-being of the patient and her fetus and were required to communicate with the neonatologist in a timely manner.

CASE EXAMPLES: CHAIN OF COMMAND

Campbell v. Pitt County Memorial Hospital, Inc. (1987), illustrates the hospital's duty to establish a mechanism for reporting and responding to any situation that is a threat to a patient's health and welfare and the nurse's obligation to use this chain of command to notify administrators of a physician's error. In

this case, the fetus had been identified as a footling breech several weeks before delivery. The patient told the admitting nurse that her physician had said the position of the fetus should be checked again at the time of labor. A physical examination and pelvimetry confirmed the presence of a footling breech, but neither the nurses nor the attending obstetrician shared this finding with the patient. The strip chart indicated that, for several hours before delivery, there were changes in the FHR indicative of fetal distress. The nurses identified the nonreassuring pattern. One nurse communicated her concern to the attending physician; however, she did not proceed to advise her supervisor or invoke an administrative chain of command when the physician failed to respond to the information given. Vaginal birth ensued approximately 2 hours later, and the neonate was diagnosed with brain damage, allegedly due to perinatal asphyxia from an entanglement of the umbilical cord with her legs. In this case, the plaintiff asserted that the hospital's failure to have in place an operational and effective mechanism to identify and respond to potentially harmful situations created a threat to the patient's welfare that was a proximate cause of the child's injuries. The court noted that the hospital has to "make a reasonable effort to monitor and oversee the treatment which is prescribed and administered by physicians practicing at the facility" (*Campbell v. Pitt County Memorial Hospital, Inc.* [1987], citing *Bost v. Riley*, 44 N.C. App. 638, 262 S.E.2d 391 [1980]). The court considered having an effective mechanism for the prompt reporting and response to any situation that creates a threat to patient health and welfare to be part of that reasonable effort.

In *Compton v. Thurston and Presbyterian Hospital of Dallas* (1996), an L&D nurse, concerned by the failure of the obstetrician to act in the face of a nonreassuring FHR pattern, went to her charge nurse for assistance. The obstetrician was approached by the charge nurse, who questioned him in regard to preparing for a cesarean birth. When the physician responded in the negative, the charge nurse failed to call for the assistance of the chief of obstetrics. The infant had profound neurologic depression at birth and died. The failure of the charge nurse to activate the chain of command process was a major factor in a $550,000 settlement paid to the parents of the deceased infant.

Documentation

One of the main issues that arise in perinatal lawsuits is documentation of the strip chart. ACOG (2005) indicates that the strip chart should be carefully labeled and retained along with the other medical records. Documentation may consist of narrative notes or the use of comprehensive flow sheets detailing periodic assessment of maternal and fetal status. Specific responses to a nonreassuring FHR pattern, such as further diagnostic procedures or therapeutic interventions, should also be documented, as well as the nature, date, and time of other pertinent events, such as the administration of medication or anesthesia. The specifics of how and where documentation is accomplished vary between institutions. It usually depends on resources and logistics, including the type of equipment used and the available method of record storage.

National guidelines for documentation of regular assessments of the strip chart include using specific, recognized nomenclature to identify the FHR patterns. This means using terms such as "late deceleration" or "variable deceleration" both in verbal and written communication (AWHONN, 2006; 2003; 1994). Periodic assessments of the strip chart are usually documented on a flow sheet and, at a minimum, should include interpretation of the baseline FHR and its variability; the presence or absence of periodic/episodic changes; the frequency and duration of uterine contractions and uterine resting tone; and maternal vital signs as designated by institutional policy. Narrative notes can be used to expound on other details, if necessary. Institutions should delineate nomenclature and devise standardized abbreviations to facilitate communication. These suggestions are applicable in reference to both computer charting and handwritten notes.

In emergency situations, when there is not sufficient time to make contemporaneous notes, late entries may be made. This is accomplished by noting the current time and date and then writing "late entry for" followed by acknowledgement of the date and time the events being described occurred. If there is not an electronic fetal monitor available for a patient or if the patient refuses to have EFM performed, these events should be documented and alternative strategies explored, such as intermittent auscultation. The care provider must be aware of the issue and participate in decisions regarding alternative monitoring. Regardless of which method of assessment is used, it is recommended that low-risk patients have the FHR evaluated and recorded every 30 minutes during the active phase of first-stage labor and every 15 minutes during second-stage labor. Accordingly, high-risk patients should have evaluation and recording of the FHR every 15 minutes during the active phase of first-stage labor and every 5 minutes during second-stage labor (ACOG, 2005; AAP & ACOG, 2002).

If a cesarean birth is indicated, it is important to continue to monitor the fetus for as long as possible. The AAP/ACOG *Guidelines for Perinatal Care* (2002, p. 148) states: "In women requiring cesarean delivery, fetal surveillance should continue until abdominal sterile preparation is begun. If internal FHR monitoring is in use, it should be continued until the abdominal sterile preparation is complete."

Central and Computerized Monitoring

Many hospitals now use computerized systems that create both a paper printout and computerized storage for electronic fetal monitor strips. A frequently asked question pertains to the storage of strip charts now that computer disk storage is available: Can the paper tracings be discarded and the electronic record used as the singular means of permanent storage? At this point in time, there are no authoritative answers to this question. From a legal defense perspective, it is best to have both the paper strip chart and the electronic record available. There are several reasons for this. There is the remote possibility that the EFM storage system may malfunction, which is similar to losing the actual strip chart and would have the same ramifications. Also, if handwritten notes were made on any portion of the original paper strip chart, they are part of the medical record. Finally, it must be kept in mind that the computer-generated FHR tracing may be a different size than the original and, to a minor extent, may affect interpretation.

Strip charts that are stored electronically are usually of high quality and accuracy, and their storage and retrieval abilities are generally quite reliable. Certainly, storage in an electronic record provides greater security and durability than paper storage. The likelihood of damage from factors such as temperature, moisture, or light is essentially eliminated, as is the possibility of tampering with the record. Most electronic archiving and charting systems have excellent tracking systems. If the record had been altered in some manner, such entries or deletions would be recognized on examination. The American Health Information Management Association (AHIMA) has developed standards for medical records that dictate that the legal medical record must record patient status, serve as a communication tool for caregivers, and provide evidence of the care given (McCartney, 2002). If a computerized system is in place, then it must meet these standards. Nurses must also be aware that state legal requirements for medical records may vary and that they should consult with hospital legal counsel when updating documentation and medical record policies and procedures to ensure compliance.

Conclusion

All clinicians who perform EFM as part of their care of patients need to know the many potential legal consequences of their actions. This knowledge needs to be accompanied by awareness that, in most states, anyone who chooses to can file suit against anyone else for any reason. If a patient suffers an adverse outcome, the nurse may be sued along with the hospital and the care provider. The best practice is to provide optimal care to every patient. Consistently meeting the standard of practice is the best legal defense.

REFERENCES

American Academy of Pediatrics and American College of Obstetricians and Gynecologists. (2002). *Guidelines for perinatal care* (5th ed.). Elk Grove Village, IL: Authors.

American College of Obstetricians and Gynecologists. (2006). *ACOG survey on professional liability results.* Washington, DC: Author.

———. (2005). *Clinical management guideline #70. Intrapartum fetal heart rate monitoring.* Washington, DC: Author.

———. (1998). *Guidelines for vaginal delivery after a previous cesarean birth* (ACOG Committee Opinion No. 64). Washington, DC: Author.

American Medical Association (AMA). (1994). *Code of medical ethics.* Chicago, IL: Author.

Association of Women's Health, Obstetric and Neonatal Nurses. (2006). *Antepartum and intrapartum fetal heart rate monitoring: Clinical competency and education guide* (4th ed.). Washington, DC: Author.

———. (2003). *Fetal heart monitoring principles and practices.* Washington, DC: Author.

———. (2000). *Fetal assessment* (position statement). Washington, DC: Author.

———. (1994). *Nursing responsibilities in implementing intrapartum fetal heart rate monitoring* (position statement). Washington, DC: Author.

———. (1980). *The nurses' role in electronic fetal monitoring.* Chicago, IL: Author.

Beckman, J. P. (1996). *Nursing negligence.* Thousand Oaks, CA: Sage.

Bentley-Lewis, R. (1996, August). Obstetrics-related claims. *Forum* [On-line serial], *17*(3), 1–4.

Board of Nurse Examiners (BNE). (1995). *Rules and regulations relating to professional nurse education, licensure and practice* (Section 217.11[5]). Austin, TX: Author.

Borgatta, L., Shrout, P. E., & Divon, M. Y. (1988). Reliability and reproducibility of non-stress test readings. *American Journal of Obstetrics and Gynecology, 159,* 554.

Campbell v. Centinella Hospital Medical Center (1994, April 29). No. YC0122–998. *Jury Verdict Weekly, 38* (17), 23–25.

Campbell v. Pitt County Memorial Hospital Inc., 352 S.E. 2d 902 (NC App, 1987).

Chauhan, S., Roach, H., Naef, R., Magann, E., Morrison, J., & Martin, J. (1997). Cesarean section for suspected fetal distress, does the decision-incision time make a difference? *Journal of Reproductive Medicine, 42*(6), 347–352.

Chez, B. F., Skurnick, J. H., Chez, R. A., & Verklan, M. T., et al. (1990). Interpretations of nonstress tests by obstetric nurses. *Journal of Obstetric, Gynecologic and Neonatal Nursing, 19,* 227.

Chez, B. F., Harvey, M. G., Harvey, C. (2000). Intrapartum fetal monitoring: past, present, and future. *Journal of Perinatal, Neonatal Nursing, 14*(3): 1–18.

Cohen, A. R., Klapholz, H., & Thompson, M. S. (1982). Electronic fetal monitoring and clinical practice—A survey of obstetric opinion. *Medical Decision Making, 2,* 79–95.

Compton v. Thurston and Presbyterian Hospital of Dallas, Dallas City (TX) Dist. Ct. Case No. 95–02288.

Devane, D., Lalor, J. (2005). Midwives visual interpretation of intrapartum cardiotocographs: intra- and inter-observer agreement. *Journal of Advanced Nursing, 52*(2): 133–141.

Fairfax Hospital System, Inc. v. McCarty, 419 SE 2d 621 VA 1992.

Feutz-Harter, S. (1994). Nursing case law update. Inexperienced nurses are high liability risks. *Journal of Nursing Law 1994, 1*, 47–52.

Fiesta, J. (1994a). Duty to communicate—"Doctor Notified." *Nursing Management, 25*, 24–25.

———. (1994b). Physician malpractice. *Nursing Management, 25*(12), 17–18.

Flamm, B. (1994). Electronic fetal monitoring in the United States. *Birth, 21*(2), 105–110.

Gimovsky, M. (1994). Electronic fetal heart rate monitoring. *Journal of Perinatology, 14*(3), 173.

Greenwald, L. (1998). *Hospital claims: A risk management overview by Pro Mutual Group.* Boston, MA: Pro Mutual Risk Management Services.

Griffin, L. P., Heland, K. V., Esser, L., & Jones, S. (1998, March/April). Overview of the 1996 professional liability survey. *ACOG Clinical Review* [On-line serial], *3*(2), 1–2, 13.

Joint Commission on Accreditation of Healthcare Organizations (JCAHO). (1996). *Comprehensive accreditation manual for hospitals.* Chicago, IL: Author.

Koniak-Griffin, D. (1999). Strategies for reducing the risk of malpractice litigation in perinatal nursing, *Journal of Obstetric, Gynecologic, and Neonatal Nursing, 28*(3), 291–299.

Mahlmeister, L. (1996, December). The perinatal nurse's role in obstetric emergencies: Legal issues and practice issues in the era of health care redesign. *Journal of Perinatal Neonatal Nursing, 10*(3), 32–46.

Mahlmeister, L. (2000). Legal implications of fetal heart assessment. *Journal of Obstetrics, Gynecologic, and Neonatal Nursing, 29*(5): 517–526.

McCartney, P. (2002). The new networking—electronic fetal monitoring and the legal medical record. *Maternal/Child Nursing, 27*(4): 249.

McMillan, et al., v. Frye Regional Medical Center et al., 89 CvS 2149 (Catawba County, November 17, 1992).

McRae, M. (1999). Fetal surveillance and monitoring: Legal issues revisited. *Journal of Obstetric, Gynecologic, and Neonatal Nursing 28*(3), 310–319.

———. (1993). Litigation, electronic fetal monitoring, and the obstetric nurse. *Journal of Obstetric, Gynecologic, and Neonatal Nursing, 22*, 410–418.

Murphy, E. (1987). The professional status of nursing: A view from the courts. *Nursing Outlook, 35*, 12–15.

Murray, M. L. (1996). Electronic fetal monitoring: role of the nurse. In Donn and Fischer (Eds.), *Risk management techniques in perinatal and neonatal practice* (pp 213–239). Armonk, NY: Futura Publishing Co.

National Institute of Child Health and Human Development Research Planning Workshop. (1997). Electronic fetal heart rate monitoring: Research guidelines for interpretation. *Journal of Obstetric, Gynecologic, and Neonatal Nursing, 26*(6), 635–640.

Nelson, K., Dambrosia, J., Ting, B. S., & Grether, J. (1996). Uncertain value of electronic fetal monitoring in predicting cerebral palsy. *New England Journal of Medicine, 334*, 613–618.

Nielsen, P. V., Stigsby, B., Nickelson, C., & Num, J. (1986). Intra- and inter-observer variability in the assessment of intrapartum cardiotocograms. *Acta Obstetricia et Gynecologica Scandinavica, 66*, 421–424.

Paul, R. H. (1994). Electronic fetal monitoring and later outcome: A thirty-year overview. *Journal of Perinatology, 14*, 393–395.

Roemer, V. M., & Rommermann-Heger, G. (1992). Emergency cesarean section: Basic data. *Zeitschrift fur Geburtschilfe und Perinatologie, 196*, 95–99.

Rommal, C. (1996). Risk management issues in the perinatal setting. *Journal of Perinatal and Neonatal Nursing, 10*(3), 1–31.

Rubsamen, D. S. (1993). *The obstetrician's professional liability: Awareness and prevention.* Hercules, CA: Professional Liability Newsletter.

Sandmire, H. (1990). Whither electronic fetal monitoring. *Obstetrics and Gynecology, 76*, 1130–1133.

Schauberger, C. W., Rooney, B. L., Beguin, E. A., et al. (1994a). Evaluating the thirty minute interval in emergency cesarean sections. *Journal of the American College of Surgeons, 179*, 151–155.

———. (1994b). The ABCs of electronic fetal monitoring. *Journal of Perinatology, 14*, 396–402.

———. (1993). Fetal surveillance during labor: The role of the expert witness. *Journal of Perinatology, 13*, 151–152.

Simpson, K. R., Knox, G. E. (2000). Risk management and electronic fetal monitoring: decreasing risk of adverse outcomes and liability exposure. *Journal of Perinatal Neonatal Nursing, 14*(3): 40–52.

Simpson, K. R. (2004). Perinatal safety: standardized language for electronic fetal monitoring. *MCN, The American Journal of Maternal/Child Nursing, 29*(5): 336.

Stolte, K., Myers, S. T., & Owen, W. L. (1994). Changes in maternity care and the impact on nurses and nursing practice. *Journal of Obstetric, Gynecologic, and Neonatal Nursing, 23*, 603–608.

Symonds, M. (1994). Fetal monitoring: Medical and legal implications for the practitioner. *Current Opinion in Obstetrics and Gynecology, 6*, 430–433.

Wood, S. H. (2003). Should women be given a choice about fetal assessment in labor? *MCN, The American Journal of Maternal/Child Nursing, 25*(5): 292–298.

7 | Electronic Fetal Monitoring Competence Validation

Kathleen Rice Simpson, PhD, RNC, FAAN

Introduction

Nursing competence can be defined as possession of the requisite knowledge and technical skills related to a specific area of professional clinical practice. Validation of competence implies both an evaluation of the nurses' level of knowledge and verification of their clinical skills. For many reasons that will be discussed in this chapter, most current methods of competence validation for nurses who use electronic fetal monitoring (EFM) fall short of achieving these goals.

Traditional written tests may be useful in determining whether the nurse has the appropriate knowledge about a specific clinical practice area but provide little or no information about technical expertise. Possession of a thorough knowledge base does not necessarily mean that the nurse has the ability to translate that knowledge into safe clinical practice. Therefore, it is important to go beyond evaluating a core knowledge in EFM. The ability to use that knowledge must also be considered as part of the overall competence validation process (Association of Women's Health, Obstetric and Gynecologic Nurses [AWHONN], 2006). Traditional skills checklists are commonly used to document clinical expertise. However, this method gives no indication whether the technically expert nurse has the ability to think critically and consider the implications of the clinical intervention. Verification of clinical skills is only one component of the competence validation process.

A more complex issue is whether competent nurses will consistently use their knowledge and clinical skills over time and for each patient interaction. Multiple factors, including nurse-to-patient staffing ratios, fatigue, interpersonal stress, and interactions with other care providers, influence the ability of competent nurses to provide safe and effective perinatal care on a routine basis. The purpose of this chapter is to review the pros and cons of current methods of competence validation for nurses who use EFM and propose an alternative approach to this process that has the potential to provide more accurate information. No one method will address all of the issues involved in competence validation, nor can one method ensure that the competent nurse will provide safe and effective care in every interaction. However, some available methods work better than others. If the goal of competence validation is to enhance the likelihood that nurses will provide safe and effective care to all women in labor, a thorough evaluation and discussion of these methods are worthwhile.

Pros and Cons of Traditional Approaches

Written Examination

Pros: Written tests about EFM content are relatively easy to develop and can be administered to many nurses in a short time frame. Knowledge about key principles of fetal heart rate (FHR) pattern interpretation, physiology, and appropriate nursing interventions can be evaluated by the use of multiple choice, fill-in-the-blank, and matching items. Most of the basic concepts can be covered in 25 to 50 test questions. Examination scoring can be accomplished easily and quickly. A minimum score can be established, and those who achieve the minimum passing score can be designated as possessing the minimum knowledge about EFM required for clinical practice. Written examination appears, at least on the surface, to provide objective data about the nurses' knowledge base. Regulatory agencies such as the Joint Commission on Accreditation of Healthcare Organizations (JCAHO) accept this method as evidence that the institution has made an appropriate effort to validate competence (JCAHO, 2004).

Cons: Although writing test questions can seem to be easy, few nurses have been educated in the rigorous process of item writing and examination development. Production of a psychometrically sound examination requires that those writing items are familiar with the process and have significant practice and experience in analyzing individual items and the examination as a whole. Without reliability and validity data about items that are used on the written examination, few conclusions can be drawn from the examination results. Obtaining reliability and validity data through the use of psychometric techniques is costly, time consuming, and beyond the scope of expertise of most nurses who develop EFM examinations in the institutional setting. Use of a poorly developed written examination as a method to validate competence can provide a false sense of assurance to the institution that the nurses who have achieved a passing score are indeed competent to provide intrapartum nursing care. A common practice is to use the same 25- to 50-item EFM examination every year. Although this may be done to conserve resources and time, another possible explanation for using the same examination each year is the limited content area of EFM. Test developers are challenged with the issue of how many ways can the same content be incorporated into a meaningful question. Thus, many perinatal nurses find themselves taking the same poorly developed written examination each year, and administrators in many institutions are led to believe that the nurses who care for women in labor have

participated in a meaningful process to validate competence in EFM.

Recommendations: If the institution chooses written examination as the preferred method for evaluation of requisite knowledge of EFM, the best approach is to use an examination that has been shown to be psychometrically sound and legally defensible. There should be reliability and validity data for individual items and the examination as a whole. The examination should be developed by nurses who are experts in both EFM content and item writing. Items should be pretested before inclusion on the examination and continually evaluated after each examination administration. A rigorous approach to examination development should provide assurance that the successful candidate does possess appropriate level and depth of knowledge in EFM content. At present, there is only one examination about EFM content that meets these criteria: The EFM examination developed by a team of content experts through the National Certification Corporation for the Obstetric, Gynecologic and Neonatal Nursing Specialties (NCC). Candidates for this examination are required to demonstrate that they are currently working in a clinical practice setting where EFM is used, but no longer have to hold one of the core NCC certifications in a specialty area of practice. Use of the NCC examination can save considerable time for the person who has been traditionally responsible for EFM examination development and allow them to pursue more valuable educational objectives. One of the added benefits of choosing NCC is the requirement for continuing education that is part of the maintenance process. Fifteen contact hours in EFM content are required every 3 years to maintain the NCC credential. There is the implied commitment to maintaining a current knowledge of EFM principles by nurses who are credentialed through the NCC examination process. Thus, this examination both evaluates knowledge using a rigorous process and promotes participation in continuing education programs. The NCC exam also is being used by many hospitals throughout the United States to validate the competency of nurse midwives, residents, and attending physicians.

Be especially wary of individuals and companies offering "certification" programs that include requirements to take their course and use their book before sitting for the examination. Not only are psychometric testing factors an issue, there also seems to be an inherent conflict that can affect quality of the process when the examination is geared to the course content. If the institution is committed to written examination, the best use of financial resources is to participate in an examination developed and supported by a national organization with expertise in the examination process.

Skills Checklists

Pros: Skills checklists are an excellent method of ensuring that all expected skills are covered during the orientation process and accuracy in implementing these skills has been observed. Refer to the AWHONN *Clinical Competencies and Education Guide: Antepartum and Intrapartum Fetal Heart Monitoring* (AWHONN, 2006) for a list of suggested clinical skills for nurses who use EFM. They can be adapted and revised based on unit practices. Comprehensive well-developed skills checklists serve as a reference to guide the preceptor during orientation and provide the orientee with a defined set of clinical expectations for the labor and birth unit. Direct observation of accurate implementation of the designated technical skills should be criteria for completion of orientation and assumption of primary responsibility for patient care. Regulatory agencies such as JCAHO accept skills checklists as evidence that the institution has attempted to verify clinical skills for professional nurses (JCAHO, 2006).

Cons: Technical skills associated with use of EFM are not complex. Once nurses have been observed performing all expected technical skills several times with accuracy during orientation, it can be assumed they maintain those skills if they are providing patient care on a routine basis unless there is evidence to suggest otherwise. Nurses who have difficulties with technical aspects of EFM are usually quickly identified by peers or through clinical situations where their deficiencies are apparent. These situations can be addressed with strategies designed for the individual nurse.

Verification of skills for experienced nurses should focus on consistency rather than a baseline evaluation. Use of skills checklists for annual clinical skills verification for experienced perinatal nurses are not helpful in truly assessing whether the nurse consistently applies technical expertise to every clinical interaction. Observer bias is a confounding issue. When an experienced nurse is observed during clinical skills implementation, more likely than not, the nurse will be on his or her "best behavior." Adherence to unit policies, sterile technique, and appropriate nurse–patient interactions is likely to be at the highest level when another nurse is directly observing clinical behavior. This method does not provide information about routine nursing interventions when the observer/evaluator is not present. Use of skills checklists for experienced nurses provides a false sense of assurance that the nurse under observation gives technically competent care on a routine basis (Simpson, 1998).

Recommendations: Use skills checklists for orientation of new nurses only as a reference to ensure that expected technical skills have been covered and directly observed by the preceptor before assuming primary responsibility for patient care. Avoid use of skills checklists for experienced nurses.

EFM Case Studies with Strip Reviews

Pros: EFM strip reviews are popular methods of competence validation because the questions are associated with a specific clinical case and a graphic display of the FHR pattern. In most cases, single items on written examinations provide little information about the clinical situation related to the topic being tested. Participants may assume more about the case than is contained in the question, which can lead to an incorrect response or frustration. Many nurses are visual learners and find it easier to relate to a picture of the FHR rather than narrative descriptions when attempting to answer questions about appropriate clinical interventions. Case studies with EFM strips are more interesting and closer to daily reality in the clinical setting than a series of single-topic examination items. Responses to case study questions are more likely to result from critical thinking and interpretation than single-topic examination items. Thus, information from a case study approach to competence validation is more valuable than scores on written examinations (Simpson, 1998). Regulatory agencies such as JCAHO accept this method as evidence that the institution has made an appropriate effort to validate competence (JCAHO, 2004).

An additional benefit of using case studies with EFM strips is the knowledge gained by those who participate in the development process. A committee of staff nurse volunteers can be recruited to develop case studies from interesting strips of actual patients. A group process can be used to review the expected responses, appropriate interpretations, and related interventions. This discussion can lead to an increased knowledge of EFM principles for all involved. Not all participants need be nurse experts with many years of clinical experience. A willingness to volunteer can be the criterion for participation. This is an excellent opportunity to mentor nurses with less experience and develop collegial relationships between unit members.

The best approach, if at all possible, is to actively seek participation from physician colleagues in the case study development process. Any opportunity for collaboration between nurses and physicians who jointly are responsible for FHR pattern interpretation and clinical interventions should be seen as a positive step toward collaboration in everyday clinical interactions. Working with physicians on developing case studies is the ideal avenue for clarifying ongoing clinical issues where interpretation and expectations of both provider groups are not in sync. Physicians may expect a series of nursing interventions for a specific FHR pattern that are not the routine of many nurses on the unit. For example, there may be clinical disagreement about what to do when uterine hyperstimulation is the result of oxytocin administration but the FHR remains reassuring. Nurses may routinely decrease the oxytocin dosage or discontinue the infusion completely, whereas physician colleagues believe the nurses are overreacting. An open discussion of the rationale based on physiologic principles and standards of care may lead to less conflict in the clinical setting (Simpson, James, & Knox, 2006).

Another common area of disagreement is description of FHR patterns. Development of case studies and accurate responses can lead to a common understanding of FHR pattern nomenclature that is mutually agreed upon and routinely used by all providers. If not already in place, this is an opportunity to suggest adoption of a common

set of definitions for FHR pattern interpretation and medical record documentation recommended by the National Institute of Child Health and Human Development (NICHD) Research Planning Workshop (NICHD, 1997). These definitions are supported by the American College of Obstetricians and Gynecologists (ACOG; 2005) and AWHONN (2005). It is important to adopt one set of definitions so all providers are speaking the same language in oral communication and written documentation in the medical record (JCAHO, 2004). A clear definition of fetal well-being should guide the majority of unit operations and can be used to simplify communication between nurses and physicians (Knox, Simpson, & Townsend, 2003). The presence of fetal well-being is the criterion for maternal discharge, maternal medications, use of oxytocin and epidural anesthesia in most clinical situations. Absence of fetal well-being necessitates direct physician evaluation with written documentation of further clinical management (Knox, Simpson, & Townsend, 2003). Coming to this agreement can be a significant outcome of joint development of EFM case studies. It is possible that this nurse–physician collaboration will have a positive spill-over effect on daily clinical operations (Simpson, James, & Knox, 2006).

Cons: EFM case studies with strip reviews have the potential to provide valuable information about core knowledge and expected clinical skills. However, many times the case studies are poorly developed and the questions evaluate content not provided in the patient history. Nurses are educated to assess the overall clinical picture including maternal history and previous and ongoing fetal status. Yet, case studies frequently provide minimal maternal data and a 10- to 15-minute graphic display of the FHR pattern. This approach is frustrating to the participant and does not approximate clinical reality. Unless the question is "What are the appropriate interventions based on this 15-minute admission strip?", a 15-minute strip is not enough for a realistic case study presentation. In the clinical practice setting, if a nurse noted a nonreassuring FHR pattern, one of the initial actions would be a quick review of the previous EFM strip and consideration of maternal factors. Thus, for case studies to be of value, enough information should be provided to simulate an actual clinical situation.

Recommendations: Develop comprehensive case studies with adequate maternal history and include at least 1 hour of an EFM strip for review. Use items that go beyond simple interpretation. Evaluate appropriate interventions and possible outcomes. Use EFM case studies as an opportunity to mentor inexperienced nurses, to strengthen relationships between nurses and physicians, and to clarify ongoing clinical issues. Promote collaboration and communication through joint development of case studies and expected responses to the clinical scenario.

An Alternative Approach to Competence Validation

Medical Record Audits

Guidelines and standards of care from professional organizations such as AWHONN, ACOG, and JCAHO provide a useful framework for validating competence of nurses who use EFM. Institutional policy and procedures, protocols, care plans, and clinical pathways should reflect practice parameters outlined in publications by these professional organizations. Therefore, it is reasonable to use this approach to develop a tool for competence validation (Simpson, 1998). The first step in the process is a thorough review of published practice guidelines and standards of care. An added benefit of assembling and reviewing all pertinent publications is the assurance that institutional policies and procedures, protocols, care plans, and clinical pathways are consistent with current guidelines and standards of care (Simpson & Knox, 2003). Some institutions have policies for frequent assessments and routine interventions that are not based on evidence or guidelines and standards of care. These policies result in unnecessary time-consuming nursing interventions that do not contribute to optimum maternal–fetal outcomes (Simpson, 2006). The medical record audit development process can serve as an opportunity to streamline clinical care and promote evidence-based practice. Fortunately, for most clinical issues, there is no need to develop policies independently because professional organizations have publications that can serve as a useful framework. Consistency with published guidelines and standards of care can decrease liability should the institution be involved in litigation related to care during childbirth (Knox, Simpson, & Townsend, 2003).

Advantages of Using Medical Record Audit Tools

Medical record audits can be designed to cover both aspects of the competence validation process. Medical record audits provide substantial data about the requisite knowledge base and essential clinical skills during the intrapartum period. Comparison of FHR and uterine activity data documented in the medical record with the electronic fetal monitor tracing provides valuable objective information about the nurses' ability to correctly interpret the patterns depicted. Medical record audits avoid observer bias inherent in the skills checklist approach.

Nursing interventions documented in the medical record related to the FHR and uterine activity displayed on the EFM tracing provide evidence of the nurses' knowledge of maternal–fetal physiology and can be used to verify clinical skills. For example, periods of uterine hyperstimulation with concurrent increases in oxytocin dosage administration may indicate that the nurse is unaware of the clinical signs of uterine hyperstimulation, the institutional policy on oxytocin administration, the pharmacokinetics of oxytocin, or the appropriate nursing interventions when there is excessive uterine activity during oxytocin administration. Prolonged periods on the EFM tracing where the FHR or uterine activity is uninterpretable may indicate that the nurse needs more information and further demonstration about Leopold's maneuvers and correct tocodynamometer placement. Inaccurate notations in the medical record about FHR patterns could be evidence that the nurse needs more practice in FHR pattern interpretation. Correct interpretation and documentation of nonreassuring FHR patterns without notations about appropriate nursing interventions suggest that the nurse could benefit from an additional clinical preceptorship and more education about how to respond when the FHR is nonreassuring. Notations about nonreassuring fetal status accompanied by entries that the physician or certified nurse midwife (CNM) is aware and not responding, with no further interventions noted, may indicate that the nurse needs to review the unit chain of command algorithm.

A well-documented medical record that is comparable with the EFM tracing and includes appropriate nursing interventions at frequencies reasonably consistent with institutional policies provides evidence that the nurse has a solid knowledge base about the physiology of FHR pattern interpretation, labor and birth, and institutional policies and standards of care, and is able to apply that knowledge in clinical practice. Selected parameters can be used to develop a medical record audit tool to review nursing care related to EFM during labor and birth.

Validation of Competence Before Completion of Orientation

Before completion of orientation, at least five randomly selected medical records and EFM strips can be reviewed with the orientee as both a learning exercise and competence validation process. The person responsible for orientation can use this session to reinforce accuracies in interpretation, documentation, and appropriate nursing interventions. This process can build confidence for nurses new to the specialty and allow a nonthreatening opportunity for the orientee to ask questions and seek clarification as needed. Nurses who need further education and clinical practice experience can be identified before completion of orientation.

Annual Ongoing Competence Validation

When medical record audits are used as a component of annual competence validation for all nurses, nurse members of a unit practice committee are ideal candidates to coordinate the program. At least three random medical records with EFM strips can be selected on an annual basis before nurses' annual performance evaluation. The committee can review the medical record and EFM strips as previously described as a group. Nurses who need further education and clinical practice experience can be identified and provided close supervision. A follow-up audit should be done that validates competence before this nurse is allowed to be the primary caregiver for a woman in labor. Reviewing at least three randomly selected medical records reflecting different days in the clinical setting for each nurse who is evaluated contributes to overall accuracy of the data collected.

Adaptation to Specific Clinical Issues

Specific unit quality care issues also can be addressed by medical record audits.

The tool should be designed based on individual unit needs. For example, if there is a consistent problem related to incomplete admission assessments, inaccuracies in medical record documentation when compared to the EFM strip, increases in oxytocin when adequate labor is established, or nurse-coached pushing during the second stage when there is evidence of nonreassuring fetal status, and so forth, the tool can be developed to evaluate these specific practice areas and provide feedback to individual nurses as needed. Heightened awareness of the importance of accurate medical record documentation and the peer review process can be incentives to enhance quality. Audits also can be useful in developing medical record forms that are more user friendly and provide cues or prompts to enter the required data. Areas for noting aspects of nursing care that are often provided but infrequently documented such as comfort measures during labor and interactions with the woman's support persons can be added to written or electronic flow sheets.

Perinatal Unit Evaluation

Medical record audits provide significant information about unit practices and adherence to unit policies. An overall culture of the unit can be evaluated by randomly selected medical records over a designated time period. For example, an audit of women who receive oxytocin for labor induction may reveal that hyperstimulation, excessive dosage and nonintervention during nonreassuring FHR patterns are characteristics of most care providers rather than individual nurses. Quality and frequency of communication between nurses and physicians can be evaluated by way of medical record audits. Trends in appropriate interventions or lack of interventions are easily identified during a comprehensive medical record audit. Inconsistencies or inaccuracies in FHR interpretation can be determined. Based on medical record audits, educational programs can be designed to enhance safe practice, and information can be provided to alert care providers of ongoing clinical issues that may contribute to unsafe care and potential patient injuries. Periodic unit evaluation through the use of medical record audits is an ideal method to verify that competent care providers are providing competent care on a routine basis.

Guidelines for Designing a Medical Record Audit Tool

Selected medical records of women during labor can be reviewed and compared to the electronic FHR tracings. Overall accuracy; consistency with established institutional policies and procedures, and AWHONN and ACOG guidelines; legibility; and clinical practice issues can be evaluated during the intrapartum period using some of the following parameters. (See Box 7–1 for suggested components of a medical record audit tool.)

Benefits of Using Medical Record Audits to Validate Competence

- Medical record audits can be used for both knowledge base evaluation and clinical skills verification.
- Medical record audits are objective and comprehensive while avoiding the observer bias inherent in using skills checklists.
- The process works well when used before completion of orientation to reinforce knowledge and clinical skills and can build confidence for nurses new to the speciality.
- The process can be incorporated into the unit's annual competence validation program for all nurses and can allow identification of nurses who could benefit from additional education and clinical practice experience.
- Tool development can be useful in ensuring that institutional policies, procedures, protocols, care plans, and clinical pathways are consistent with published guidelines and standards of care from professional organizations.
- Audit process can lead to redesign and enhancements of current medical record forms.
- Feedback can heighten awareness of the importance of accurate documentation on the medical record.

- Results can be used as part of the unit quality improvement process.
- Improvements in documentation and clinical practice can lead to decreased institutional liability. (Simpson & Knox, 2003)

Complex Issues Related to Competence Validation

Professional Responsibility

Maintaining and validating competence is a shared responsibility. Regulatory agencies such as JCAHO mandate periodic competence validation for care providers (JCAHO, 2004). The institution as the employer has responsibility to make a reasonable attempt to validate competence of the professional nursing staff. Areas of clinical competence are outlined by professional organizations such as AWHONN and ACOG and can be used as a framework for developing comprehensive programs. Institutions also have responsibility for providing continuing education programs so nurses can have the opportunity to review basic concepts and learn about new trends and techniques.

Nurses have an individual responsibility to maintain competence in clinical practice. Most states' nurse practice acts have statements or standards that address requirements for nurses to keep current in nursing practice. AWHONN *Standards and Guidelines for Professional Nursing Practice in the Care of Women and Newborns* (AWHONN, 2003) outline expectations for maintaining competence. If the nurse believes the institution's programs fall short in providing continuing education programs that promote knowledge about current practice, there is a responsibility to seek outside educational opportunities while advocating for improvements in institutional programs.

Clinical Errors by Competent Care Providers

Perinatal care providers are expected by their communities, patients, and society in general to provide competent care. Perinatal units are expected to operate essentially without clinical errors or mistakes over long periods (Knox, Simpson, & Townsend, 2003). A clinical error during labor

Box 7–1. Suggested Components of a Medical Record Audit

- Are the times noted on the Admission Assessment, Labor Flow Chart, and initial electronic fetal monitoring (EFM) strip consistent with each other within a reasonable time frame?
- If elective labor induction, is gestational age of at least 39 weeks confirmed?
- Is there documentation of physician notification of admission within the time frame outlined in the policies and procedures?
- Is fetal well-being established on admission?
- Is fetal well-being established prior to ambulation?
- Is fetal well-being established prior to medication administration?
- Does the EFM fetal heart rate (FHR) baseline rate match the FHR baseline documented?
- Does the EFM FHR baseline variability match the FHR baseline variability documented?
- If there is evidence of absent or minimal FHR variability, is it documented?
- If there is evidence of absent or minimal FHR variability, are appropriate interventions documented?
- If there are FHR decelerations on the EFM strip, are they correctly documented?
- Are appropriate interventions documented during nonreassuring FHR patterns?
- Is there documentation of physician or nurse-midwife notification during nonreassuring FHR patterns?
- If FHR accelerations are documented, are they on the EFM strip?
- Are maternal assessments documented according to policy?
- If there is evidence of a nonreassuring FHR pattern, is oxytocin dosage increased?
- If there is evidence of a nonreassuring FHR pattern, is oxytocin dosage discontinued?
- If there is evidence of uterine hyperstimulation, are appropriate interventions documented?
- If there is evidence of adequate labor, is oxytocin dosage increased?
- If there is evidence of uterine hyperstimulation, is oxytocin dosage increased or decreased?
- Does the frequency of uterine contractions on the EFM strip match what is documented?
- Is the uterine activity monitor (external tocodynamometer or intrauterine pressure catheter [IUPC]) adjusted to maintain an accurate uterine activity baseline?
- Are oxytocin dosage increases charted when there is an inaccurate uterine baseline tracing or an uninterpretable FHR tracing?
- Is the physician's or nurse-midwife's documentation of fetal status consistent with the nurse's documentation?
- Are automatically generated data from the blood pressure device accurate?
- Does documentation continue during the second stage of labor?
- Are women in the second stage of labor encouraged to push before they feel the urge to push?
- Are women in the second stage of labor encouraged to push with contractions when the FHR is nonreassuring (ie, there are variable or late FHR decelerations occurring with each contraction)?
- When the FHR is nonreassuring during the second stage of labor, is pushing discontinued or encouraged with every other or every third contraction to maintain a stable baseline rate and minimize decelerations?
- If the FHR is nonreassuring during the second stage of labor, is oxytocin discontinued?
- Are uterine contractions continuously monitored during the second stage of labor via external tocodynamometer or IUPC?
- Does the time of birth on the medical record match the time of birth at the end of the EFM strip?
- If the woman had regional analgesia/anesthesia, is a qualified anesthesia provider involved in the decision to discharge from postanesthesia care unit (PACU) care?
- If the woman had regional analgesia/anesthesia, is the discharge from PACU care scoring evaluation documented?
- Are maternal assessments documented during the immediate postpartum period every 15 minutes for the first hour?
- Are newborn assessments documented during the transition to extrauterine life at least every 30 minutes until the newborn's condition has been stable for 2 hours?

and birth can be devastating to the infant and family. Competent care providers make clinical errors that lead to adverse maternal–fetal outcomes. One of the limitations of even the most comprehensive and rigorous competence validation programs is the inability to ensure that competent care providers will give competent care to every patient every day. Although clinical judgment disagreements can also lead to adverse patient outcomes, basic clinical errors should not occur and are not well tolerated by patients and society in general especially when they result in patient injury.

Clinical errors by competent care providers are common. Most errors are the result of faulty systems and poorly designed processes that set providers up to make mistakes by putting them in situations where errors are more likely to be made.

Perinatal units are prone to error due to multiple factors (Knox, Simpson, & Townsend, 2003). Unit operations are routine and usually successful in achieving good patient outcomes. However, successful operations are potentially dangerous because success leads to oversimplification, shortcuts, and a "normalization of deviance" (Vaughan, 1996). The concept of normalization of deviance is important in understanding the potential for error in perinatal unit operations. In Vaughan's (1996) analysis of the Challenger disaster, she concluded that all work groups continually redefine risk in the context of accidents that do not occur. Competent care providers can unknowingly let professional and technical standards degrade over time. Incrementally, the unit culture can become less safe over time because "they get away with it" (Vaughan, 1996). For example, in some units, understaffing is the routine. On most days, nurses may be responsible for more than two women in active labor receiving oxytocin. Nurses may be mandated to work extra shifts, resulting in fatigue, stress, and burnout. After months of not having adequate nurses to care for women in labor with no adverse outcomes, administrators may begin to believe this is a cost-effective way of doing business. Nurses and physicians can become desensitized to hyperstimulation patterns related to oxytocin because the healthy fetus can usually tolerate this stress for a period of time before demonstrating a nonreassuring FHR pattern. Aggressive pushing techniques during which the fetus demonstrates a variable deceleration with each contraction are many times the

norm because most healthy fetuses can tolerate this stress temporarily. Use of a vacuum for operative vaginal birth when the fetus is too high for forceps does not usually result in fetal injury. A consistent problem with physicians not being present during birth may be accepted because most babies do well when they are born into the hands of experienced labor nurses. Ongoing conflict between nurses and physicians in a culture where the expected behavior is to comply with physician orders without initiating the chain of command when appropriate may be tolerated because of the negative implications for nurses who try to change the system.

Most childbearing women are healthy, most fetuses are resilient to iatrogenic stress, and, thus, most errors do not result in patient injury. Because injuries are rare, there is no immediate or apparent consequence for not strictly adhering to policies or protocols designed to prevent adverse outcomes. Because there are usually good outcomes even in the case of errors, near misses are frequently not viewed by competent care providers as opportunities to learn or improve unit behavior. Given the predominance of good outcomes and overall normality of perinatal practice, perinatal units are especially prone to normalizing deviance (Knox, Simpson, & Townsend, 2003). Competent care providers new to the unit are sometimes amazed at potentially unsafe practices and routines. This is an ideal opportunity to reevaluate that unit practice. Instead, what usually happens is, 6 months later, these same professionals are just as amazed when another newcomer questions the safety of the same practices with which they themselves have now grown comfortable (Knox, Simpson, & Townsend, 2003). Thus, unsafe clinical practices can become accepted by those who have been designated as competent because of unit cultural factors and the fact that most errors do not result in adverse outcomes, not because they are lacking appropriate knowledge and clinical skills.

Where Do We Go from Here?

The goal of any competence validation program is to ensure that competent caregivers will consistently provide competent care. However, competence validation of individual nurses is only one component of safe and effective perinatal nursing care. Characteristics of units that promote safe care and minimal patient injuries have been described in the literature (Knox, Simpson, & Townsend, 2003). Unit culture contributes to the ability of competent nurses to consistently provide safe care. Nurse-to-patient ratios, nurse–physician interactions, and routine practices not based on evidence or standards and guidelines for care are important factors (Simpson & Knox, 2003). The future of competence validation should be directed toward evaluating the consistent competence of teams of perinatal care providers and reviewing adverse outcomes related to clinical errors. Currently, the only method for this type of approach is an analysis of claims data from perinatal units. But there are inherent flaws in a simple claims analysis approach because of data to suggest that six patient injuries occur for every one claim filed (Localio, Lawthers, & Brennan, 1991). More research is needed to develop effective methods of validating clinical competence and promoting safe patient care. For now, the best approach is use of medical record audits to evaluate individual care providers and to analyze overall unit practices and culture that contribute to the best possible outcomes for childbearing women.

REFERENCES

American College of Obstetricians and Gynecologists. (2005). *Intrapartum fetal heart rate monitoring*. (Practice Bulletin No. 62). Washington, DC: Author.

Association of Women's Health, Obstetric, and Neonatal Nurses. (2006). *Clinical competencies and education guide: Antepartum and intrapartum fetal heart rate monitoring* (4th ed.). Washington, DC: Author.

———. (2005). *Fetal heart monitoring program*. Washington, DC: Author.

———. (2003). *Standards and guidelines for professional nursing practice in the care of women and newborns*. Washington, DC: Author.

Joint Commission on Accreditation of Healthcare Organizations. (2004). *Preventing infant death and injury during delivery*. (Sentinel Event Alert No. 30). Oak Brook, IL: Author.

———. (2001). *Comprehension accreditation manual for hospitals*. Oak Park, IL: Author.

Knox, G. E., Simpson, K. R., & Townsend, K. E. (2003). High reliability perinatal units: Further observations and a suggested plan for action. *Journal of Healthcare Risk Management, 23*(4), 17–21.

Localio, A. R., Lawthers, A. G., & Brennan, T. A. (1991). Relation between malpractice claims and adverse events due to negligence: Results of the Harvard Medical Practice Study III. *New England Journal of Medicine, 325*, 245–251.

National Institute of Child Health and Human Development Research Planning Workshop. (1997). Electronic fetal heart rate monitoring: Research guidelines for interpretation. *Journal of Obstetric, Gynecologic, and Neonatal Nursing, 26*(6), 635–640.

Simpson, K. R. (1998). Using guidelines and standards from professional organizations as a framework for competence validation. In K. R. Simpson & P. A. Creehan (Eds.), *AWHONN's competence validation for perinatal care providers: Orientation, continuing education and evaluation*. Philadelphia: PA: Lippincott-Raven.

Simpson, K. R., James, D. C., & Knox, G. E. (2006). Nurse-physician communication during labor and birth: Implications for patient safety. *Journal of Obstetric, Gynecologic and Neonatal Nursing, 35*(4), 547–556.

Simpson, K. R., & Knox, G. E. (2003). Common areas of litigation related to care during labor and birth: Recommendations to promote patient safety and decrease risk exposure. *Journal of Perinatal and Neonatal Nursing, 17*(1), 94–109.

Vaughan, D. (1996). *The Challenger launch decision: Risky technology, culture and deviance at NASA*. Chicago, IL: University of Chicago Press.

8 | Electronic Fetal Monitoring and Information Technology

Patricia Robin McCartney, RNC, PhD, FAAN

Despite controversy, the use of electronic fetal monitoring (EFM) technology in birth is escalating and obstetric care providers must understand the nature and capabilities of the tools in use. As a technology, EFM is not only a biophysical and electronic engineering tool used to capture the fetal heart rate (FHR) signal but, in many cases, also a component of a digital health information tool. A solid understanding of the information technology capabilities of EFM is necessary for providers to harness the information benefits and use EFM appropriately and effectively for optimum birth outcomes. This chapter will provide a brief introduction on how EFM relates to the electronic health record, computerized clinical information systems, and informatics. Clinicians are encouraged to access the chapter references for additional learning.

The Electronic Health Record

The Institute of Medicine (IOM) report *Crossing the Quality Chasm* called for elimination of handwritten data and set a goal to implement a paperless electronic health record (EHR) before the end of the decade, citing evidence that the EHR improves health care quality, safety, and efficiency (IOM, 2001). The electronic format provides a record of clinical data that are legible, organized, complete, and accessible by multiple users across sites of care and episodes of care. In addition, the electronic records enable a database of clinical information that can be automatically analyzed.

The IOM goal immediately reinforced and promoted the present efforts by the government, health care agencies, professional organizations, and industry partners to develop the EHR. The U.S. Department of Health and Human Services (DHHS) established two goals for the effective use of health information technology that are particularly relevant to obstetric patients and fetal monitoring: (a) informing clinical practice and (b) interconnecting clinicians (U.S. DHHS, 2006). Informing clinical practice aims to bring electronic data directly to the front-line providers, to reduce duplicative work, and to provide access to clinical data immediately (e.g., one-time entry of the mother's expected delivery date that flows to all parts of the medical record simultaneously; immediate access to interpret and document on a fetal tracing). Interconnecting clinicians aims to promote sharing of data with interoperable standards, so information is portable and travels with the patient (such as immediate access to prenatal FHR assessments and diagnostics). The DHHS identified several key strategies to achieve these goals: adoption of the EHR, development of a Nationwide Health Information Network (NHIN) as the interoperable system for the secure exchange of health care information, and development of Regional Health Information Organizations (RHIOs) for local health information exchange. Collectively, these strategies will deliver the right information to the right person at the right time.

The transition to an EHR poses education and practice challenges for currently practicing obstetric care providers, which can overwhelm the provider and subsequently compromise successful implementation. A multidisciplinary summit sponsored by the American Health Information Management Association addressed such training needs and listed specific actions for not only health care workers, but also employers, vendors, educators, and the government to promote workforce competencies (2006). This panel recommended that health care workers themselves identify knowledge gaps and seek ongoing professional development. Obstetric clinicians must recognize how the national agenda will shape EFM practice with clinical information systems and informatics.

> **S T O R K   B Y T E :**
>
> Don't let the EHR train pass you by; jump on board!

EFM and Clinical Information Systems

Clinical information systems (CISs) are networks of computers that share clinical data in a digital format, typically bedside computer workstations connected to a central server. The CIS is the backbone or architecture for the paperless EHR. The use of CISs in obstetrics expanded in the 1990s with "perinatal systems" capable of transmitting and displaying the fetal tracings recording from all the bedside stations in the system on all the screens in the system (*surveillance*), and storing the tracings in an electronic format on an optical disk (*archiving*). Networks expanded to include remote transmission of the fetal tracings through an Internet connection or wireless device to and from settings outside the labor and delivery unit, such as antepartum testing units and ambulatory offices, on a desktop or hand-held device. Clinicians began documenting on the computer tracing. Gradually, the monitor paper was used less or turned off. This conversion from the traditional fetal monitor paper to a digital perinatal system challenges and changes the actual clinical workflow and requires substantial staff effort. Clinicians need to see direct benefits from the system. Initially, clinicians were most interested in the risk management benefit of what came to be known as "central monitoring," or the display of all fetal tracings at a centrally located station. With central monitoring, clinicians could monitor tracings when a care provider could not be at the bedside. Quality assurance projects reported less loss of tracings with electronic storage. And soon, clinicians recognized the value of the CIS *database* functions, including documentation or data entry, data analysis (such as aggregation and trending), and data reporting.

Perinatal systems are niche systems, developed to meet the unique clinical needs in a specialty area. These small systems are generally not integrated or interoperable with the main CIS in the health care organization; however, industry engineers are addressing this constraint. These niche systems are needed as few general CISs have perinatal-specific documentation forms. Some unique issues to consider with perinatal CISs are the following: a direct application of the device on the patient (FHR monitor) requires approval by the U.S. Food and Drug Administration, one admission actually generates at least two admissions, all patients are transferred between units, and the litigation risk is high.

Perinatal Information System Functions

State-of-the-art perinatal systems provide a comprehensive and longitudinal EHR, with surveillance, archiving, documentation, and database applications in use across the care continuum: from prenatal primary care to inpatient birth, newborn, and postpartum care and then, to postpartum primary care. This overview focuses on the applications, benefits, and limitations to consider in using computerized systems with EFM tracings (Table 8–1).

Surveillance

Effective surveillance, communication, and response to potential risk promote patient safety. The safety goal with EFM is to correctly recognize, communicate, and intervene with a nonreassuring FHR tracing. Computerized EFM surveillance systems are intended to promote this safety goal and reduce risk. Computer surveillance can certainly help clinicians assess, but there are some limitations to consider.

Table 8–1. BENEFITS AND LIMITATIONS OF PERINATAL ELECTRONIC CLINICAL INFORMATION SYSTEMS

Function	Benefit	Limitation
For all functions	Benefits of electronic health record: legible, complete, accessible through digital transmission, federal requirements for privacy and security, improved charge capture and positive financial return on investment	Costs of system implementation and maintenance Computer downtime Inability to interface with other systems
Surveillance	Accessibility of fetal tracing on connected workstations and mobile devices provides viewing from remote locations Effective communication of fetal heart rate (FHR) data promotes safety, rapid identification, and response to a nonreassuring FHR	Visual appearance of fetal tracing displays differences that could result in interpretation differences Remote viewing may replace or reduce assessment at the bedside Computer clock may not be synchronized with wall clocks
Archiving	Less loss of fetal tracing data than with monitor paper and microfiche Federal standards mandate data security (retrievable and reproducible)	Data loss or corruption despite federal mandates Retrieval barriers with older tracings and older technology Long statutes of limitations requirements to retrieve and reproduce the tracings High litigation risk
Documentation-database	Maternal–fetal–newborn data is entered once and immediately populates the entire record Record is simultaneously accessible to multiple providers, at multiple sites, over time Effective access to clinical data identifies risks and promotes safety Database is available for data analysis and outcomes reporting Electronic record can link with other electronic safety technologies (provider order entry, electronic medication administration record, bar code medication administration, decision support, knowledge portals)	Workforce training for documentation Database management analyst needed

Central displays assist with the recognition and communication aspects of safety. Although central displays can provide extra "eyes" for clinicians, a commonly voiced concern is the potential for the caregivers to focus their attention on the computer screens and assess the mother and fetus "from the desk" rather than at the bedside. Most perinatal systems have visual or auditory alarm functions to assist with recognition by notifying the clinician when the FHR is outside preset parameters (such as signal loss or a change in baseline rate). However, when central displays and alarms are used, clinicians must acknowledge and respond for the safety process to be complete.

FHR interpretation and discrimination between a reassuring and nonreassuring tracing is a learned skill built from practicing visual analysis of patterns. So any distortion in the visual image (the scale of the grid underlying the fetal waveform or in the speed of the grid underlying the fetal waveform) could distort the appearance of the pattern and affect interpretation. A chief concern with use of the digital tracing is the visual match between the traditional monitor paper printout and (a) the computer screen display (for interpreting the tracing during care), (b) the computer paper printout (for interpreting the tracing generated from a computer printer), and (c) the archived tracing (for interpreting the tracing retrieved later from the archive) (Fig. 8–1). In some cases, the computer screen, printout, or stored pattern is not comparable to the actual monitor paper pattern and suggests different interpretations of the FHR status. The standards of speed and scale must be identical. Presently, there is not an agreed-upon standard. Additional issues to consider with electronic displays is the clarity of the waveform and grids, the length of the tracing segment visible on the screen at one time, and the ergonomics of viewing the screen (brightness, height, angle, position of the screen, split screens competing for visual attention).

The time stamp on the EFM tracing is the legal medical record and must accurately correspond to the time of interventions. Since computer clocks and wall clocks are seldom synchronized, clinicians must have a clear policy regarding the time source, documentation of time, and documentation of discrepancies (McCartney, 2003b).

Archiving

Fetal monitoring tracings are a part of the medical record described as "patient identifiable source data," or data from which interpretations are derived, and must be stored and retrievable (McCartney, 2002). Many settings that use computer displays and archiving no longer run monitor paper during care or save monitor paper. However, when patient care is documented on the monitor paper tracing, the paper becomes a record of care and must be stored and retrievable. Some settings store both laser and paper records because of concern about retrieving archived tracings. Each health care agency should have a policy describing the medical record components and particular storage media.

The security of electronic health records is now protected by the Health Insurance Portability and Accountability Act (HIPAA) standards (which pertain only to patient data in electronic form; the paper forms do not have this security protection) (McCartney, 2003a). The security requirements protect electronic records from wrongful access, alteration, and loss through safeguards such as electronic user identification, audit trails of who has accessed a file, and a data backup plan for network failure. To attain HIPAA compliance, the system must demonstrate that EFM tracings are retrievable and reproducible.

Documentation and Databases

CIS documentation or data entry is done with a variety of user input devices (keyboard, mouse, light pen, touch screen) at a bedside or mobile computer workstation. Data is also automatically entered from biophysical monitoring devices (EFM, maternal blood pressure, pulse oximeter). With a fully electronic record, FHR data and any electronic charting entered on the tracing automatically flow to all parts of the EHR, so there is no need for duplicate charting or "double-documenting." Eliminating duplicate documentation reduces the risk of transcription inconsistencies. The computer screens used for documentation (forms) are usually customizable and should be designed to match obstetric workflow and standard of care. Studies report that electronic obstetric records improve the accuracy and completeness of data entry and improve the collection of outcome data (Dombrowski, Tomlinson, Bottoms, Johnson, & Sokol, 1995; Nielson, Thomson, Jackson, Kosman, & Kiley, 2000). In addition, the privacy of electronic health records is protected by HIPAA standards (McCartney, 2003a).

Although obstetric providers constantly collect and document valuable patient data in the medical record and the unit log book, the later analysis and reporting of this data is not efficient in a paper-based record system (Ivory, 2005). Efficient data analysis is a necessity in today's data-driven health care system. Documentation is the actual recording of clinical data in the patient's record, database management is the software program for data analysis, and the database is the collected data. All

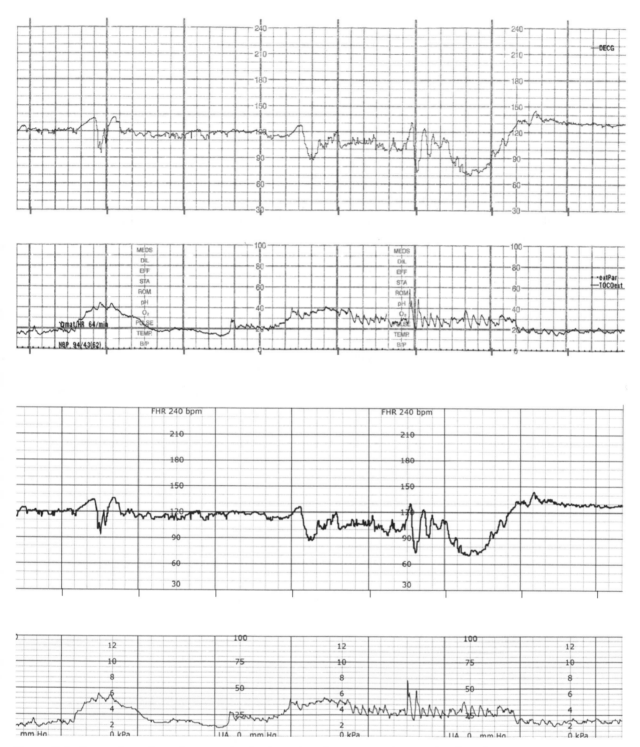

Figure 8–1. Comparison of monitor paper tracing (upper) and computer printer tracing (lower).

three components are necessary to build information from collected data. The database software in a CIS does facilitate more efficient clinical data collection, analysis, and reporting (Bakken, 2001). The perinatal database software can store, aggregate, and analyze individual patient data, such as the FHR, labor events, and birth outcomes. However, clinical experts must be involved with the design of the database so that relevant perinatal data elements are defined and collected and meaningful analysis is accomplished. Data definitions must be clear, quantifiable, and agreed upon. Standardized terminology should be used so that data entries are consistent and can be compared over encounters and settings (such as FHR pattern definitions constructed by the National Institute of Child Health and Human Development Research Planning Workshop [NICHD, 1997]).

A major benefit of perinatal database management is outcomes reporting. A well-designed database can generate reports (paper printouts of data tables, graphs, tracking, trends, audits, summaries) tailored for obstetric department needs, such as census, monthly and vital statistics, quality assurance, national standards compliance, and regulatory agency requirements (Ivory, 2005; Kelly, 1999). Specific obstetric data can be part of the larger agency-wide database if the perinatal system interfaces or is compatible with the larger health care system.

A carefully planned database can be searched to answer clinical research questions about FHR, interventions, and birth outcomes. A retrospective analysis of the database of one unit's records (log books) provided evidence to guide staffing decisions (Ivory, 2005). The individual patient data from daily practice can be transferred to a separate, larger repository of clinical data (data warehouse) where investigators can analyze the aggregated data using a research technique called data mining. A retrospective analysis of perinatal data in a data warehouse was used to identify relationships between demographic data and preterm birth outcomes (Goodwin et al., 2001).

Perinatal System Life Cycle

CIS implementation is best described as a phase in the overall system life cycle. As a phase, implementation is not an independent task, but part of an ongoing process that links to the other phases. Informaticists illustrate the system life cycle with various models, but the typical phases include needs assessment, system selection, implementation, and maintenance (Fig. 8–2). The system life cycle is a process that is never completed, especially as the

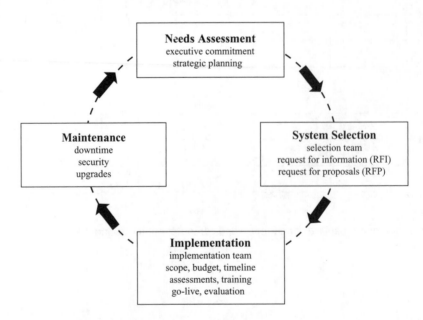

Figure 8–2. Perinatal clinical information system life cycle. Adapted from Barnes, J. (2006). Implementing a perinatal clinical information system: A work in progress. *Journal of Obstetric, Gynecologic and Neonatal Nursing, 35*(1), 134–140; and Hunt, E., Sproat, S., & Kitzmiller, R. (2004). *The nursing informatics implementation guide.* New York: Springer-Verlag.

expected lifespan of hardware and software grows shorter. While any one implementation phase is occurring, there may be other technology implementations occurring or competing priorities that interrupt or delay implementation. Too often, a perinatal clinical specialist or manager without previous informatics education or experience is assigned to lead the implementation of an EFM CIS. Sound, systematic project management is essential for successful implementation. The project leader can optimize the process for all stakeholders—and avoid trial-and-error implementation—by reading the literature, attending conferences, and networking with colleagues (McCartney, 2004). Hunt, Sproat, and Kitzmiller provided practical strategies for accomplishing each phase of the life cycle (2004). Unfortunately, not enough perinatal systems managers publish about their work. Generally, the information systems (IS) staff provides support through the system life cycle, but this is less common with specialty niche systems like EFM.

STORK BYTE:

Don't reinvent the wheel; read the literature on CIS implementation.

Needs Assessment

The needs assessment begins with executive commitment to resources and strategic planning with primary stakeholders participating. The overall vision and information needs must be clear and agreed upon throughout all phases. A clear description of the organization's needs will focus the selection phase.

System Selection

Wilhoit, Mustain, and King explained how the system vendor in essence becomes a strategic business partner for years to come and must be deliberately chosen (2006). These authors provided a detailed account of a selection process involving front-line nurses and scoring tools for demonstrations and site visits. The selection team should be multidisciplinary and include representation from management, IS, and front-line users. Team members must collectively reflect the organization,

possess sound knowledge about the organization and clinical practice, and demonstrate strong communication skills. One of the major causes for implementation failure is a lack of user involvement and ownership. The team is responsible for completing the request for information (RFI) (general information about the product and the vendor), the request for proposal (RFP) (detailed information about the vendor), vendor product demonstrations, site visits, product decisions, and contract negotiations.

Implementation

Implementation may include the initial installation of computerized EFM surveillance and archiving, or expansion of a current system to include documentation. Barnes (2006) used a case study to illustrate in detail how seven key implementation factors were considered in a project to add intrapartum nursing documentation (admission assessment, delivery summary, and labor, recovery, and triage flow sheets) to an existing EFM surveillance and archiving system. The implementation team is led by the project manager and should represent stakeholders, especially front-line users. This team is responsible for focusing the scope of the project, clarifying and monitoring the budget, and projecting the timeline. The team must identify goals that are precise and measurable for evaluation. A comprehensive assessment is done on the documentation systems, workflow analysis, and training needs. Documentation screens and data reports may need to be customized by the IS design team. Trainers and superusers (staff serving as an on-site resource for other staff) are identified. An individualized work plan for training and the actual start date ("go-live" date) are determined based on the assessments. Successful implementation depends on a sound plan that is effectively communicated. Support for the staff is critical. As workflow changes, productivity will initially slow down during the learning curve. Staff needs to see tangible benefits (such as not having to enter gravidity and parity repeatedly on forms). Although an entire system may be implemented for everyone at once ("big bang"), more often the new system is implemented in phases (one unit at a time or one documentation form at a time). Evaluation includes measuring

Table 8–2. INFORMATICS AND LEVELS OF COMPUTER ANALYSIS OF FHR

Informatics Concept	Informatics Definition	EFM	Clinical Example
Data	An objective measurement of a variable	Electronic or paper tracing of the FHR signal	Recording of the FHR at a specific bpm rate, eg, 110bpm
↓	↓	↓	↓
Information	An interpretation of organized data	FHR pattern interpretation, per standardized definitions	Recognition that this 110bpm rate is an abrupt decrease from the baseline FHR (occurring in <30 seconds) and identification of this change as a variable deceleration
↓	↓	↓	↓
Knowledge	A synthesis of information with a clinical knowledge base to make a decision	Synthesis of FHR interpretation, electronic knowledge tools, and the clinician's knowledge base for decision-making and planning care	Clinical decision-making ensues.

outcomes against original goals and identifying any unintended consequences.

Maintenance

Key components of the maintenance phase are processes to prevent downtime, maintain data security, implement upgrades, and generally improve use of the system. System expansion or new software versions are likely as health care processes, standards, and information needs are dynamic. System vendors may offer maintenance contracts for unanticipated needs such as software patches for viruses and security upgrades. Investment in maintenance can ensure the performance of the system. Vendor-specific user groups offer electronic mailing lists and conferences with valuable information to answer questions and generally help clinicians to optimize the use of their system. Many clinicians are not aware of or do not take advantage of the full range of clinical information system tools.

S T O R K   B Y T E :
Don't be an island; reach out and network with other perinatal CIS users.

Informatics and Electronic Fetal Monitoring Knowledge Tools

The use of informatics concepts and knowledge tools with computerized information systems can inform decision making and promote quality clinical care. These informatics concepts and specialty tools can support, not replace, human decision making with EFM.

Informatics

Health care informatics integrates clinical practice, information science, and computer technology to better communicate and manage data (an objective measurement of a variable), information (an interpretation of organized data), and knowledge (a synthesis of information with the clinician's knowledge base to make a decision) (American Nurses Association, 2001) (Table 8–2). In terms of EFM, the goal of effectively communicating and managing data, information, and knowledge would focus on surveillance for reassuring or nonreassuring fetal tracings and responding with appropriate interventions (intrauterine resuscitation). Computers can assist human skill in this process by improving data collection (FHR tracing surveillance), improving objective interpretation of collected data (computer analysis of the FHR and alerts), and providing knowledge resources for the clinician (expert knowledge base and knowledge portals). While surveillance applications address the data collection, decision support applications have been constructed to address the interpretation and knowledge resource functions.

Decision Support

A clinical decision support tool is a software program that integrates information rules (algorithms, flow charts, decision trees) with the collected patient data in the computer system, and is sometimes called a "smart chart," "intelligent EHR," or "expert system." Decision support facilitates the interpretation of data to produce information and provides resources for knowledge. Decision support is widely recognized as an application to improve patient safety. The program might provide interpretation of patient data with alarms when findings are outside normal parameters (FHR alarms and alerts), prompt the user for missing clinical data or guide what documentation is needed (maternal blood pressure during epidural administration), bring reference resources to the point of care (FHR monitoring policy during oxytocin infusion or epidural administration), recommend standard treatments, and generally reduce reliance on memory and the opportunity for clinical error. Support tools can be automatically presented to the user or be optional to the user. Automatic tools ("push" technology) present information to the user, including alerts, reminders, prompts, and recommendations. Optional tools are often links to references, such as an online library (knowledge portals).

Resource content for either approach can consist of practice standards from professional organizations, evidence-based clinical guidelines, policies, treatment protocols, procedures, an online library or Internet links for references, a drug library, and calculation tools. Collectively, the information is called an *expert knowledge base* and is constructed from the input of clinical experts, practice standards (NICHD pattern definitions), research evidence, and the statistical analysis of a large volume of clinical cases (computer analysis of the FHR). The expert knowledge base generates the decision an expert would make and recommends but does not execute a decision. The software rules can be customized and updated with changes in practice standards.

The benefits of decision support include more complete care, standardized care, a double-check that can avoid errors, and immediate access to up-to-date references right at the point of care. More complete documentation may lower malpractice insurance premiums for the health care organization and increase revenue with improved charge capture. Limitations of decision support include clinician noncompliance, overrides of alerts or recommendations, and disagreement on treatment protocols. One decision support tool specifically designed for obstetrics is integrated with EFM and claims to improve documentation (Kranz, 2005).

Computer Analysis of the FHR

Computer analysis of the FHR is a decision support tool that facilitates the interpretation of FHR data to produce information for the clinician. The objective, electronically quantified interpretation of the FHR tracing aids the subjective interpretation of the human eye. Even experts show low rates of agreement in visual interpretation of the EFM tracing. Study after study has confirmed that clinician visual interpretation of the FHR tracing is not consistent; there is poor agreement between clinicians' interpretations (interobserver reliability) and poor agreement when one clinician interprets the same tracing at different times (intraobserver reliability) (McCartney, 2000). Recent multidisciplinary and international investigations continue to demonstrate poor agreement with visual analysis (Devane & Lalor, 2005: Figueras et al., 2005). A key limitation in the visual analysis study designs has been the absence of standardized, quantified, or sometimes even identified FHR pattern definitions. That being said, findings in one recent study suggested that intensive clinician training with the NICHD four categories of variability resulted in a high level of accuracy and agreement (Tongsong et al., 2005).

Computer software for the analysis of the FHR performs objective mathematical analysis based on predetermined criteria for both antepartum testing (nonstress testing) and labor settings. Programs have been used in patient care and research and are available in commercial fetal monitoring products. The FHR software contains rules that detail the pattern features to detect, measure, and interpret. Software rules can be customized by the user. In addition to pattern features, some rules may include patient characteristics such as gestational age. The computations are developed and tested from archives of thousands of tracings and clinical cases. Computer output may be an auditory or visual alarm when the FHR is outside normal parameters or a printout of the measurement and interpretation. The benefit of computer analysis is objectivity based on mathematical rules. However, there must be agreement on which FHR features are assessed, how patterns are defined, and the criteria for a reassuring tracing. The most common automated FHR feature is baseline rate; additional features might include variability, accelerations, and decelerations.

Investigators have compared clinician visual analysis of the fetal tracing to computer mathematical analysis and found better reliability with computer analysis (McCartney, 2000). Because computer analysis is an objective and reliable measure, the technology has been used frequently in research on relationships between clinical variables and FHR response.

The Sonicaid monitoring tool (Sonicaid Monitor, Oxford Medical Lt, United Kingdom), using the Dawes-Redman criteria for pattern interpretation, has been reported most frequently in the literature (McCartney, 2000). The Dawes-Redman criteria for interpretation include a measure of baseline "variation," not variability. Variation is a purely mathematical measure of the FHR fluctuations around the baseline, measured in pulse intervals as precise as milliseconds, for determining long-term variation and short-term variation by external ultrasound measure. The Sonicaid software is designed for antepartum analysis of the nonstress test (NST), not for use in labor. The analysis alerts the clinician as soon as predetermined criteria for FHR normality are achieved and prints a graphic summary of the test results (Huntleigh Healthcare, 2005). The efficiency of the analysis and alerting can reduce the duration of monitoring for the average NST. Because digital FHR data are captured and stored, this software can trend serial NSTs in the prenatal period to identify subtle changes in baseline variation over time. The U.S. Food and Drug Administration approved this analysis program for use in the Sonicaid FetalCare monitor (Pardey, Moulden, & Redman, 2002). Clinical validation of the power

to predict hypoxemia and acidemia with the Sonicaid tool has been accomplished by comparing the computer NST findings with cordocentesis for cord blood analysis immediately following the NST or with umbilical cord blood analysis in a scheduled cesarean delivery without labor following the NST (Pardey et al., 2002, includes printout examples).

A multicenter international study used the SisPorto software program for computer analysis of the NST to compare automated analysis with neonatal outcomes (umbilical blood gas analysis, Apgar scores, neonatal hypoxic-ischemic encephalopathy) in scheduled cesarean deliveries (Ayers-de-Campos, Costa-Santos, & Bernardes, 2005). Researchers found that the analysis of FHR variability and accelerations were predictive of Apgar scores and less predictive of umbilical artery gas analysis, and did detect both cases of neonatal hypoxic-ischemic encephalopathy in the sample of 345 cases.

Computer intelligence can help clinicians process EFM data, information, and knowledge. The unique qualities of human intelligence and machine intelligence must continue to be debated, researched, and distinguished.

Balancing Information Technology

Obstetric clinicians must understand the informatics concepts, benefits, and limitations of the EHR, perinatal systems, and knowledge tools to lead integration in care and advocate for women. Clinicians must ensure that the information technology supports care during labor and birth and does not interfere with this process or introduce unintended risk.

REFERENCES

American Health Information Management Association. (2006). *Building the workforce for health information transformation*. Retrieved July 15, 2006, from http://www.ahima.org/

American Nurses Association. (2001). *Scope and standards of nursing informatics practice*. Washington, DC: Author.

Ayers-de-Campos, D., Costa-Santos, C., & Bernardes, J. SisPorto Multicentre Validation Study Group. (2005). Prediction of neonatal state by computer analysis of fetal heart rate tracings: The antepartum arm of the SisPorto multicentre validation study. *European Journal of Obstetrics and Reproductive Biology, 118*(1), 52–60.

Bakken, S. (2001). An informatics infrastructure is essential for evidence-based practice. *Journal of the American Medical Informatics Association, 8*(3), 199–201.

Barnes, J. (2006). Implementing a perinatal clinical information system: A work in progress. *Journal of Obstetric, Gynecologic and Neonatal Nursing, 35*(1), 134–140.

Devane, D., & Lalor, J. (2005). Midwives' visual interpretation of intrapartum cardiotocographs: Intra- and interobserver agreement. *Journal of Advanced Nursing, 52*(2), 133–141.

Dombrowski, M., Tomlinson, M., Bottoms, S., Johnson, M., & Sokol, R. (1995). Obstetrics computer-generated admission forms have greater accuracy. *American Journal of Obstetrics and Gynecology, 173*(3), 847–848.

Figueras, F., Albela, S., Bonino, S., Palacio, M., Barrau, E., Hernandez, A., et al. (2005). Visual analysis of antepartum fetal heart rate tracings: Inter and intra-observer agreement and impact of knowledge of neonatal outcome. *Journal of Perinatal Medicine, 33*(3), 241–245.

Goodwin, L., Iannacchione, M., Hammond, W., Crockett, P., Maher, S., & Schlitz, K. (2001). Data mining methods find demographic predictors of preterm birth. *Nursing Research, 50*(6), 340–345.

Hunt, E., Sproat, S., & Kitzmiller, R. (2004). *The nursing informatics implementation guide.* New York: Springer-Verlag.

Huntleigh Healthcare. (2005). Sonicaid Fetalcare antepartum analysis: Clinical application guide. Retrieved July 15, 2006, from http://www.sonicaidfetalcare.com/downloads/application_uk.pdf

Institute of Medicine. (2001). *Crossing the quality chasm: A new health system for the 21st century.* Washington, DC: National Academy Press.

Ivory, C. (2005). Finding buried treasure in unit log books: Data mining. *AWHONN Lifelines, 9*(1), 62–66.

Kelly, C. S. (1999). Perinatal computerized patient record and archiving systems: Pitfalls and enhancements for implementing a successful computerized medical record. *Journal of Perinatal & Neonatal Nursing, 12*(4), 1–14.

Kranz, J. (2005). *Clinical decision support system.* Retrieved July 15, 2006, from http://www.e-and-c.com/docs/articles/AlphaSightsF_W05p14-17.pdf

McCartney, P. (2004). Leadership in nursing informatics. *Journal of Obstetric, Gynecologic and Neonatal Nursing, 33*(4), 371–380.

——— (2003a). HIPAA and electronic health information security. *MCN: The American Journal of Maternal/Child Nursing, 28*(5), 333.

——— (2003b). Synchronizing with standard time and atomic clocks. *MCN: The American Journal of Maternal/Child Nursing, 28*(1), 51.

——— (2002). Electronic fetal monitoring and the legal medical record. *MCN: The American Journal of Maternal/Child Nursing, 27*(4), 249.

——— (2000). Computer analysis of the fetal heart rate. *Journal of Obstetric, Gynecologic and Neonatal Nursing, 29*(5), 527–536.

National Institute of Child Health and Human Development Research Planning Workshop. (1997). Electronic fetal heart rate monitoring research guidelines for interpretation. *American Journal of Obstetrics and Gynecology, 177*(6), 1385–1390.

Nielson, P., Thomson, B., Jackson, R., Kosman, K., & Kiley, K. (2000). Standard obstetric record charting system: Evaluation of a new electronic medical record. *Obstetrics & Gynecology, 96*(6), 1003–1008.

Pardey, J., Moulden, M., & Redman, C. (2002). A computer system for the numerical analysis of nonstress tests. *American Journal of Obstetrics and Gynecology, 186*(5), 1095–1103.

Tongsong, T., Iamthongin, A., Wanapirak, C., Piyamongkol, W., Sirichotiyakul, S., Boonyanurak, P., et al. (2005). Accuracy of fetal heart-rate variability interpretation by obstetricians using the criteria of the National Institute of Child Health and Human Development compared with computer-aided interpretation. *Journal of Obstetrics and Gynecology Research, 31*(1), 68–71.

U.S. Department of Health and Human Services. (2006). *Office of the National Coordinator for Health Information Technology.* Retrieved July 15, 2006, from http://www.hhs.gov/healthit/

Wilhoit, K., Mustain, J., & King, M. (2006). The role of frontline RNs in the selection of an electronic medical record business partner. *CIN: Computers, Informatics, Nursing, 24*(4), 188–195.

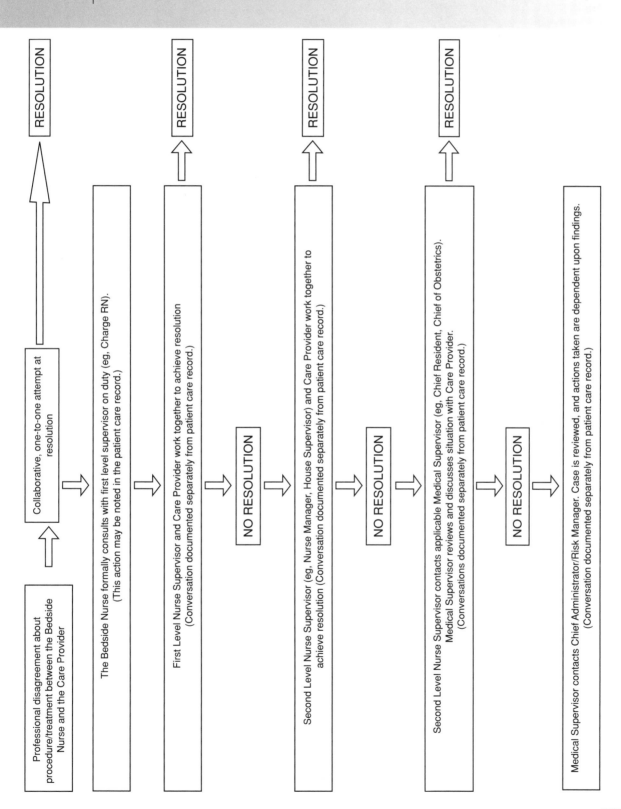

Algorithm for Management of Antepartum Testing

Starting with the NST or CST, this chart outlines options for managing antepartum test results. It is meant to be used as a guide to assist the clinician. Each patient should be evaluated and treated on an individual basis.

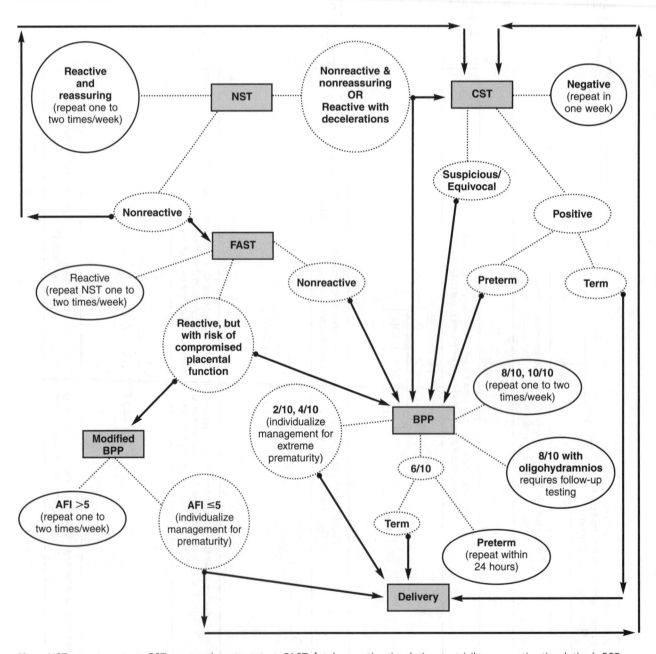

Key: NST, nonstress test; CST, contraction stress test; FAST, fetal acoustic stimulation test (vibra-acoustic stimulation); BPP, biophysical profile; AFI, amniotic fluid index.

Intrapartum Assessment of Electronic Fetal Monitoring

Examples of Components of a Reassuring FHR Tracing (No Intervention Necessary)

Baseline	Variability	Accelerations	Decelerations	Uterine Activity
Stable; within normal range	Moderate	Present	None	Appropriate; no hyperstimulation
Stable; within normal range	Moderate	Present	Early	Appropriate; no hyperstimulation

Examples of Components of FHR Tracing Requiring Further Observation and/or Preventive Intervention

Baseline	Variability	Accelerations	Decelerations	Uterine Activity
Stable; within normal range	Moderate	Present	None or early	Hyperstimulation
Stable; within normal range	Moderate	None	None	Appropriate; no hyperstimulation
Stable; within normal range	Minimal/absent	None	None	Appropriate; no hyperstimulation
Stable; within normal range	Moderate	Present	Variable	Appropriate; no hyperstimulation
Within normal range, but rising	Moderate	Present	None	Appropriate; no hyperstimulation
Within normal range, but rising	Minimal/absent or marked	Present	None	Appropriate; no hyperstimulation

Examples of Components of a Nonreassuring FHR Tracing (Requires Investigation and Remedial Intervention)

Baseline	Variability	Accelerations	Decelerations	Uterine Activity
Stable, within normal range	Moderate	None	None	Hyperstimulation
Stable, within normal range	Moderate	Present	Late or prolonged	With or without hyperstimulation
Stable, within normal range	Moderate	Present	Late, variable, and/or prolonged	With or without hyperstimulation

(*continued*)

Examples of Components of a Nonreassuring FHR Tracing (Requires Investigation and Remedial Intervention)

Baseline	Variability	Accelerations	Decelerations	Uterine Activity
Stable, within normal range	Minimal/absent or marked	None	None	Hyperstimulation
Stable, within normal range	Minimal/absent or marked	Present	Late, variable, and/or prolonged	With or without hyperstimulation
Stable, within normal range	Minimal/absent or marked	None	Late, variable, and/or prolonged	With or without hyperstimulation
Within normal range, but rising	Moderate	Present	Late, variable, and/or prolonged	With or without hyperstimulation
Within normal range, but rising	Moderate	None	Late, variable, and/or prolonged	With or without hyperstimulation
With normal range, but rising	Minimal/absent or marked	Present	None	Hyperstimulation
Within normal range, but rising	Minimal/absent or marked	None	None	With or without hyperstimulation
Within normal range, but rising	Minimal/absent or marked	Present	Late, variable, and/or prolonged	With or without hyperstimulation
Tachycardic	Moderate	Present	None	With or without hyperstimulation
Tachycardic	Moderate	None	None	With or without hyperstimulation
Tachycardic	Moderate	Present	Late, variable, and/or prolonged	With or without hyperstimulation
Tachycardic	Moderate	None	Late, variable, and/or prolonged	With or without hyperstimulation
Tachycardic	Minimal/absent or marked	Present	None	With or without hyperstimulation
Tachycardic	Minimal/absent or marked	None	None	With or without hyperstimulation
Tachycardic	Minimal/absent or marked	Present	Late, variable, and/or prolonged	With or without hyperstimulation
Tachycardic	Minimal/absent or marked	None	Late, variable, and/or prolonged	With or without hyperstimulation

Examples of Components of a Nonreassuring FHR Tracing (Requires Investigation and Remedial Intervention)

Baseline	Variability	Accelerations	Decelerations	Uterine Activity
Bradycardic	Moderate	Present	None	With or without hyperstimulation
Bradycardic	Moderate	None	None	With or without hyperstimulation
Bradycardic	Moderate	Present	Late, variable, and/prolonged	With or without hyperstimulation
Bradycardic	Moderate	None	Late, variable, and/or prolonged	With or without hyperstimulation
Bradycardic	Minimal/absent or marked	Present	None	With or without hyperstimulation
Bradycardic	Minimal/absent or marked	None	None	With or without hyperstimulation
Bradycardic	Minimal/absent or marked	Present	Late, variable, and/or prolonged	With or without hyperstimulation
Bradycardic	Minimal/absent or marked	None	Late, variable and/or prolonged	With or without hyperstimulation

The Role of the Nurse-Midwife in the Management of Electronic Fetal Monitoring

It is a fundamental responsibility of the nurse-midwife to assess fetal status. Assessment of maternal/fetal/placental status may include, but is not limited to, the following:

On Admission

Subjective Data	Objective Data	
• Review maternal history; determine gestational age • Maternal report of the presence of a usual amount of fetal movement • Maternal report of well-being • Maternal report of adequate coping	• Observation and/or palpation of fetal movement • Maternal vital signs • Prenatal course and current gestational age • Length of time in labor, cervical status • Coping mechanisms being used by the patient • Color, consistency, and odor of any discharge, bleeding, or amniotic fluid present • Palpation of contractions: contractions should last <60–90 seconds and number ≤5 in 10 minutes, with a minimum of a 1-minute period of uterine relaxation between contractions **Reassuring Fetal Status** • Auscultation of FHR: regular rate and rhythm within normal baseline range; remaining stable between, during, and after contractions; audible accelerations of the FHR that rise from the baseline and return to the baseline OR • Reassuring electronic fetal monitor strip chart: stable baseline FHR within normal limits, moderate variability, and the presence of accelerations ≥15 bpm above the baseline lasting ≥15 seconds occurring within a continuous, 20-minute recording	⌖ In the event that fetal status is nonreassuring on admission, the following steps should be considered: 1. Promote intrauterine resuscitation (eg, alter maternal position, administer IV fluids and oxygen, decrease stress of contractions on the fetus) 2. Notify backup physician 3. Vaginal examination, as appropriate (check for progress of labor, presence of cord, and so forth) 4. Consider continuous electronic fetal monitoring/internal monitoring, depending on the circumstances 5. Initiate adjunct measures of fetal assessment, as appropriate and available (scalp stimulation, sonographic evaluation, fetal scalp blood sampling) 6. Prepare the patient for transport, if necessary 7. Prepare the patient for operative intervention, if necessary

During Labor

Subjective Data	Objective Data	

Subjective Data

- Review maternal history; determine gestational age
- Maternal report of the presence of fetal movement
- Maternal report of well-being (relative to her laboring condition)
- Maternal report of adequate coping (relative to her laboring condition)

Objective Data

- Observation and/or palpation of fetal movement
- Maternal vital signs
- Length of time in labor, cervical status
- Coping mechanisms being used
- Color, consistency, and odor of any discharge, bleeding, or amniotic fluid present
- Palpation of contractions: contractions should last <60–90 seconds and number ≤5 in 10 minutes, with a minimum of a 1-minute period of uterine relaxation between contractions

Reassuring Fetal Status
- Auscultation of FHR: regular rate and rhythm within normal baseline range; remaining stable between, during, and after contractions; audible accelerations of the FHR that rise from the baseline and return to the baseline
  OR
- The presence of a reassuring continuous recording of the FHR: stable baseline FHR within normal limits, moderate variability present; accelerations present; and the absence of variable, late, and prolonged decelerations

🔔 In the event that fetal status becomes nonreassuring during labor, the following steps should be considered:

1. Promote intrauterine resuscitation (eg, alter maternal position, administer IV fluids and oxygen, decrease stress of contractions on the fetus)
2. Notify backup physician
3. Vaginal examination, as appropriate (check for progress of labor, presence of cord, and so forth)
4. Consider continuous electronic fetal monitoring/internal monitoring, depending on the circumstances
5. Initiate adjunct measures of fetal assessment, as appropriate and available (scalp stimulation, sonographic evaluation, fetal scalp blood sampling)
6. Prepare the patient for transport, if necessary
7. Prepare the patient for operative intervention, if necessary

Examples of FHR Baseline Variability

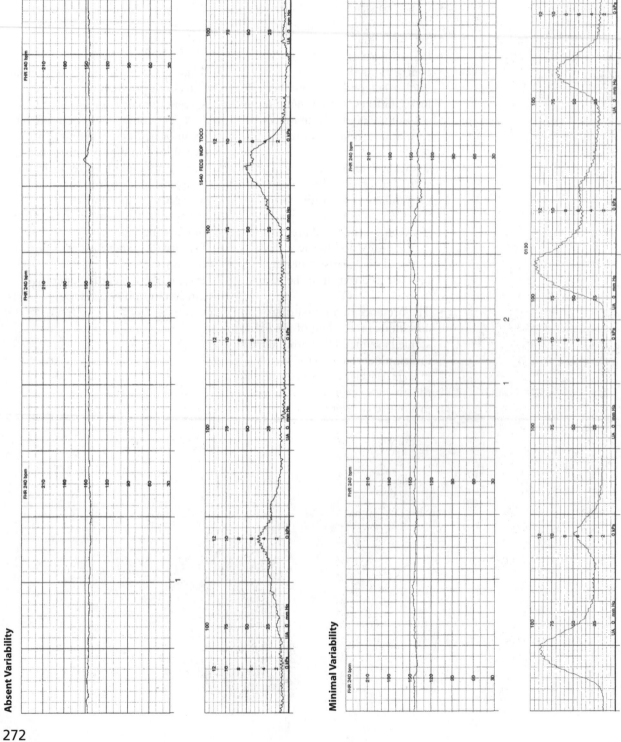

Absent Variability

Minimal Variability

Moderate Variability

Marked Variability

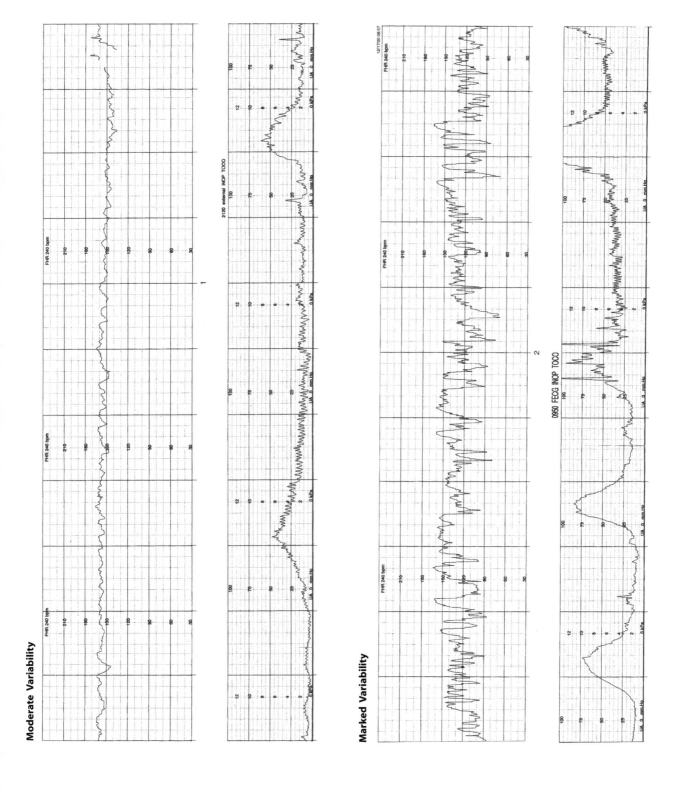

Terminology

Acidosis	Pathologic condition marked by an increased concentration of hydrogen ions in tissue
Acidemia	Increased concentration of hydrogen ions in the blood
Asphyxia	Hypoxia with clinically significant metabolic acidosis
Baroreceptor	Receptor that senses a change in pressure; also known as a pressoreceptors
Chemoreceptor	Cells in the carotid body that are stimulated by chemical substances and cause a reflex change in heart rate
Confidence Level	Chance that the result is correct; the risk associated with not being 100% confident
False Negative	Test result is negative (reassuring), but the outcome is poor
False Positive	Test result is positive (nonreassuring), but the outcome is good
Hyoxemia	Decreased oxygen content in blood
Hypoxia	Pathologic condition marked by a decreased level of oxygen in tissue
Inter-observer reliability	Differences in interpretation of a phenomenon due to variations in perception
Negative Predictive Value	The chances that a negative test is truly negative
Positive Predictive Value	The chances that a positive test is truly positive
Vagus Nerve	Tenth cranial nerve; acts as a messenger between the brain and the heart, influencing cardiac function

INDEX

Page numbers followed by *b* refer to text in boxes; page numbers followed by *f* refer to figures; page numbers followed by *t* refer to tables.